Oscillator-Amplifier Free Electron Lasers an Outlook to Their Feasibility and Performances

Oscillator-Amplifier Free Electron Lasers an Outlook to Their Feasibility and Performances

Editors

Giuseppe Dattoli
Alessandro Curcio
Danilo Giulietti

MDPI • Basel • Beijing • Wuhan • Barcelona • Belgrade • Manchester • Tokyo • Cluj • Tianjin

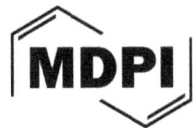

Editors

Giuseppe Dattoli
ENEA Fusion department
Frascati Research Center
Italy

Alessandro Curcio
Centro de LaseresPulsados
(CLPU)
Spain

Danilo Giulietti
Physics Department of the Pisa University
Largo Bruno Pontecorvo
Italy

Editorial Office
MDPI
St. Alban-Anlage 66
4052 Basel, Switzerland

This is a reprint of articles from the Special Issue published online in the open access journal *Applied Sciences* (ISSN 2076-3417) (available at: https://www.mdpi.com/journal/applsci/special_issues/Oscillator-Amplifier_Free_Electron_Lasers).

For citation purposes, cite each article independently as indicated on the article page online and as indicated below:

LastName, A.A.; LastName, B.B.; LastName, C.C. Article Title. *Journal Name* **Year**, *Volume Number*, Page Range.

ISBN 978-3-0365-5807-3 (Hbk)
ISBN 978-3-0365-5808-0 (PDF)

© 2023 by the authors. Articles in this book are Open Access and distributed under the Creative Commons Attribution (CC BY) license, which allows users to download, copy and build upon published articles, as long as the author and publisher are properly credited, which ensures maximum dissemination and a wider impact of our publications.

The book as a whole is distributed by MDPI under the terms and conditions of the Creative Commons license CC BY-NC-ND.

Contents

About the Editors vii

Giuseppe Dattoli, Alessandro Curcio and Danilo Giulietti
Preface to "Oscillator-Amplifier Free Electron Lasers an Outlook to Their Feasibility and Performances"
Reprinted from: *Appl. Sci.* 2022, *12*, 9444, doi:10.3390/app12199444 1

Emanuele Di Palma, Silvio Ceccuzzi, Gian Luca Ravera, Elio Sabia, Ivan Spassovsky and Giuseppe Dattoli
Radio-Frequency Undulators, Cyclotron Auto Resonance Maser and Free Electron Lasers
Reprinted from: *Appl. Sci.* 2021, *11*, 9499, doi:10.3390/app11209499 3

Andrea Doria
Hybrid (Oscillator-Amplifier) Free Electron Laser and New Proposals
Reprinted from: *Appl. Sci.* 2021, *11*, 5948, doi:10.3390/app11135948 21

Peter van der Slot and Henry Freund
Three-Dimensional, Time-Dependent Analysis of High- and Low-Q Free-Electron Laser Oscillators
Reprinted from: *Appl. Sci.* 2021, *11*, 4978, doi:10.3390/app11114978 33

Michele Opromolla and Vittoria Petrillo
Two-Color TeraHertz Radiation by a Multi-Pass FEL Oscillator
Reprinted from: *Appl. Sci.* 2021, *11*, 6495, doi:10.3390/app11146495 81

Alessandro Curcio
Recirculated Wave Undulators for Compact FELs
Reprinted from: *Appl. Sci.* 2021, *11*, 5936, doi:10.3390/app11135936 91

Georgia Paraskaki, Sven Ackermann, Bart Faatz, Gianluca Geloni, Tino Lang, Fabian Pannek, Lucas Schaper and Johann Zemella
Advanced Scheme to Generate MHz, Fully Coherent FEL Pulses at nm Wavelength
Reprinted from: *Appl. Sci.* 2021, *11*, 6058, doi:10.3390/app11136058 105

Michele Opromolla, Alberto Bacci, Marcello Rossetti Conti, Andrea Renato Rossi, Giorgio Rossi, Luca Serafini, Alberto Tagliaferri and Vittoria Petrillo
High Repetition Rate and Coherent Free-Electron Laser Oscillator in the Tender X-ray Range Tailored for Linear Spectroscopy
Reprinted from: *Appl. Sci.* 2021, *11*, 5892, doi:10.3390/app11135892 127

Elio Sabia, Emanuele Di Palma and Giuseppe Dattoli
Two-Beam Free-Electron Lasers and Self-Injected Nonlinear Harmonic Generation
Reprinted from: *Appl. Sci.* 2021, *11*, 6462, doi:10.3390/app11146462 137

Giuseppe Dattoli, Emanuele Di Palma, Silvia Licciardi and Elio Sabia
Free Electron Laser High Gain Equation and Harmonic Generation
Reprinted from: *Appl. Sci.* 2021, *11*, 85, doi:10.3390/app11010085 153

About the Editors

Alessandro Curcio

Dr. Alessandro Curcio started his career at the University of Pisa with a Master's Degree thesis on ultra-compact and ultra-bright laser-based X-ray sources. Afterwards, he obtained a position in the Ph.D. school of accelerator physics at the University of Rome La Sapienza, concluding with a thesis on innovative concepts for ultra-bright radiation sources and particle acceleration based on the laser–matter interaction at relativistic intensities.

In November 2017, he won a Research Fellowship at the CERN Linear Accelerator for Research (CLEAR), in which he was responsible for the scientific activity on the generation of high accelerating gradients via the emission of coherent radiation from ultra-short electronbeams and on ultra-short particle diagnostics via THz radiation.

At the beginning of 2020, he joined the National Polish Synchrotron SOLARIS, in Krakow, as Section Leader in beam diagnostics and instrumentation. Currently, he is Senior Scientist at CLPU with the main role of designing and developing beamlines and diagnostics for particles and radiation produced in laser-plasma accelerators.

Giuseppe Dattoli

Giuseppe Dattoli was born in Lagonegro, Italy, in 1953. He received the Ph.D. degree in physics from La Sapienza University of Rome, Italy, in 1976. He is an ENEA Researcher and has been involved in different research projects, including high energy accelerators, free electron lasers, and applied mathematics networks, since 1979. Dr. Dattoli has taught in Italian and Foreign universities and has received the FEL Prize Award for his outstanding achievements in the field.

Danilo Giulietti

Danilo Giulietti received a degree in Physics (cum laude) at Pisa University and a Ph.D. at Scuola Normale di Pisa in 1979. He has developed scientific and teaching activity in the Physics Department of Pisa University, where he is at the present professor and lecturer of Classical Electrodynamics and Quantum Optics. The research fields in which he has been mainly involved are laser-produced plasmas, the physics of the Inertial Confinement Fusion, the particle acceleration in plasmas, and innovative laser-induced nuclear-fusion reactions. D.G. is the author of more than 200 publications in international journals and over 300 communications in national and internationals congresses, some of them as invited talks. D.G. has been in charge of the management of some scientific international initiatives and the chair of international conferences devoted to the topics of his research activity. Due to his activity in the field of particle acceleration in plasmas, he is associated with the Istituto Nazionale di Fisica Nucleare. He has been the National Representative of the INFN Strategic Project PLASMONX: plasma acceleration and monochromatic, tunable X-ray radiation, the European Projects ELI (Extreme Light Infrastructure), and HiPER (High Power laser Energy Research facility).

Editorial

Preface to "Oscillator-Amplifier Free Electron Lasers an Outlook to Their Feasibility and Performances"

Giuseppe Dattoli [1,*], Alessandro Curcio [2] and Danilo Giulietti [3]

[1] ENEA Dipartimento FSN Frascati, Via Enrico Fermi 45, Frascati, 00044 Rome, Italy
[2] Centro de Laseres Pulsados (CLPU), Edificio M5. Parque Cientifico, C. del Adaja, 8, 37185 Villamayor, Spain
[3] Dipartimento di Fisica, "E. Fermi", Università di Pisa and INFN, Largo B. Pontecorvo, n.3, 56127 Pisa, Italy
* Correspondence: pinodattoli@libero.it

Free Electron Lasers (FELs) are certainly among the most interesting devices, belonging to the realm of coherent radiation sources. These lasers are now widely used all over the world and are the highest performing in terms of brilliance, monochromaticity, coherence, directionality and polarization control.

Despite their undoubted success and reliability as experimental devices, their wider use is still hampered by their size and cost, which require large laboratories and significant financial efforts.

It would be therefore desirable to develop more compact and economical FELs with, e.g., higher repetition rates and larger average brightness.

A future prospect, pursued by many worldwide research institutions, would be to build FEL facilities in the VUV-X region, using compact accelerators and shorter undulator sections.

Within this context, the most natural solutions are those of designing high gradient accelerating devices, capable of providing high-quality electron beams and non-standard undulator lines.

Both solutions might concur with the reduction in either the size or the cost, but although these are the most obvious, they are not the only ones.

"Alternative" undulator lines should be studied to prevent the use of hundred meters of magnetic devices, necessary to provide the saturation length, in standard FEL architecture. However other solutions can be adopted, including a combination of non-linear harmonic generation, seeding, hybrid devices, coupled oscillators amplifier systems, etc.

This Special Issue is devoted to "non-conventional" FEL architectures and describes different strategies, which have been proposed in the past and examines both the underlying physics and the different aspects of the relevant design, with particular reference to feasibility and relevant performance.

The ideas and the proposals described here have reached some level of maturation and can be employed in the near or middle future as the paradigm for the design of compact FEL architectures.

The Special Issue contains nine contributions which can be grouped into the following topics:

(A) Discussion of FEL devices based on the design of wave undulators.

Wave undulators are undulating devices provided by electromagnetic waves aimed at reducing the size of the undulator line.

In particular, in [1], the design of a CARM-type microwave source is described along with the relevant use for the operation of FEL devices. In [2], an FEL design employing a recirculated electromagnetic undulator provided by a high-power laser in a resonator cavity is described in detail.

(B) Design of combinations of seeding and non-linear harmonic devices.

Ref. [3] deals with the design of an FEL device driven by the e-beam from a Super-Conducting and producing tunable radiation from 100 to 2 micrometers. Ref. [4] describes the use of two beam energies' harmonic generation and self-seeding schemes. The theoretical aspects and design formulae for SASE/higher order harmonic FEL are described in [5].

(C) Hybrid and oscillator/amplifier devices

The article in [6] focuses on the possibility of coupling different emission mechanisms (Cerenkov, Smith–Purcell, etc.) to provide a high-performance, small-size FEL-type devices. High-repetition-rate X-ray FELs are described in [7,8] within the context oscillator/amplifier architectures. Ref. [9] describes an accurate modelling of the coupling of low/high-gain undulators.

Author Contributions: All the authors have equally contributed. All authors have read and agreed to the published version of the manuscript.

Funding: The authors declare that no external funding have been received.

Institutional Review Board Statement: Not applicable.

Informed Consent Statement: Not applicable.

Data Availability Statement: Not applicable.

Conflicts of Interest: The authors declare no conflict of interest.

References

1. Di Palma, E.; Ceccuzzi, S.; Ravera, G.L.; Sabia, E.; Spassovsky, I.; Dattoli, G. Radio-Frequency Undulators, Cyclotron Auto Resonance Maser and Free Electron Lasers. *Appl. Sci.* **2021**, *11*, 9499. [CrossRef]
2. Curcio, A. Recirculated Wave Undulators for Compact FELs. *Appl. Sci.* **2021**, *11*, 5936. [CrossRef]
3. Opromolla, M.; Petrillo, V. Two-Color Tera-Hertz Radiation by a Multi-Pass FEL Oscillator. *Appl. Sci.* **2021**, *11*, 6495. [CrossRef]
4. Sabia, E.; Di Palma, E. Two-Beam Free-Electron Lasers and Self-Injected Nonlinear Harmonic Generation. *Appl. Sci.* **2021**, *11*, 6462. [CrossRef]
5. Dattoli, G.; di Palma, E.; Licciardi, S.; Sabia, E. Free Electron Laser High Gain Equation and Harmonic GenerationDoria Hybrid (Oscillator-Amplifier) Free Electron Laser and New Proposals. *Appl. Sci.* **2020**, *11*, 85. [CrossRef]
6. Doria, A. Hybrid (Oscillator-Amplifier) Free Electron Laser and New Proposals. *Appl. Sci.* **2021**, *11*, 5948. [CrossRef]
7. Opromolla, M.; Bacci, A.; Conti, M.R.; Rossi, A.R.; Rossi, G.; Serafini, L.; Tagliaferri, A.; Petrillo, V. High Repetition Rate and Coherent Free-Electron Laser Oscillator in the Tender X-ray Range Tailored for Linear Spectroscopy. *Appl. Sci.* **2021**, *11*, 5892. [CrossRef]
8. Paraskaki, G.; Ackermann, S.; Faatz, B.; Geloni, G.; Lang, T.; Pannek, F.; Schaper, L.; Zemella, J. Advanced Scheme to Generate MHz, Fully Coherent FEL Pulses at nm Wavelength. *Appl. Sci.* **2021**, *11*, 6058. [CrossRef]
9. Van der Slot, P.J.; Freund, H.P. Three-Dimensional, Time-Dependent Analysis of High- and Low-Q Free-Electron Laser Oscillators. *Appl. Sci.* **2021**, *11*, 4978. [CrossRef]

Article

Radio-Frequency Undulators, Cyclotron Auto Resonance Maser and Free Electron Lasers

Emanuele Di Palma *,†, Silvio Ceccuzzi †, Gian Luca Ravera †, Elio Sabia †, Ivan Spassovsky † and Giuseppe Dattoli †

ENEA—Frascati Research Center, Via Enrico Fermi 45, 00044 Rome, Italy; silvio.ceccuzzi@enea.it (S.C.); gianluca.ravera@enea.it (G.L.R.); elio.sabia@gmail.com (E.S.); ivan.spassovsky@enea.it (I.S.); pinodattoli@libero.it (G.D.)
* Correspondence: emanuele.dipalma@enea.it; Tel.: +39-06-9400-5709
† These authors contributed equally to this work.

Abstract: We discuss a hybrid Free Electron Laser (FEL) architecture operating with a RF undulator provided by a powerful Cyclotron Auto-Resonance Maser (CARM). We outline the design elements to operate a compact X-ray device. We review the essential aspects of wave undulator FEL theory and of CARM devices.

Keywords: gyrotron; CARM; free electron laser; compton scattering

1. Introduction

The interest in Free Electron Laser (FEL), during the last decade, has moved toward devices producing X-ray beams with high brilliance matching the requirements for many applications such as nuclear materials detection [1], small-angle X-ray scattering [2], phase contrast imaging [3], macromolecular X-ray crystallography for drug discovery [4] and X-ray microscopy [5].

The Linac Coherent Light Source (LCLS) at SLAC National Accelerator Laboratory [6], FLASH at DESY Deutsches Elektronen-Synchrotron [7] with other advanced X-ray FEL [8–13] provide, or have been designed to provide, high-brightness X-ray beams, but size, cost and operational complexity are the main drawbacks for a widespread use in small laboratories, hospitals, universities.

The X-FEL technology is based on two pillars, high-energy (multi-GeV) high-quality electron beam Linacs and hundred-meters-long undulators. A high-brilliance X-ray device demands, accordingly, large facilities and therefore any progress towards "compact" X-ray FELs requires technological improvements in terms of high-gradient accelerators and/or short "wavelength" undulators. The last possibility will be considered in this paper.

The availability of powerful electromagnetic sources (lasers or RF sources) offers the possibility of replacing magnetic with electromagnetic undulators. The advantage would be that of reducing both the size of the undulator and the energy of the e-beam (electron beam).

In Figure 1 we sketch out the scaling of the beam energy and of the undulator length, with magnetic or RF wave undulators. The last option comprises either laser and RF solutions.

The use of an electromagnetic undulator pumped by a GHz RF field allows, for the same FEL wavelength, to reduce the energy of the electron beam by several units and the length of the magnet by more than one order of magnitude.

We provide below a preliminary idea of how electron beam and Radio Frequency Undulators (RFU) combine to drive an X-ray FEL Self-Amplified Spontaneous Emission (SASE) device. It is evident, as underscored below, that the price to be payed to exploit RFU, in a FEL-SASE operation, is that of employing high intensity fields. We do not specify, for the moment, any electromagnetic source, we fix a reference RF power and the relevant operating wavelength to specify electron beam parameters suitable for FEL SASE X-ray operation.

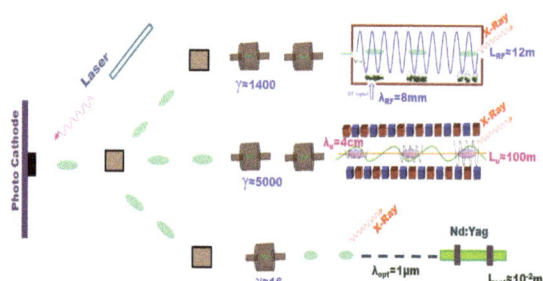

Figure 1. Comparison between Laser Wave (or optical), magnetic and RF undulators from bottom right to top right, respectively, for an output of X-ray radiation with $\lambda_r = 1$ nm. The figure reports an electron beam emitted from the photocathode to the "undulator", after a suitable acceleration. The expected undulator lengths and the e-beam energies necessary to reach the SASE-FEL performances are underlined too.

It is well known that, from the conceptual point of view, wave or magnetic undulators do not change the FEL physics and the associated design criteria. In both cases, the emission process can be traced back to Compton/Thomson backscattering and after establishing the suitable correspondence, in terms of FEL strength parameter, most of the design strategy and scaling properties work as in the case of "ordinary" magnetostatic undulators [14,15].

One of the pivotal parameters ruling the electron dynamics inside the undulator is the so-called strength K which measures the amount of electron transverse momentum, acquired inside the undulator, allowing the coupling between the e-beam and a transverse co-propagating wave. The parameter K is specified

(a) for the magnetostatic case with on-axis field intensity B_0 and period λ_u, by [16]

$$K_m = \frac{eB_0\lambda_u}{2\pi m_e c^2} \quad (1)$$

(b) for a RF/wave undulator with the microwave field power density I_w, by [17]

$$K_w = 8.5 \times 10^{-15} \cdot \lambda_w[nm]\sqrt{I_w[W/m^2]} \quad (2)$$

where the subscripts m, w stand for magnetic and wave, respectively, while e, m_e denote the electron charge and mass, respectively, λ_w—the RF wavelength and c is the speed of light.

The electron relativistic factor γ is linked to the K parameter, FEL operating wavelength λ_r and undulator period by

$$\gamma = \frac{1}{2}\sqrt{\frac{\lambda_w}{\lambda_r}(1+K^2)}. \quad (3)$$

being $K = K_w/\sqrt{2}$, for a linearly polarized RF wave.

In Figure 2 we report γ vs λ_w for two different values of the FEL wavelength ($\lambda_r = 1$ nm and $\lambda_r = 5$ nm). The corresponding K_w values are apparently small, for a safe FEL operation (below 0.5 for the region of interest). The choice of a sufficiently large ρ (with a suitable combination of energy and current values) ensures the saturation in a reasonable saturation length.

The key quantity of FEL dynamics is the so-called Pierce parameter [18]

$$\rho \approx \frac{8.36 \times 10^{-3}}{\gamma}\left(J \cdot (K_w f_b \lambda_w)^2\right)^{1/3}, \qquad (4)$$

where $J = I/\Sigma$, with $\Sigma = 2\pi\sigma_x\sigma_y$, is the electron beam current density, namely the current I divided by the transverse area of the electron beam (with section $\sigma_{x,y}$) and f_b the Bessel function factor (which for circular polarized wave can be taken to be 1 [15]).

In Figure 3 we report the beam current density, necessary to support a Pierce parameter of around 5×10^{-4} for two different FEL operating wavelengths, following from Equation (4).

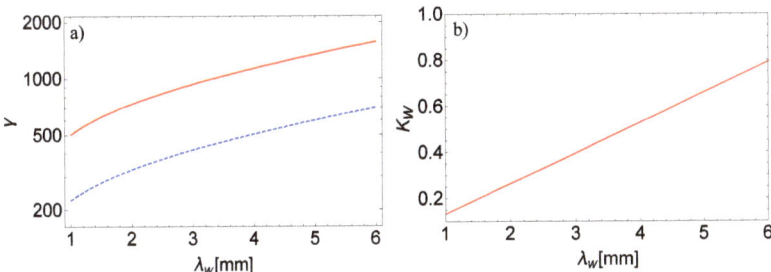

Figure 2. (a) Electron relativistic factor vs. the undulator wavelengths for $\lambda_r \equiv 1$ nm (continuous line) and $\lambda_r \equiv 5$ nm (dashed line). (b) K_w values vs. λ_w used to plot the graphs in (a) assuming $I_w = 2.4 \times 10^{14}$ W/m².

$$J = 1.71 \times 10^6 \frac{(\gamma\rho)^3}{(K_w f_b \lambda_w)^2}. \qquad (5)$$

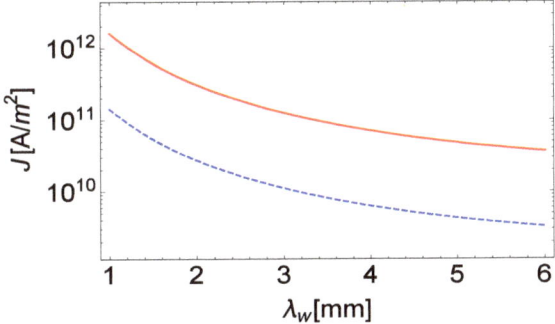

Figure 3. Electron beam current density (A/m²) vs. the undulator wave length for $\lambda_r \equiv 1$ nm (continuous line) and $\lambda_r \equiv 5$ nm (dashed line).

The importance of ρ stems from the fact that it controls all the significant parameters for the SASE FEL, like the gain length specified in [18],

$$L_g = \frac{\lambda_w}{4\pi\sqrt{3}\rho}, \qquad (6)$$

which in turns defines the saturation length L_s, which can be quantified as [18]

$$L_s \simeq 20 L_g. \qquad (7)$$

The nonideal beam qualities (finite relative energy spread and emittance) determine a dilution of the gain and a consequent increase of the saturation length. The ρ parameter is helpful to quantify these detrimental contributions. The effect of the relative energy spread on the saturation length is, e.g., negligible if [18]

$$\sigma_\epsilon < \frac{\rho}{2}, \tag{8}$$

with the chosen value of ρ we expect an undulator length (for $\lambda_w = 1$ mm) of about 2 m and a beam with relative energy spread around 0.25‰.

The request on the electron beam parameters in terms of energy and current does not appear challenging. If we consider a beam with a normalized emittance of 1 mm·mrad and assume that it is focused with an average transverse section of less than 60 μm (for $\lambda_r \in [1, 5]$ nm), along the interaction region, the request on the necessary peak current are constrained within reasonable limits (see Figures 4 and 5).

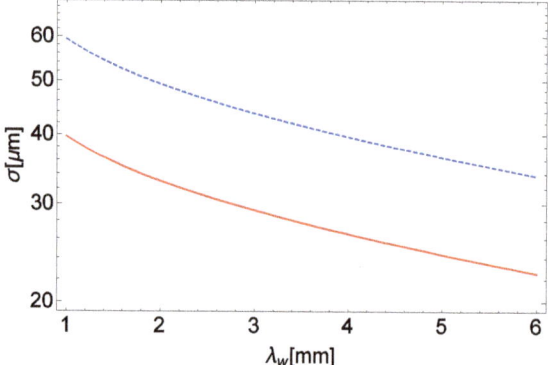

Figure 4. Electron beam cross section (μm) vs. the undulator wavelength for $\lambda_r \equiv 1$ nm (continuous red line) and $\lambda_r \equiv 5$ nm (dashed blue line); assuming a normalized emittance value of 1 mm mrad with a $\beta_{x,y}$ Twiss value of $5 \text{ m}/2\pi$ and using the Equation 3 with the same parameters reported in Figure 2.

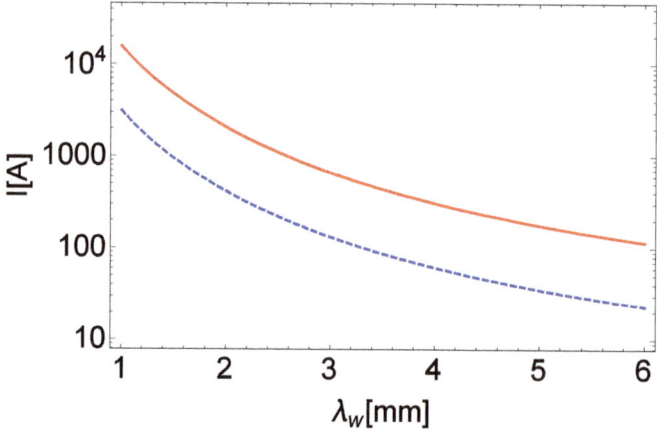

Figure 5. Electron beam current vs. the undulator wavelength for $\lambda_r \equiv 1$ nm (continuous line) and $\lambda_r \equiv 5$ nm (dashed line); derived from Equation (5) using the parameters values reported in Figure 4 and assuming $\sigma_x = \sigma_y$.

The request, regarding the electron beam parameters, becomes challenging (in terms of peak current) for the operation at short FEL wavelength and relax with increasing λ_w. A large amount of power density necessary to obtain reasonable strength undulator values is not a secondary issue and will be carefully discussed in the concluding section.

The scientific literature on the subject of RF undulators has significantly grown in the past and a partial list can be found in [19–29].

We would like to underscore that the design numbers we have foreseen can be made more accessible at short λ_w if we consider FEL operation in the VUV-X region, which requires low-energy electron beams. We have not specified yet the type of source providing the RFU. The region above 1–9 mm can be achieved with gyrotrons, gyro-klystrons or any other device (see below). Even though all these sources are candidates for RFU, a few elements of discussion are necessary to decide in favor of one or the other.

Gyrotrons work as oscillators and the only way to drive several undulator sections is to be phase locked. The drawback of this configuration is that stable phase locking oscillator operates at 10% only of the locked power. Such an efficiency drop makes this solution scarcely appealing and therefore will not be discussed here. The gyroklystron is a promising source [30]. It operates at 3 mm wavelength, however, for shorter wavelength the size of the rf cavity has to be reduced too, which will reduce the output power due to the breakdown problems. The peak power of those amplifiers is around 100 kW and the duty factor is about 10%. It is possible to use the gyro-TWT [31]. Its peak power is 80–100 kW at 60–80 GHz.

The Cyclotron Auto Resonance Maser (CARM) [32,33] promises good performances in the region 1–5 mm, therefore we choose it as RFU candidates in the forthcoming discussion. In Section 2, we summarize the physics of CARM and fix the design conditions to get sufficient power for RFU operation. In Section 3 we discuss an actual RFU configuration and discuss the associated critical issues.

2. CARM as a Source of RF Undulator

The CARM is a Free Electron device representing the transition element between microwave tubes and FELs, as nowadays conceived.

The key elements to understand the CARM FEL dynamics are sketched out in Figure 6, which displays a moderately relativistic e-beam, with a relativistic factor γ, moving inside the waveguide of a resonant cavity, along an axial static magnetic field B_0, executing helical trajectories with a period

$$\Lambda_{CH} = \frac{2\pi c}{\Omega_{CH}} \tag{9}$$

where $\Omega_{CH} = eB_0/(\gamma m_e)$, the cyclotron relativistic frequency.

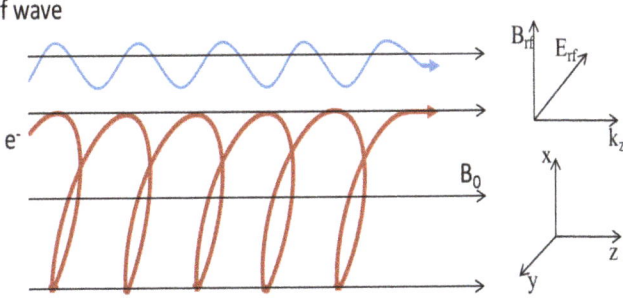

Figure 6. Geometry of the CARM interaction.

The "behavioural" paradigm of CARM is the same as for any free electron radiation generator, namely, the electrons are expected to lose energy in favor of a selected operating mode, if appropriate matching conditions are satisfied. The way in which the energy exchange occurs is traced back to the standard mechanisms of the e-beam energy modulation and bunching. The last effect is characterized by transverse and longitudinal contributions.

Going back to Figure 6, we note that the underlying dynamics can be described as follows. The electrons with longitudinal velocity v_z are propagating in a longitudinal magnetic field in the presence of a co-propagating electromagnetic field characterized by a wavevector k_z which in terms of frequency and phase velocity (v_p) reads

$$k_z = \frac{\omega}{v_p}. \tag{10}$$

We can now establish an analogy between CARM and magnetic undulator FEL (U-FEL) using only kinematics arguments.

The electron velocity inside the cavity is specified by its longitudinal and vertical components, linked to the relativistic factor by

$$\beta_z^2 + \beta_\perp^2 = 1 - \frac{1}{\gamma^2}$$

$$\beta_{z,\perp} = \frac{v_{z,\perp}}{c}, \tag{11}$$

and

$$\gamma_z = \frac{1}{\sqrt{1-\beta_z^2}} = \frac{\gamma}{\sqrt{1+(\gamma\beta_\perp)^2}}. \tag{12}$$

The electron and the radiation move, inside the cavity, at different speeds. We expect that after each helical path the following slippage is accumulated

$$\delta = (v_p - v_z)\frac{\Lambda_{CH}}{c}. \tag{13}$$

This is the phase advance of the electromagnetic wave after each helical path with respect to the electrons. Constructive interference of the wavefront of the emitted radiation at the next period is ensured if

$$\delta = \lambda \tag{14}$$

with λ being the wavelength of the field propagating with the electrons. Putting together Equations (9), (14) and (11), we end up with the matching condition.

The transverse component of the velocity $\beta_\perp$ is the key parameter allowing the coupling with the wave transverse field. In terms of the analogy we are suggesting it plays the same role as the undulator strength parameter being $K \equiv \gamma \beta_\perp$.

In the relativistic regime and assuming that $v_p \simeq c$ Equation (13) reduces to

$$\delta \cong (1-\beta_z)\Lambda_{CH} \simeq \frac{\Lambda_{CH}}{2\gamma^2}(1+K^2) \tag{15}$$

where the trajectory helical path is understood to play the same role of the undulator period (for further comments see [18,34]).

The Equation (15), derived under the assumption of (ultra) relativistic regime, provides a brief idea of how CARM and U-FEL can be viewed within a common framework. In the following we will develop a more appropriate treatment valid for the nonrelativistic regime.

The discussion might be misleading if not properly commented. Therefore, we underscore that the interaction occurs in a waveguide, whose dispersion relation needs to be included to derive the matching conditions, specifying the CARM operating wavelength. The interaction can be viewed as an intra waveguide Compton backscattering, the associated frequency up-shift is written as

$$\omega - s\Omega_{CII} + k_z v_z. \qquad (16)$$

and the matching to the waveguide conditions is ensured by the coupling with the dispersion relation

$$\omega^2 = \omega_c^2 + c^2 k_z^2 \qquad (17)$$

where s and ω_c are the harmonic index and cutoff frequency (see below), respectively.

Unlike the free space FEL, the intersection between the curves of Equations (16) and (17) admits (see Figure 7, for a geometric interpretation in the Brillouin (ω, k) space) two solutions, corresponding to gyrotron (lower frequency) and CARM (higher frequency) operations modes

$$k_{z+,-} = \frac{s\Omega_{CH}\gamma_z^2}{c}(\beta_z \pm \sqrt{1-\Psi}), \qquad (18)$$

$$\omega_{+,-} = s\Omega_{CH}\gamma_z^2(1 \pm \beta_z\sqrt{1-\Psi}),$$

being

$$\Psi = \frac{\omega_c^2}{s^2 \gamma_z^2 \Omega_{CH}^2} \qquad (19)$$

The cutoff frequency in Equation (18) ($\omega_c = c\chi_{m,n}/R$) is defined in terms of the eigenvalues $\chi_{m,n}$ of the wavenumber characterizing the $TE_{m,n}$ mode excited by the FEL CARM interaction. The relevant physical role is that of controlling the "nature" of the roots in Equations (18), determined by the intersection of the curves of Equations (16) and (17).

The "wave parameter" Ψ is lower than 1, in order to ensure two distinct intersections and is assumed to be greater than $1/\gamma_z^2$, to avoid a backward wave root.

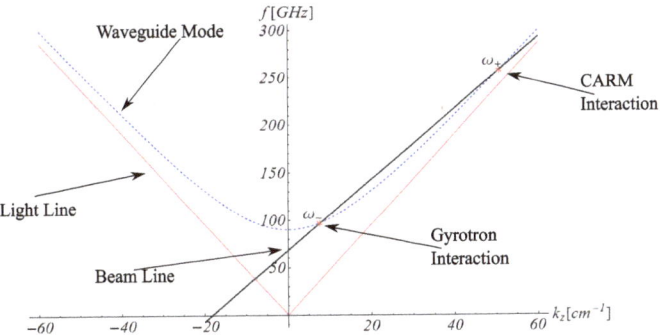

Figure 7. Brillouin diagram for the different conditions of electron cyclotron resonance selections corresponding to the intersections of the beam line (straight line) with the dispersion curve of the operating cavity mode (dotted line).

Before introducing more specific details, let us further comment on the presence of both gyrotron and CARM modes. This is a distinctive feature with respect to the magnetic undulator configuration. In principle, both modes have a chance to grow. Particular care should therefore be devoted to the suppression of the ω_- counterpart.

The theoretical analysis of CARM has been developed in the past in a number of authoritative papers [32,33,35–41] and will not be reported here. We note simply that the set of equations ruling the CARM interaction, even though characterized by a more complicated phenomenology than the ordinary magnetic FEL, can be viewed in a way not dissimilar from the pendulum-like equations, adopted in the description of FEL undulator devices.

In Figure 8 we report the growth of the CARM power for the set of parameters specified in the caption. We have included a comparison with the (analytical) small signal approximation (SSA), obtained in [42].

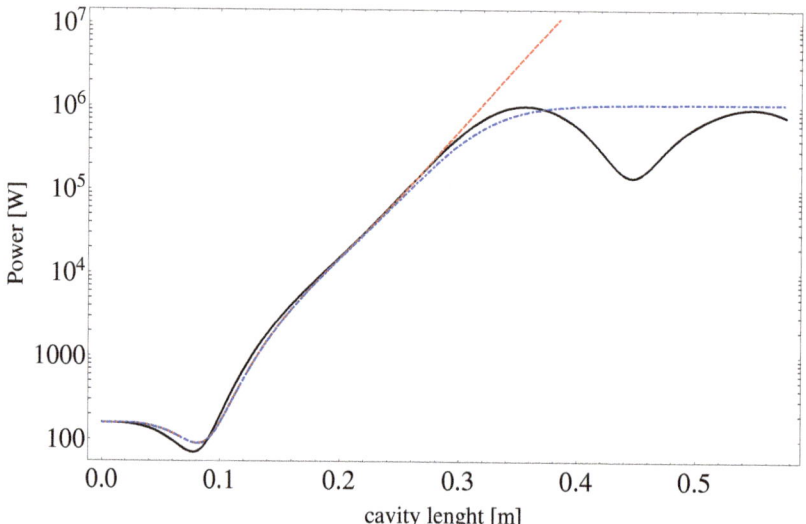

Figure 8. Numerical simulation of the CARM growth signal (continuous line), analytical solution (dashed line) with the logistic curve (dot-dashed line) reproducing the saturation. The simulation was performed with a beam energy of 700 keV, current 60 A and pitch factor $\alpha = v_\perp/v_\parallel = 5.3$ interacting at the resonance frequency of 260 GHz with the mode TE_{53} of a cylindrical tube with radius of 7.5 mm embedding an on-axis field of intensity $B_0 = 5.3$ T. An input signal of 130 W was used to seed the CARM interaction.

The power growth exhibits the same S-shaped logistic behavior of high-gain SASE FEL devices (see the superimposed dot-dashed curve), which is analytically reproduced (till the onset of the saturation) by

$$P_{sat}(z) = P_0 \frac{\overline{P}(z)}{1 + \frac{P_0}{P_F}\left(\overline{P}(z) - 1\right)} \quad (20)$$

where $\overline{P}(z) = P_l(z)/P_0$ with $P_l(z)$ being the analytical linear solution of the growth signal, P_0—the input signal power and P_F the final CARM power given by

$$P_F = \eta P_{beam} \quad (21)$$

being η the efficiency of the device, which will be commented on later in this section.

The inspection of Figure 8 confirms that the power growth consists of three distinct phases:

(a) lethargy, where the system organizes coherence;
(b) linear regime;
(c) saturation.

We consider in the following a specific configuration of parameters (see Table 1) capable of providing sufficiently large power in the region below 3 mm wavelength. In Figure 9 we show the frequency selection on the Brillouin diagram. The chosen parameters realize the CARM interaction in a region with $k_z/k_c \approx 2-3$ allowing to select the operating mode without exciting the parasitic modes, and with $\omega/\omega_c \approx 3$ by the use of a moderately relativistic beam.

Table 1. Main parameters settings to generate a CARM RF wave at ≈ 150 GHz with output power of ≈ 5 MW.

	CARM Wave Generation
beam energy	420 kV ($\gamma = 1.82$)
beam current	60 A
pitch factor	$\alpha = 0.55$
magnetic field	$B_0 = 2.99$ T
cavity radius	1 cm
operating mode	TE_{23}

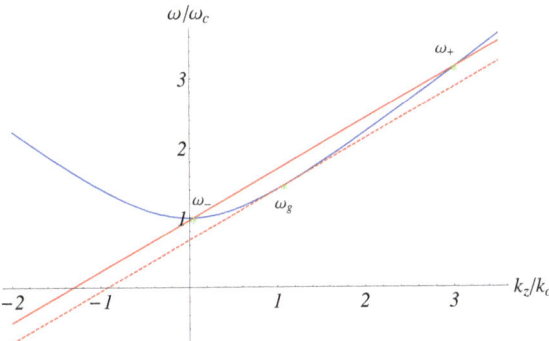

Figure 9. Beam-wave cold cavity interaction in the Brillouin diagram (ω, k) normalized to the cutoff frequency (ω_c) and to the wave vector (k_c) using the parameters reported in Table 1. The transition from the condition of two operating frequency (two intersections ω_-, ω_+ continuous line) to that of grazing incidence ($\omega_- = \omega_+ = \omega_g$ dashed line) is obtained by changing, i.e., the magnetic field intensity from $B_0 = 2.99$ T to 2.1 T.

Figure 10 shows the associated power growth for two frequencies (153–154) GHz close to the CARM resonance (ω_+), which displays a maximum output power of 4.8–6.4 MW and thus an efficiency of 19–25%, respectively.

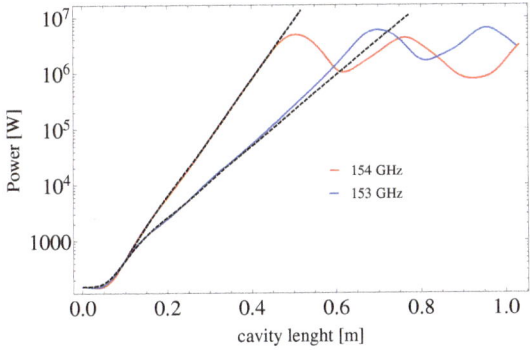

Figure 10. Analytical solution in SSA regime (dashed line) overlapped at the numerical solution (continuous line) obtained using the parameters in Table 1.

The linear regime is characterized by the small signal gain, which exhibits, along the longitudinal coordinate the transition from low- to high-gain regime, displayed in Figure 11. The gain curve vs. the normalized detuning Δ,

$$\Delta = 2(1 - \beta_z/\beta_p)/(\beta_\perp^2(1-\beta_p)^{-2})\delta_0, \qquad (22)$$

where $\beta_p = v_p/c$ and $\delta_0 = 1 - \beta_z/\beta_p - \Omega_{CH}/\omega_+$, exhibiting the characteristic bell-shaped form.

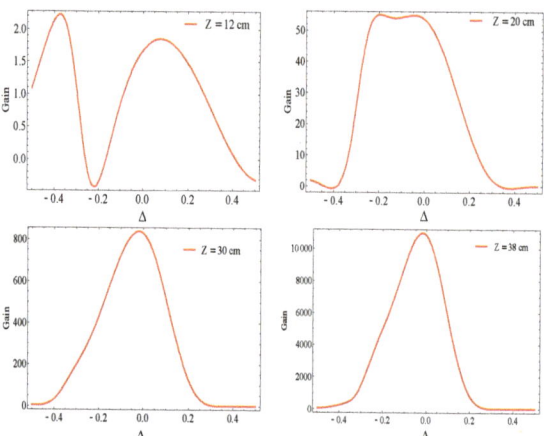

Figure 11. Gain vs. the normalized detuning Δ at different z-position for the ω_+ resonance calculated using the analytical solution in the SSA regime with the parameters reported in Table 1.

Before concluding this section, we would like to clarify two points we have just touched on. We mention that the gyrotron mode may grow too. In Figure 12 we report the temporal growth rate vs. the wave vector k_z, using the parameters reported in Table 1, exploring the two resonances at ω_+ and ω_-.

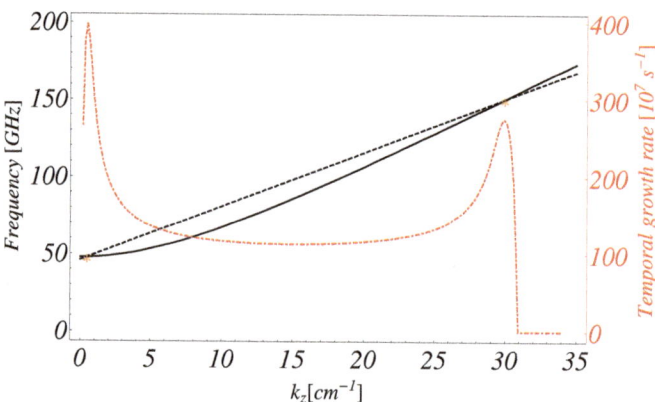

Figure 12. Frequency value (left axis) corresponding to the interaction of the beam (dashed line) with the dispersion curve of the operating mode TE_{23} (continuous line) and growth rate (dot-dashed line) using the the parameters reported in Table 1.

In Figure 13, we report the low-frequency mode ω_-, at different z-values inside the waveguide. The gain is significantly larger and could be dominant with respect to the

CARM mode. The associated power growth can be suppressed by suitably seeding the up-shifted mode.

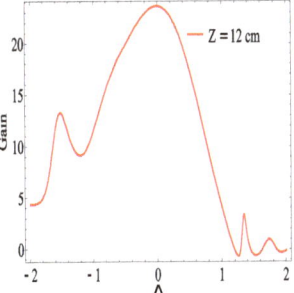 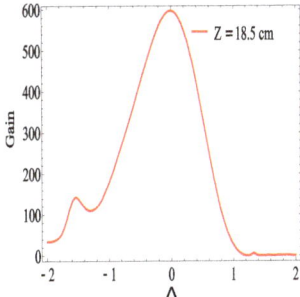

Figure 13. Gain vs. the normalized detuning Δ at different z-position for the ω_- resonance calculated using the analytical solution in the SSA regime with the parameters reported in Table 1.

The second point concerns the evaluation of the CARM efficiency, which, unlike the magnetic case is significantly larger and reaches values around tens of percent. The reasons underlying these large values are the characteristic feature of the device itself. The interaction occurs in such a way that the gain curve is larger and the interaction is resonant for a longer time [33] thus following a behavior not dissimilar by tapered FEL device [43].

3. CARM, RFU and VUV Soft X-ray FEL Operation

In the introductory section of this paper, we set out the general conditions to be fulfilled by a RF wave in the millimeter region, to sustain the operation of a RFU. The requirements in terms of power, power density, wavelength...of the RF field ensuring a FEL SASE operation have shown some criticalities, which relax with increasing FEL wavelength.

The conclusions we have drawn apply to any RF device (Gyrotron, Gyro-klystron, Magnetron, etc.) CARM is suited to operate in the region above 100 GHz ($\lambda_w < 3$) mm, where the other sources exhibit a breakdown in terms of maximum achievable power. We will therefore discuss a few specific issues for the use of 1–3 mm CARM-RFU.

In the introductory section, we have a RF power density larger than $I_{rf} \approx 10^{15}$ W/m^2 in order to achieve values of the strength parameter (K_w see Figure 2b) not far from unity (the subscript w has been replaced by rf to underscore that it refers to radio frequency intensity). The CARM power, namely, the amount of power transferred from the electron beam to the RF field, is expected to be about $P_{rf} \approx 5.4$ MW, which should accordingly be transported along a pipe with a radius $r = 1/\pi(\sqrt{P_{rf}/I_{rf}}) \approx 22$ µm, small to transport radiation in the microwave range and for any realistic mechanical handling.

In Figure 14, we have reported the electron beam energy, the electron beam current density, the electron beam transverse section and the peak current vs. the RF wavelength, assuming a significantly reduced value of the RFU power density ($I_{rf} \approx 5.3 \cdot 10^{13}$ W/m^2) and FEL wavelengths in the VUV-X range (10 ~ 20) nm .

We should underscore that, even with these relaxed numbers, it is not an easy task to transport this amount of power density. In order to enhance the RF power density we can proceed by increasing CARM output power, using, e.g., a suitable compression of the associated pulse.

We remind that the CARM is driven by an e-beam sustained by a pulse forming system, with a flat top of the order of microseconds [44]. The RF pulse has accordingly a comparable length. The power can be enhanced by compressing the pulse, by reducing it to a length comparable with the saturation length, namely tens of ns.

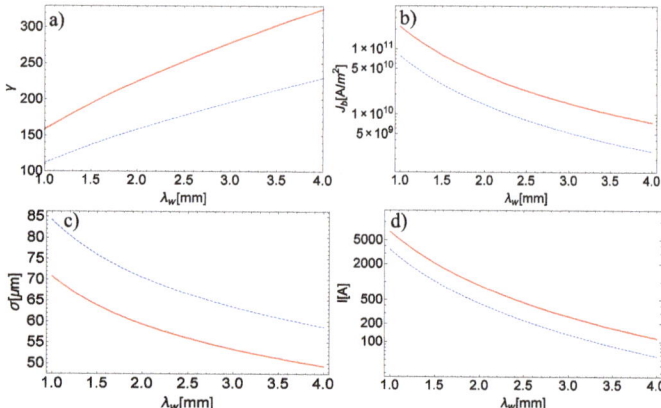

Figure 14. Electron beam energy (**a**), electron beam current density (**b**), the electron beam transverse section (**c**) and the peak current (**d**) vs. the RF wavelength λ_w for two FEL radiation $\lambda_r = 10$ nm (continuous line) and $\lambda_r = 20$ nm (dashed line).

According to the previous discussion, the CARM pulse compression to a duration of tens of ns (few meters, approximately the saturation length foreseen for RFU operation) is sufficient to ensure CARM peak power level near the GW level.

The possibility of achieving these results has been suggested in refs. [45,46], in which the use of a dispersive corrugated metal waveguide was proposed. The crucial idea put forward in these articles is that of exploiting a swept frequency modulated train of pulses that propagate inside the waveguide, with a monotonically increasing group velocity. Accordingly, the tail of the pulse will overtake its head, thus providing either a shortening of its duration and an increase (in absence of significant losses) of the relevant amplitude.

Most of the compression process occurs at the end of the waveguide, where all the frequency components are present at the same time and the compression ratio (C) can be expressed as [46]

$$C = \frac{\Delta f}{f_0} \frac{L}{\lambda_0} \left(\frac{1}{k_1} - \frac{1}{k_2} \right) e^{-\gamma_0 L} \qquad (23)$$

being $k_{1,2} = v_{g,1,2}/c$, with $v_{g,1,2}$ the group velocities at the beginning and at the end frequencies of the RF pulse, $\Delta f / f_0$—the fractional bandwidth, L—the waveguide length, $\lambda_0 = c/f_0$—the CARM wavelength and γ_0—the waveguide losses. The compression factor, summarized by Equation (23), is one of the central point of the discussion. It requires a careful design of the radiation transport in the corrugated waveguide, that follows the "active" waveguide where the CARM amplification and growth occurs. The physical mechanism beyond Equation (23) is fairly straightforward; the helically corrugated waveguide is designed with a dispersion relation ensuring a significant dependence of the group velocity on the frequency, accordingly, if a pulse is modulated from one frequency to a frequency with a higher group velocity the pulse will be compressed. The simulations and the experimental results of the aforementioned paper [46,47] report compression ratios around 25, for tens of GHz RF with a bandwidth of 5%. In accordance with our simulation the bandwidth of the RF generated by the CARM amplifier is sufficiently large (around 5.3%), and can be be eventually increased by using an input seed in the CARM cavity with larger bandwidth in order to compensate any major losses in the compression factor. Finally, the cavity length must be adjusted to contain the highest flat power of the signal to be compressed. This could be a limitation for the pulse length which in principle cannot be more than hundreds of ns for a reasonable cavity length (a couple of meters assuming a group velocity value $1/10$ of light speed). A long CARM RF pulse ($\sim \mu$s) can be also used by modulating the input signal in the CARM cavity in order to produce a conveniently chopped signal.

According to our preliminary calculations, we can foresee an analogous behavior for RF CARM around 150 GHz; we have been conservative regarding the maximum CARM output power and we would like to underscore that even a factor two larger is within the realm of the present technology.

Considering a reduction of the pulse duration by two orders of magnitude and assuming a power loss of 50% we can foresee an amount of power, available for wave-undulator operation, 250 MW. The required power density is accordingly obtained by confining the RFU over a surface of $0.7 \sim 1$ mm radius (reasonably large to transport radiation in the wavelength region of our interest).

The next step is to specify how the RF transport cavity should be designed.

The conclusion we may draw, from the inspection of the plots, is that the CARM RFU FEL is conceivable, at least in the soft X-ray region. The RFU power should be confined over a small surface to ensure the required density power level, warranting K_w values suitable for FEL SASE operation.

The following analysis is limited to RF wavelength within 1–3 mm. The requests on the electron beam are not particularly challenging, with respect to those of the RFU power transport waveguide, which according to the prescription of ref. [24] requires the selection of $TE - TM$ modes combination, characterized by a small transverse section, ensuring the required large intensity.

Regarding the electron–radiation interaction schemes, several solutions have been foreseen, as illustrated in Figure 15 where the "standard" RFU standing wave undulator is reported on the left, while the flying undulator concepts on the right with phase and group velocity are directed in the opposite electron direction.

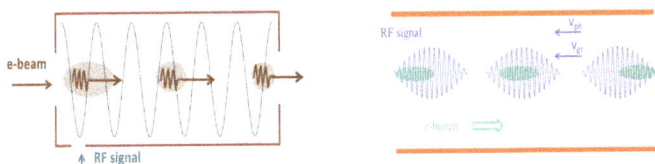

Figure 15. Compton backscattering with a standing wave (**left**). Compton scattering with a short pulse (**right**). The cavity filling time (lasting few ns) can be synchronized with repetition rate of the e-beam injection.

There is a natural drawback affecting the counter propagating scheme, namely the effective interaction length. If the RF wave propagates inside the guide with group velocity v_g and if the RFU pulse has a duration τ, the effective interaction length is [24]

$$L_{eff} = \frac{v_g \tau}{1 + \frac{v_g}{c}} \qquad (24)$$

for $v_g \approx c$. In other words, the effective length becomes a factor two lower than the pulse length itself, which means only half of the undulator is exploited. On the other side, the "co-propagating" scheme in Figure 16 (left) does not suffer the same problem. The cavity is indeed designed with corrugated helical ripples [24] which allow the pulse train to move with group velocity pointing in the same direction of the electrons and the phase velocity opposite. The effective interaction length is therefore

$$L_{c,eff} = \frac{v_g \tau}{1 - \frac{v_g}{c}} \qquad (25)$$

greater than the head-on case by a factor $(1 + v_g/c)(1 - v_g/c)$.

It might be thought that for the co-propagating scheme, the Compton backscattering up-shift does not occur. This is not true because the waveguide structure ensures the up-shift, according to what is shown in Figure 16 (right) where the effective intra-guide RF propagation is displayed. The radiation follows a kind of reflection, at each ripple, allowing multiple reflections pushing its "center of mass" in the forward direction. The head-on interaction occurs in the region where electrons and radiation overlaps (brown disk in Figure 16 (left)).

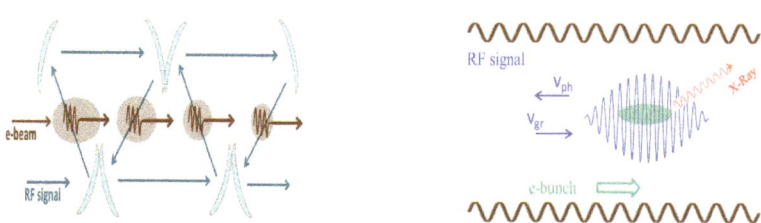

Figure 16. Mirror model of the intra-guide RFU propagation (**left**) and helical ripple waveguide and flying RFU pulse (**right**).

The use of a standing wave backscattering configuration is, however, feasible, at the price of operating the device with a longer waveguide.

Both configurations require the necessity of a pulse compression and the transport through a waveguide supporting hybrid mode structures, whose detailed design will be presented elsewhere. The solution foreseen in Figure 16 seems to be more appealing for the architecture we consider.

In Figure 17 we report a sketch of the whole device, indicating the RF CARM injected inside the corrugated waveguide (with a mode converter/mirror) and after the compression delivered in the second corrugated waveguide where the FEL SASE interaction occurs.

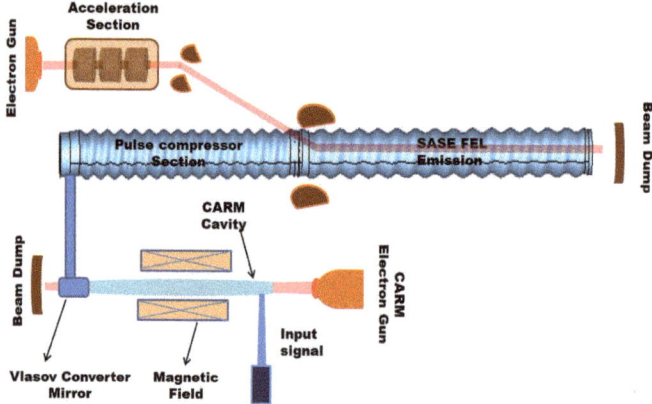

Figure 17. CARM-Undulator, SASE-FEL layout. Lower part: CARM generator and radiation transport system. Upper part: consecutive helical waveguides, the first acts as RF power compressor, the second, fed with an external e-beam, realizes the SASE interaction region.

In this paper, we consider the possibility of operating a FEL SASE device using a RFU pumped by a CARM device. The microwave CARM is a nearly mature technology, useful to develop "compact" FELs operating in the VUV and soft X-ray region. The intrinsic limitations of these devices are, as previously underscored, associated with the maximum CARM available power (limiting the K_w strength parameter) and with the physical dimensions of the radiation transport vacuum pipe radius, limiting the cutoff frequency of the propagated radiation. The combination of these two limiting factors has indicated a threshold of 10 nm as the minimum operating wavelength. It should furthermore be stressed that, although we have indicated a pulse compression method as a useful device to enhance the microwave power, we did not underscore enough that it is still at the level of experimental studies, not yet conducted in the frequency range above 100 GHz. This solution, if viable, would provide a real step towards the realization of compact X-ray FEL devices. The construction of this type of short FEL wavelength device is a challenging promising task, which foresees the use and merging of high-level technologies, within the present or next future capabilities.

Author Contributions: The E.D.P., S.C., G.L.R., E.S., I.S. and G.D. made the same contributions in terms of conceptualization, writing, data control and critical reading. All authors have read and agreed to the published version of the manuscript.

Funding: This research received no external funding.

Institutional Review Board Statement: Not applicable.

Informed Consent Statement: Not applicable.

Acknowledgments: The Authors like to express their sincere appreciation to an anonymous Referee, whose challenging comments improved the quality of the paper.

Conflicts of Interest: The authors declare no conflict of interest.

References

1. Gilbert, A.J.; McDonald, B.S.; Robinson, S.M.; Jarman, K.D.; White, T.A.; Deinert, M.R. Non-invasive material discrimination using spectral X-ray radiography. *J. Appl. Phys.* **2014**, *115*, 154901, doi:10.1063/1.4870043. [CrossRef]
2. Settens, C.; Bunday, B.; Thiel, B.; Kline, R.J.; Sunday, D.; Wang, C.; Wu, W.-L.; Matyi, R. Critical dimension small angle X-ray scattering measurements of FinFET and 3D memory structures. *Proc. SPIE Int. Soc. Opt. Eng.* **2013**, *8681*, 86810L, doi:10.1117/12.2012019. [CrossRef]
3. Wen, H.; Gomella, A.A.; Patel, A.; Lynch, S.K.; Morgan, N.Y.; Anderson, S.A.; Bennett, E.E.; Xiao, X.; Liu, C.; Wolfe, D.E. Subnanoradian X-ray phase-contrast imaging using a far-field interferometer of nanometric phase gratings. *Nat. Commun.* **2013**, *4*, 2659. [CrossRef]
4. Carvalho, A.L.; Trincão, J.; Romão, M.J. X-ray crystallography in drug discovery. *Methods Mol. Biol.* **2009**, *4*, 572.
5. Sakdinawat, A.; Attwood, D. Nanoscale X-ray imaging. *Nat. Photonics* **2010**, *4*, 480. [CrossRef]
6. Emma, P.; Akre, R.; Arthur, J.; Bionta, R.; Bostedt, C.; Bozek, J.; Brachmann, A.; Bucksbaum, P.; Coffee, R.; Decker, F.-J.; et al. First lasing and operation of an ångstrom-wavelength free-electron laser. *Nat. Photonics* **2010**, *4*, 641–647, doi:10.1038/nphoton.2010.176 [CrossRef]
7. Ackermann, W.; Asova, G.; Ayvazyan, V.; Azima, A.; Baboi, N.; Bähr, J; Balandin, V.; Beutner, B.; Brandt, A.; Bolzmann, A.; et al. Operation of a free-electron laser from the extreme ultraviolet to the water window. *Nat. Photonics* **2007**, *1*, 336–342, doi:10.1038/nphoton.2007.76 [CrossRef]
8. Allaria, E.; Appio, R.; Badano, L.; Barletta, W.A.; Bassanese, S.; Biedron, S.G.; Borga, A.; Busetto, E.; Castronovo, D.; Cinque-grana, P.; et al. Highly coherent and stable pulses from the FERMI seeded free-electron laser in the extreme ultraviolet. *Nat. Photonics* **2012**, *6*, 699–704, doi:10.1038/nphoton.2012.233 [CrossRef]
9. Milne, J.C.; Schietinger, T.; Aiba, M.; Alarcon, A.; Alex, J.; Anghel, A.; Arsov, V.; Beard, C.; Beaud, P.; Bettoni, S.; et al. SwissFEL: The Swiss X-ray Free Electron Laser. *Appl. Sci.* **2017**, *7*, 720, doi:10.3390/app7070720. [CrossRef]
10. Yun, K.; Kim, S.; Kim, D.; Chung, M.; Jo, W.; Hwang, H.; Nam, D.; Kim, S.; Kim, J.; Park, S.-Y.; et al. Coherence and pulse duration characterization of the PAL-XFEL in the hard X-ray regime. *Sci. Rep.* **2019**, *9*, 3300, doi:10.1038/s41598-019-39765-3. [CrossRef]
11. Huang, Z.; Lindau, I. SACLA hard-X-ray compact FEL. *Nat. Photonics* **2012**, *6*, 505–506. doi:10.1038/nphoton.2012.184 [CrossRef]
12. Zhao, Z.; Wang, D.; Gu, Q.; Yin, L.; Gu, M.; Leng, Y.; Liu, B. Status of the SXFEL Facility. *Appl. Sci.* **2017**, *7*, 607, doi:10.3390/app7060607. [CrossRef]
13. Huang, N; Deng, H.; Liu, B.; Wang, D. Physical Design and FEL Performance Study for FEL-III Beamline of SHINE. In Proceedings of the 39th International Free Electron Laser Conference, Hamburg, Germany, 26–30 August 2019, doi:10.18429/JACoW-FEL2019-TUP063. [CrossRef]
14. Madey John, M.J. Stimulated emission of bremsstrahlung in a periodic magnetic field. *J. Appl. Phys.* **1971**, *42*, doi:10.1063/1.1660466. [CrossRef]
15. Dattoli, G.; Renieri, A. *Experimental and Theoretical Aspects of the Free-Electron Laser*; Chapter in Laser Handbook; Stitch, M.L.; Ball, M.S., Eds.; North-Holland: Amsterdam, The Netherlands, 1985; Volume IV, doi:10.1016/B978-0-444-86927-2.50005-X. [CrossRef]
16. Saldin, E.; Schneidmiller, E.V.; Yurkov, M.V. *The Physics of Free Electron Lasers*; Springer: Berlin/Heidelberg, Germany, 2000; doi:10.1007/978-3-662-04066-9. [CrossRef]

17. Ciocci, F.; Dattoli, G.; Torre, A.; Renieri, A. *Insertion Devices for Synchrotron Radiation and Free Electron Laser*; Series on Synchrotron Radiation Techniques and Applications; World Scientific: Singapore, 2000; Volume VI, doi:10.1142/4066. [CrossRef]
18. Dattoli, G.; Di Palma, E.; Pagnutti, S.; Sabia, E. Free Electron coherent sources: From microwave to X-rays. *Phys. Rep.* **2018**, *739*, 1–51, doi:10.1016/j.physrep.2018.02.005 [CrossRef]
19. Bratman, V.L.; Ginzburg, N.S.; Petelin, M.I. Energy feasibility of a relativistic Compton laser. *JEPT Lett.* **1978**, *28*, 190.
20. Shintake, T.; Huke, K.; Tanaka, J.; Sato, I.; Kumabe, I. Development of Microwave Undulator. *Jpn. J. Appl. Phys.* **1983**, *22*, 844–851, doi:10.1143/jjap.22.844. [CrossRef]
21. Tantawi, S.; Shumail, M.; Neilson, J.; Bowden, G.; Chang, C.; Hemsing, E.; Dunning, M. Experimental Demonstration of a Tunable Microwave Undulator. *Phys. Rev. Lett.* **2014**, *112*, 164802, doi:10.1103/PhysRevLett.112.164802. [CrossRef]
22. Kuzikov, S.V.; Jiang, Y.; Marshall, T.C.; Sotnikov, G.V.; Hirshfield, J.L. Configurations for short period rf undulators. *Phys. Rev. ST Accel. Beams* **2013**, *16*, 070701, doi:10.1103/PhysRevSTable16.070701. [CrossRef]
23. Savilov, A.V. Compression of complicated rf pulses produced from the super-radiant backward-wave oscillator. *Appl. Phys. Lett.* **2010**, *97*, 093501, doi:10.1063/1.3484963. [CrossRef]
24. Kuzikov, S.V.; Savilov, A.V.; Vikharev, A.A. Flying radio frequency undulator. *Appl. Phys. Lett.* **2014**, *105*, 033504, doi:10.1063/1.4890586. [CrossRef]
25. Gaponov, A.V.; Miller M.A. On the Potential Wells for Charged Particles in a High-Frequency Electromagnetic Field. *J. Exp. Theor. Phys.* **1958**, *7*, 168.
26. Bandurkin, I.V.; Kuzikov, S.V.; Savilov, A.V. Cyclotron-undulator cooling of a free-electron-laser beam. *App. Phys. Lett.* **2014**, *105*, 073503, doi:10.1063/1.4893455. [CrossRef]
27. Bandurkin, I.V.; Kuzikov, S.V.; Plotkin, M.E.; Savilov, A.V.; Vikharev, A.A. Terahertz FEL based on Photoinjector Beam in RF Undulator. In Proceedings of the 36th International Free Electron Laser Conference (FEL-2014), Basel, Switzerland, 25–29 August 2014; p. TUP046. Available online: https://accelconf.web.cern.ch/FEL2014/posters/tup046_poster.pdf (accessed on 1 December 2015).
28. Zhang, L.; He, W.; Clarke, J.; Ronald, K.; Phelps, A.D.R.; Cross, A.W. Microwave Undulator Using a Helically Corrugated Waveguide. *IEEE Trans. Electron Devices* **2018**, *65*, 5499–5504. doi:10.1109/TED.2018.2873726. [CrossRef]
29. Toufexis, F.; Tantawi, S.G. Development of a millimeter-period rf undulator. *Phys. Rev. Accel. Beams* **2019**, *22*, 120701, doi:10.1103/PhysRevAccelBeams.22.120701. [CrossRef]
30. Danly, B.G.; Blank, M.; Calame, J.P.; Levush, B.; Nguyen, K.T.; Pershing, D.E.; Parker, R.K.; Felch, K.L.; James, B.G.; Borchard, P.; et al. Development and testing of a high-average power, 94-GHz gyroklystron. *IEEE Trans. Plasma Sci.* **2000**, *28*, 713–726. doi:10.1109/27.887710. [CrossRef]
31. Sinitsyn, O.V.; Nusinovich, G.S.; Nguyen, K.T.; Granatstein, V.L. Nonlinear theory of the gyro-TWT: Comparison of analytical method and numerical code data for the NRL gyro-TWT. *IEEE Trans. Plasma Sci.* **2002**, *30*, 915–921. doi:10.1109/TPS.2002.801569. [CrossRef]
32. Petelin, M.I. On the theory of ultrarelativistic cyclotron self-resonance masers. *Radiophys. Quantum Electron.* **1974**, *17*, 902–908, doi:10.1007/BF01038662. [CrossRef]
33. Bratman, V.L.; Ginzburg, N.S.; Nusinovich, G.S.; Petelin, M.I.; Strelkov, P.S. Relativistic gyrotrons and cyclotron autoresonance maser. *Int. J. Electron.* **1981**, *13*, 541–567. doi:10.1080/00207218108901356. [CrossRef]
34. Bratman, V.L.; Ginzburg, N.S.; Petelin, M.I. Common properties of free electron lasers. *Opt. Commun.* **1979**, *30*, 409–412, doi:10.1016/0030-4018(79)90382-1. [CrossRef]
35. Yulpatov, V.K. Nonlinear theory of the interaction between a periodic electron beam and an electromagnetic wave. *Radiophys. Quantum Electron.* **1967**, *10*, 846–856, doi:10.1007/BF01089857. [CrossRef]
36. Gaponov, A.V.; Petelin, M.I.; Yulpatov, V.K. The induced radiation of excited classical oscillators and its use in high-frequency electronics. *Radiophys. Quantum Electron.* **1967**, *10*, 794–813. doi:10.1007/BF01031607. [CrossRef]
37. Ginzburg, N.S. Nonlinear theory of electromagnetic wave generation and amplification based on the anomolous Doppler effect. *Radiophys. Quantum Electron.* **1979**, *22*, 323–330, doi:10.1007/BF01035358. [CrossRef]
38. Fliflet, A.W. Linear and non-linear theory of the Doppler-shifted cyclotron resonance maser based on TE and TM waveguide modes. *Int. J. Electron.* **1986**, *61*, 1049–1080, doi:10.1080/00207218608920939. [CrossRef]
39. Chen, C.; Wurtele, S. Linear and non linear theory of cyclotron autoresonance masers with multiple waveguide modes. *Phys. Fluids B* **1991**, *3*, 2133, doi:10.1063/1.859626. [CrossRef]
40. Sabchevski, S.; Idehara, T. Cyclotron autoresonance with TE and TM guided waves. *Int. J. Infrared Millim. Waves* **2005**, *26*, 669–689, doi:10.1007/s10762-005-4977-6. [CrossRef]
41. Nusinovich, G. *Introduction to the Physics of Gyrotrons*; The Johns Hopkins University Press: Baltimore, MD, USA, 2004.
42. Ceccuzzi, S.; Dattoli, G.; Di Palma, E.; Doria, A.; Sabia, E.; Spassovsky, I. The High Gain Integral Equation for CARM-FEL Devices. *IEEE J. Quantum Elect.* **2015**, *51*, 1–9. doi:10.1109/JQE.2015.2432719. [CrossRef]
43. Dattoli, G.; Pagnutti, S.; Ottaviani, P.L.; Asgekar, V. Free electron laser oscillators with tapered undulators: Inclusion of harmonic generation and pulse propagation. *Phys. Rev. ST Accel. Beams* **2012**, *15*, 030708, doi:10.1103/PhysRevSTable15.030708. [CrossRef]

44. Artioli, M.; Aquilini, M.; Campana, E.; Cappelli, M.; Carpanese, M.; Ceccuzzi, S.; Ciocci, F.; Dattoli, G.; De Meis, D.; Di Giovenale, S.; et al. *Conceptual Design Report. A 250 GHz Radio Frequency CARM Source for Plasma Fusion*; Enea Publisher: Rome, Italy, 2016; ISBN 978-88-8286-339-5. Available online: https://www.enea.it/it/seguici/pubblicazioni/pdf-volumi/v2016-cdr-carm.pdf (accessed on 1 December 2018).
45. Samsonov, S.V.; Phelps, A.D.; Bratman, V.L.; Burt, G.; Denisov, G.G.; Cross, A.W.; Ronald, K.; He, W.; Yin H. Compression of frequency-modulated pulses using helically corrugated waveguides and its potential for generating multigigawatt rf radiation. *Phys. Rev. Lett.* **2004**, *92*, 118301, doi:10.1103/PhysRevLett.92.118301. [CrossRef]
46. Zhang, L.; Mishakin, S.V.; He, W.; Samsonov, S.V.; McStravick, M.; Denisov, G.G.; Cross, A.W.; Bratman, V.L.; Whyte, C.G.; Robertson, C.W.; et al. Experimental Study of Microwave Pulse Compression Using a Five-Fold Helically Corrugated Waveguide. *IEEE Trans. Microw. Theory Tech.* **2015**, *63*, 1090–1096. doi:10.1109/TMTT.2015.2393882. [CrossRef]
47. McStravick, M.; Samsonov, S.V.; Ronald, K.; Mishakin, S.V.; He, W.; Denisov, G.G.; Whyte, C.G.; Bratman, V.L.; Cross, A.W.; Young, A.R.; et al. Experimental results on microwave pulse compression using helically corrugated waveguide. *J. Appl. Phys.* **2010**, *108*, 054908, doi:10.1063/1.3482024. [CrossRef]

Article

Hybrid (Oscillator-Amplifier) Free Electron Laser and New Proposals

Andrea Doria

ENEA, Fusion Physics Division, C.R. Frascati, via E. Fermi 45, I-00044 Frascati (Rome), Italy; andrea.doria@enea.it

Abstract: The present work analyses a hybrid free electron laser (FEL) scheme where the oscillator is based on a radiation source operating with a slow-wave guiding structure as, for instance, a Cerenkov FEL or a Smith–Purcell FEL. Such devices, often running in transverse magnetic (TM) modes, present a longitudinal electric field which can easily affect the longitudinal electrons' velocities, inducing an energy modulation on the beam. Such a modulation, properly controlled, can induce a strong radiation emission in a magnetic undulator properly designed to operate as a radiator. General considerations will be exposed together with a practical numerical example in the far infrared region of the spectrum.

Keywords: free electron laser; Oscillator-Amplifier; TeraHertz

1. Introduction

Free electron lasers (FELs) are widely acknowledged as the most versatile generators of coherent electromagnetic radiation. Since the first studies in the late 1960s [1] and their "official" invention in 1977 [2], it has been clear that FELs are capable of bridging the gap between conventional electron-based sources (such as klystrons, magnetrons, travelling wave tubes) that are limited to the high frequency direction, and the lasers that, with some exceptions, generate single frequency radiation with a power that is limited by the nature of the active medium. FELs can be designed, in principle, to operate at any frequency and with a time structure and related power suitable for any kind of experiment. This kind of flexibility comes from the fact that many of the parameters involved, such as the electron energy and the magnetic field, can be adjusted with continuity. Moreover, many dynamical regimes can be exploited for FEL design; from the low-gain regime, suitable for oscillator devices [3], to the high gain regime ideal for the self-amplified spontaneous emission (SASE) scheme [4]. Furthermore, FEL offers significant potential options to combine different schemes in sequence in order to increase the performances of some specific features without overly stressing the project parameters. One of the most relevant FEL structures arrangements, among others, is a modulator at a synchronous frequency followed by a frequency multiplier that exploits the harmonic content in the modulated beam [5,6]. Such an arrangement may be reproduced several times, creating a kind of cascade [7] that results in final beam degradation.

This study presents one of the possible arrangements based on a Cerenkov FEL oscillator as a modulator and a magnetic undulator as a radiator: this solution can be considered a hybrid FEL scheme device [8]. The reason why the term hybrid can be ascribed to such a scheme is not only due to the fact that the modulator and radiator present two different mechanisms of radiation generation, but mainly because in Cerenkov-like FEL devices [9] (as is the case for Smith–Purcell gratings [10]), the coupling between electrons and field is longitudinal, while the magnetic undulator induces a transverse motion to the electrons and accordingly, to the coupling. This circumstance, combined with the fact that Cerenkov (and Smith–Purcell) FELs operate with slow-wave guiding structures, has a relevant effect on the differences, for "synchronism condition" [9,11], that links the spontaneous emission wavelength with the most relevant parameters of the experiment, between Cerenkov and undulator FELs.

The paper is arranged in four sections: after the present Introduction, Section 2 is dedicated to the study of the Cerenkov-based modulator. Section 3 will introduce the hybrid system as a whole, highlighting the value of the main parameters. Section 4 will describe the effects of the modulation on the emission from a magnetic undulator exploited as a radiator; this analysis includes the ballistic effects of a variable drift space. Section 5 is devoted to final conclusions.

2. The Hybrid System

The hybrid FEL system can be assumed to be composed of three main elements: (1) an electron beam accelerator; (2) a Cerenkov slow-wave guiding structure, with an adequate radiation resonator for the saturation regime accomplishment; and lastly, (3) a magnetic undulator acting as a radiator after the velocity modulation induced by an electric field associated with the radiation stored in the Cerenkov oscillator (see Figure 1).

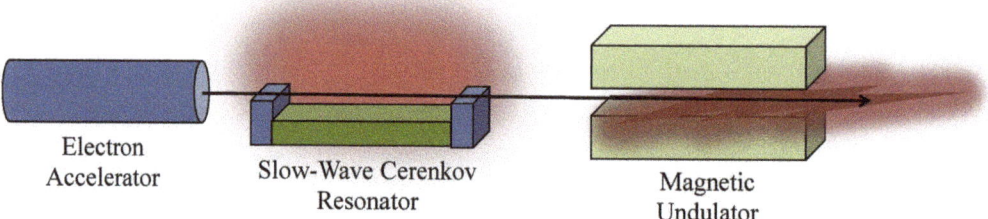

Figure 1. Schematic drawing of the hybrid FEL under study. The accelerated electron beam generates radiation interacting with the Cerenkov resonator. The electric beam associated with the stored radiation modulates the electrons' velocities in order to obtain the most efficient emission in the magnetic undulator radiator.

The first problem to face is related to the energy of the electron beam that will be common to both generating structures. As discussed in the introduction, the synchronism conditions for Cerenkov and undulator FELs are rather different and can be summarised as follows (see Refs. [9,11]), where the subscript U and C indicate the undulator and Cerenkov, respectively:

$$\lambda_U = \frac{\lambda_w}{2\gamma^2}\left(1 + K^2\right); \lambda_C = 2\pi\gamma d\left(\frac{\varepsilon - 1}{\varepsilon}\right) \quad (1)$$

where λ_w indicates the undulator period, K is the undulator parameter, d is the dielectric thickness of the Cerenkov guiding structure, ε is its dielectric constant and γ is the Lorentz parameter of the electrons. All these parameters will be more deeply described in the following sections.

In order to obtain an efficient modulation of the electron beam, it is required that the radiation generated from the Cerenkov oscillator and from the Undulator radiator be "correlated"; a way to achieve this target is to obtain the condition: $\lambda_U = \lambda_C/n$ where $n = 1, 2, \ldots$ specifies the harmonic number. Such a relation, with the use of Equation (1), becomes:

$$\frac{\lambda_w}{2\gamma^2}\left(1 + K^2\right) = \frac{2\pi\gamma}{n}d\left(\frac{\varepsilon - 1}{\varepsilon}\right) \Leftrightarrow \gamma^3 = \frac{\lambda_w}{4\pi}n\left(1 + K^2\right)\frac{\varepsilon}{d(\varepsilon - 1)} \quad (2)$$

Equation (2) gives the value of the electron energy as a function of all the parameters involved in both the Cerenkov and undulator FELs. In order to have an idea about the numbers, we can assign some reasonable values for the involved parameters in Equation (2) such as: λ_w = 2.5 cm, K = 1, d = 5 μm, n = 1, ε = 5 (dielectric constant of quartz [12]) from which we obtain a result, for the electron energy, $\gamma \sim 10$, that corresponds to a moderate relativistic energy. By inserting these values into Equation (1), we conclude that such a source would operate in the so-called far-infrared (FIR) spectral region (also called TeraHertz (THz)-region) because $\lambda_U \sim \lambda_C \sim 250$ µm.

Another approach can be obtained by rearranging Equation (2) as follows:

$$d\left(\frac{\varepsilon - 1}{\varepsilon}\right) = \frac{\lambda_w}{4\pi\gamma^3}\left(1 + K^2\right)n \tag{3}$$

from which it is possible to obtain the Cerenkov parameters values starting from the undulator FEL ones. Let us suppose we have an FEL source with $\lambda_w = 2.5$ cm, $K = 1$, $\gamma = 20$ and again working on the fundamental harmonic $n = 1$, Equation (3) gives: $[d(\varepsilon - 1)/\varepsilon] \sim 5 \cdot 10^{-7}$ µm. Such a value may be obtained in several ways since, for instance, $\varepsilon = 2$ and $d = 1$ µm. Using all these values for the hybrid FEL parameters, we eventually obtain from Equation (1) the value for the emitted wavelength from both the elements of the hybrid FEL: $\lambda_U \sim \lambda_C \sim 60$ µm.

3. The Cerenkov FEL Oscillator

A well-known class of waveguides is characterised by having open boundaries and the possible presence of an electromagnetic (e.m.) field outside the boundary; these guides support propagating modes called "surface waves" [13]. Dielectric films deposited over conducting plates are devices that fall into the aforementioned category; the surface waves, in this case, present an exponential behaviour, normal to the dielectric surface, that decays when moving away. Such a waveguide category is the relevant one for the realisation of the Cerenkov FEL device because the field–particle interaction occurs in the region of the space where the "evanescent" e.m. field is present.

These propagating devices present field distributions associable with transverse electric (TE) or transverse magnetic (TM) modes. The case of TM modes is more favourable for the FEL use due to the presence of a longitudinal electric field component related to them. The vector potential for the TM modes of a single slab geometry waveguide is expressed by [9,13]

$$\begin{cases} A_x = A_0 \frac{ck}{\omega q} e^{-qx} \sin(kz) e^{-i\omega t} \\ A_y = 0 \\ A_z = A_0 \frac{c}{i\omega} e^{-qx} \sin(kz) e^{-i\omega t} \end{cases} \tag{4}$$

where k indicates the longitudinal momentum, while q is the transverse momentum in vacuum and p is the transverse momentum in the dielectric of thickness d. All these parameters are linked by two coupled "dispersion relations" that can be deduced by the field continuity along the vacuum–dielectric interface and dielectric–conductor interface:

$$\begin{cases} qd = \frac{pd}{\varepsilon} \tan(pd) \\ (pd)^2 + (qd)^2 = d^2\left(\frac{\omega}{c}\right)^2(\varepsilon - 1) \end{cases} \text{and} \begin{cases} p = \sqrt{\varepsilon\left(\frac{\omega}{c}\right)^2 - k^2} \\ q = \sqrt{k^2 - \left(\frac{\omega}{c}\right)^2} \end{cases} \tag{5}$$

In order to obtain the electric and magnetic fields from Equation (4), we can adopt the Coulomb gauge ($\mathbf{E} = -\partial \mathbf{A}/\partial t$; $\mathbf{B} = \nabla \times \mathbf{A}$) which is useful for evaluating the fields in absence of charges and currents, as for the free modes in a guiding structure. Neglecting the coupling between the electrons and the transverse electric field E_x (due to the small values of the electrons' velocities in the x direction), we obtain for the longitudinal field:

$$E_z = -cA_0 e^{-qx} \sin(kz) e^{-i\omega t} \tag{6}$$

In order to achieve the maximum field intensity, it is necessary to reach the saturation regime inside the Cerenkov waveguide resonator. The dynamics of the emission process in Cerenkov FEL has been established in the past as far as the spontaneous emission process [9,14] is concerned and with regard to the stimulated emission mechanism and the gain coefficient calculation [14,15]. Let us, therefore, consider the case discussed in Section 2 while discussing Equation (2); the relevant parameters are summarised in Table 1.

Table 1. Cerenkov FEL Parameters @ λ = 250 µm.

Cerenkov FEL Parameters @ λ = 250 µm					
Electron Energy	Dielectric Thickness	Dielectric Constant	Resonator Length	Resonator Width	Double Slab Height
γ = 10.0	d = 50 µm	ε = 5.0	L = 35.0 cm	W = 1.0 cm	D = 2 cm

Table 1 reports the parameters for both a single slab geometry device [9] and for the double slab one [16] adequate for an operation around λ_C = 250 µm. The behaviour of the spontaneous emission for a single-electron beam with a transverse size of σ_x = 1 mm (r.m.s.), as a function of frequency and beam centroid distance from the dielectric surface, is reported in Figure 2a). The same analysis for the double slab geometry and a beam size of σ_x = 1 cm (r.m.s.) is reported in Figure 2b):

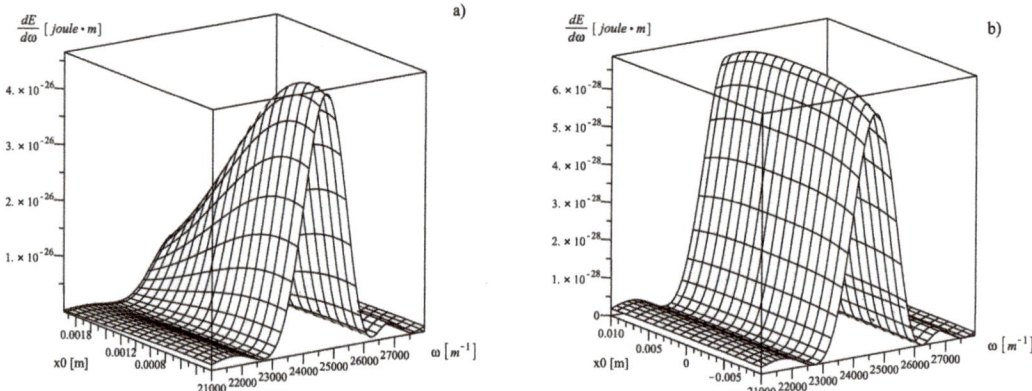

Figure 2. Spontaneous emission spectra as a function of the beam centroid distance from the dielectric surface: (**a**) single slab waveguide geometry; and (**b**) double slab waveguide geometry.

The one-dimensional stimulated emission process, until saturation, can be studied by means of semi-analytical techniques [17] (three-dimensional theory can be found in [18]). The saturation mechanism in free electron devices is quite similar to that occurring in conventional lasers, as has been derived by Rigrod approximately sixty years ago [19] and is also present in the theory of passive saturable absorber for laser mode-locking [20]. Two different but similar approaches can be applied; the first technique starts from the application of the Ginzburg–Landau equation to FEL systems [21] and leads to the $G_I(I)$ expression in Equation (7). The second method is based on the logistic equation approach [22] and ends up the $G_{II}(I)$ expression in Equation (7):

$$\begin{cases} G_I(I_n) = 0.849 \cdot g_{0MAX} \dfrac{1-\exp\left(-\frac{\pi}{2}\frac{I_n}{I_{SAT}}\right)}{\frac{\pi}{2}\frac{I_n}{I_{SAT}}} \\ I_{SAT} = \dfrac{\gamma I_0 I_{AV}}{4 g_{0MAX} N_{eq} c} \\ I_{n+1} = [I_n + G_I(I_n)I_n](1-\Gamma) \end{cases} ; \begin{cases} G_{II}(n) = \dfrac{I(n)-I(n-1)}{I(n-1)} \\ I(n) = I_{SP} \dfrac{\exp\{[g_{0MAX}(1-\Gamma)-\Gamma]n\}}{1+(I_{SP}/I_{e,i})[\exp\{[g_{0MAX}(1-\Gamma)-\Gamma]n\}-1]} \\ I_{e,i} = \dfrac{2}{\pi}\dfrac{1-\Gamma}{\Gamma} g_{0MAX}\left\{1-\exp\left[-\dfrac{1.8}{1+g_{0MAX}}\dfrac{g_{0MAX}(1-\Gamma)-\Gamma}{\Gamma}\right]\right\} I_{SAT} \end{cases} \quad (7)$$

where $N_{eq} = L/(2\gamma^2\lambda_C) \sim 7.3$ represents the equivalent value of the number of undulator periods in Cerenkov FELs; $I_{SAT} \sim 7.4 \cdot 10^6$ [W] expresses the saturation power value related to the gain of the device (conventionally, the intensity is used instead of power, however, in this case, the radiation transverse cross-section is a constant due to the presence of a waveguide, making power and intensity interchangeable); n indicates the round-trip number; $I_{AV} \sim 17,000$ A indicates the Alfven current; Γ represent the total losses in the radiation resonator; I_{SP} expresses the spontaneous emission power of all the electrons in the bunch and integrated over the bandwidth; $I_{e,i}$ refers to the intracavity equilibrium power, and finally, g_{0MAX} indicates the maximum value of the small-gain, small-signal gain coefficient as a function of frequency [15]. The relevant parameters for the gain calculation are reported in Table 2.

Table 2. Cerenkov FEL Gain Parameters @ λ = 250 μm.

Cerenkov FEL Gain Parameters @ λ = 250 μm					
Electron Bunch Current	Angular Distribution	Transverse Distribution	Peak Gain Coefficient	Total Resonator Losses	Intracavity Equilibrium Power
$I_0 = 20.0$	$\sigma' = 5 \times 10^{-4}$ (r.m.s.)	$\sigma_x = 1$ mm (r.m.s.)	$g_{0MAX} = 0.4$	$\Gamma = 0.042$	$I_{e,i} = 7.22 \times 10^7$ W

The behaviour of Equation (7) is reported in Figure 3a) for the gain expressions, G_I and G_{II}, as a function of the round trip number n, and in Figure 3b) for the ongoing power radiation, I_n and $I(n)$, again with respect to the round trip. The main result, as can be deduced from Figure 3, is that saturation is reached after about n = 100 round trips considering both methods reported in Equation (7). Considering the resonator length, as indicated in Table 1, we can deduce that saturation is gained in about $T_{SAT} \sim 200$ ns, which is quite a short time with respect to the conventional macro-bunch duration of electron pulses generated by RF accelerators in the S-band (~3 GHz), which of the order of several microseconds. This will be relevant for the analysis of the velocity modulation induced on the remaining part of the macro-bunch itself.

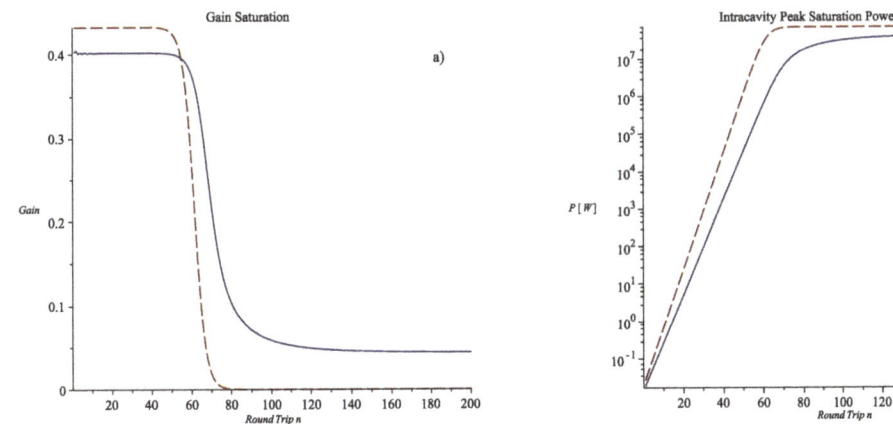

Figure 3. Saturation behaviour: (**a**) gain as a function of the round-trip number; and (**b**) intracavity power as a function of the round-trip number.

The peak intra-cavity peak power, as deduced by Figure 3b), is about $P_{SAT} \sim 4.2 \times 10^7$ W; considering an average transverse radiation dimensions, obtained from the data reported in Table 1, of about $\Sigma_L = 1$ cm^2, the electric field associated to the intracavity radiation at saturation is:

$$E_{SAT} = \sqrt{2 I_{SAT}/(\varepsilon_0 c \Sigma_L)} \approx 1.782 \cdot 10^7 \, [\text{V/m}]$$

Before analysing the dynamical process, it is worth briefly addressing the question of the longitudinal modes in the Cerenkov FEL resonator. The wavenumber mode separation, as evident from Equation (6), is $(\Delta\omega/c) = \pi/L$. The relative gain bandwidth is [11,15]:

$$\frac{\Delta\omega_G}{\omega} \approx \frac{1}{4N_{eq}} = \frac{\gamma^2 \lambda_C}{2L} \Rightarrow \frac{\Delta\omega_G}{c} = \frac{\omega_C}{c}\frac{\gamma^2 \lambda_C}{2L} \approx \frac{\pi\gamma^2}{L}$$

The number of modes contained in the gain bandwidth is therefore: $\Delta\omega_G/\Delta\omega = \gamma^2$. It is well known [11] that any FEL based on the RF accelerator locks all the longitudinal modes in a natural way. The result of such mode-locking is that a single short pulse of radiation travels back and forth inside the tuned resonator with a group velocity that is slightly smaller than that of the electron beam, causing a kind of anti-lethargic effect [23], unlike what happens for undulator FELs.

4. Electron Beam Modulation and Undulator Emission

At the end of the previous section, we saw how an intense electromagnetic pulse, that can be generated inside an optical resonator in about 200 nanoseconds, needs to be saturated. For electron macro-bunches, as long as few microseconds we will have thousands of micro-bunches available interacting with the electromagnetic field. If we analyse each of these electron micro-bunches, we recognise that, at the resonator entrance, each of them superimposes with a correspondent radiation micro-pulse as illustrated in Figure 4a). In such a situation, the electrons of the bunch, generally equally spaced in phase, will experience the oscillating longitudinal electric field E_z (Equation (6)) with a spatial periodicity of λ_C, as showed in Figure 4b). The situation represented in Figure 4 is quite similar to that of an electron beam accelerated by a series of RF cavities such as those of a standing-wave Linac [11,24]. The number of cavities can be estimated by calculating the number of the electric field oscillations "contained" within the electron micro-bunch length $(\delta z \sim \tau_e \beta_e c)$ divided by the wavelength λ_C: $N_c \sim (\delta z/\lambda_C)$. The most widely used accelerators for FELs operate in the so-called S-band $(\nu_{RF} \sim 3$ GHz$)$ and generate micro-bunches of a typical duration of $\tau_e \sim 15$ ps, which corresponds to a bunch length of about $\delta z \sim 5$ mm. Considering a radiation wavelength of $\lambda_C \sim 250$ μm, as for the example discussed in the previous sessions, we obtain $N_c \sim 20$.

It is possible, therefore, to imagine any optical cycle acting on the electrons in a way similar to that of the accelerating cavities of a Linac. We know, in fact, that electrons undergo to an energy variation that is connected to the particle-radiation relative phase. Such an energy variation will be positive for electrons close to the so-called accelerating phase and negative for those with an opposite phase. The result is a bunching of the electrons into N_c "slices".

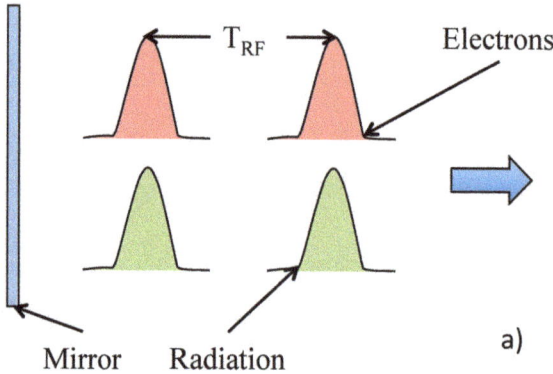

Figure 4. Cont.

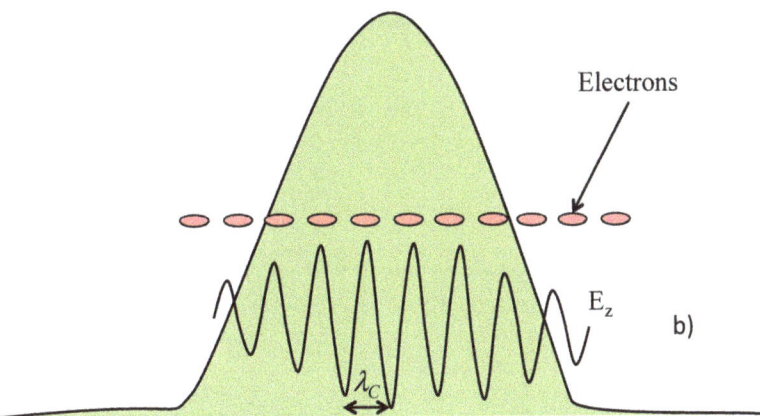

Figure 4. Electron bunch and radiation pulse interaction: (**a**) phase locking; and (**b**) electrons and radiation electric field interaction.

To properly evaluate the energy variation of a single electron, let us consider that the energy exchange occurs along the time needed for the electron, to cross the resonator length L. The particle, during this time $T = L/(c\beta_e)$, experiences a quasi-static electric field due to the fact that, even with small differences, its speed is almost synchronous with the electromagnetic pulse that travels with its group velocity $\beta_g = d(\omega/c)/dk$ (see Equation (5)), and therefore, $\beta_g \sim \beta_e$. The energy variation, for each electron, is consequently:

$$\Delta\gamma = \frac{\Delta E}{m_0 c^2} = \frac{\mathbf{F} \cdot \mathbf{s}}{m_0 c^2} = \int_0^T \frac{e\mathbf{E}(t)}{m_0 c^2} \cdot \mathbf{v}_e dt = \frac{eE_{0z}}{m_0 c^2} c\beta_e \int_0^T \cos(\omega t + \phi) dt \quad (8)$$

where the longitudinal electric field has been derived from Equation (6) and the constant term E_{0z} contains the transverse coupling between the electron and the evanescent field in the x direction. Before getting an explicit form for Equation (8), it is worth underlining that the phase φ usually refers to the RF field, at an angular frequency ω_{RF}, that accelerates the electron beam in the accelerator (Linac, for instance). In the present case, the phase φ should be referred to as the Cerenkov radiation field in the optical resonator, and therefore, ought to be "normalised" by means of the frequency ratio ω_C/ω_{RF}: $\phi \Rightarrow \phi(\omega_C/\omega_{RF}) = \phi(\lambda_{RF}/\lambda_C)$. After some algebra, we obtain:

$$\Delta\gamma = \frac{eE_{0z}}{m_0 c^2} L \left[\frac{\sin\left(\frac{\omega}{c}\frac{L}{\beta_e}\right)}{\left(\frac{\omega}{c}\frac{L}{\beta_e}\right)} \cos\left(\phi\frac{\lambda_{RF}}{\lambda_C}\right) + \frac{\cos\left(\frac{\omega}{c}\frac{L}{\beta_e}\right)}{\left(\frac{\omega}{c}\frac{L}{\beta_e}\right)} \sin\left(\phi\frac{\lambda_{RF}}{\lambda_C}\right) \right] \quad (9)$$

The result of what has been discussed is that the energy modulation expressed by Equation (9) can be exploited to generate powerful radiation inside a magnetic undulator utilised as a radiator. The discussion after Equation (2) in Section 2 leads to a set of parameters, summarised in Table 3, for an undulator synchronous with the fundamental Cerenkov emission.

Table 3. Undulator–Radiator FEL Parameters @ λ_U = 250 µm.

Undulator–Radiator FEL Parameters @ λ_U = 250 µm					
Electron Energy	Undulator Period	Undulator Parameter	Number of Periods	Waveguide Width	Waveguide Height
γ = 10.0	λ_w = 2.5 cm	=1.0	N_U = 50	W = 0.5 cm	H = 0.5 cm

The emission of radiation from a radiator by means of an ensemble of charged particles distributed in the phase space has been faced in the recent past [25,26]. To summarise some concepts, we can say that the electron beam, after the interaction, carries a modulation of the current $\vec{J}$ that can be expressed as a Fourier expansion in terms of the harmonics l of the RF. Moreover, the electromagnetic field can be expanded in terms of the transverse modes, expressed by the aggregate index λ, of the waveguide that is needed to confine the radiation in the far infrared spectral range, and expressing the expansion coefficients as $A_{l,\lambda}$. Finally, the power $P_{l,\lambda}$, emitted due to the energy exchange between the electron beam and the radiation field in the magnetic field of the undulator, can be evaluated by means of the flux of the Poynting vector. Equation (10) summarises all the above in an extensive demonstration which can be found in [25] and the references therein:

$$\vec{J} = \sum_{l=1}^{\infty} \vec{J}_l \exp(-i\omega_l t) \ ; \ \omega_l = 2\pi \frac{l}{T_{RF}}$$
$$A_{l,\lambda} = -\frac{Z_0}{2\beta_g} \frac{e}{T_{RF}} \frac{KL}{\sqrt{\Sigma_\lambda}} \sum_{j=1}^{N_e} \frac{1}{\beta_{z,j}\gamma_j} \frac{\sin(\theta_{l,\lambda,j}/2)}{\theta_{l,\lambda,j}/2} i \exp\left(\frac{\theta_{l,\lambda,j}}{2} + l\psi_j\right) \ ; \ \theta_{l,\lambda,j} = \left(\frac{\omega_l}{c\beta_{z,j}} - \frac{2\pi}{\lambda_w} - k_\lambda\right) \quad (10)$$
$$P_{l,\lambda} = \frac{\beta_g}{2Z_0}|A_{l,\lambda}|^2$$

where e is the electron charge, Z_0 is the vacuum impedance, Σ_λ is the radiation transverse mode size, N_e is the number of electrons contained in the bunch, $\beta_{z,j}$ is the longitudinal velocity of the j-th electron, β_g is the radiation group velocity and k_λ is the transverse mode momentum.

A brief analysis of Equation (10) tells us that the expansion coefficient $A_{l,\lambda}$ plays a significant function in the determination of the radiation formation. It is, in fact, the role of each electron in the bunch is relevant because it carries a specific energy γ_j and a specific phase ψ_j. In particular, the electron phase ψ_j, together with the interaction phase $\theta_{l,\lambda,j}$ enter in a more general phase term in $A_{l,\lambda}$ that, when summing up all of the contributions of the N_e electrons of the bunch, may generate constructive or destructive interactions. The maximum radiated power in the undulator is obtained when all the electrons contribute to the radiation formation with the same phase term (only depending on the harmonic number l), therefore, with an adequate distribution of the electrons in the phase-space.

What has been discussed, so far, about Equation (10), refers to the longitudinal properties of the particle–wave interaction, which concur with the undulator parameter K and period λ_w and the electron longitudinal velocities $\beta_{z,j}$. The transverse characteristics of the radiation emission are summarised by the mode aggregate index λ. It is evident, however, that the transverse space can play a role when the electron beam emittance values could be relevant for the radiation wavelength to be generated. A deeper and exhaustive analysis can be found in [27].

With such a mathematical background, an appropriate computational code was set up for the evaluation of the coherent generation of radiation in the undulator–radiator. The code is capable of evaluating the impact of an electron bunch, with a specific distribution in the phase-space, for the radiation generation, calculating the contribution of any electron, integrated along the interaction length. The code, at the moment, does not take into account saturation effects. The effect of the energy modulation introduced by the electron–field interaction inside the Cerenkov FEL optical resonator can be assessed by comparing the emission from an electron distribution $D(\gamma_j, \psi_j)$ and the same distribution to which an energy modulation is added $D(\gamma_j + \Delta\gamma(\psi_j)_j, \psi_j)$, where the contribution $\Delta\gamma(\psi_j)_j$ is calculated from Equation (9) for each electron. To this aim, an ad hoc electron distribution was generated in the phase-space having a uniform partitioning in energy with a total $\Delta\gamma = 0.2$ around $\gamma = 10$ (see Table 3) corresponding to a $\sigma_\gamma \approx 5 \cdot 10^{-3}$ r.m.s. The phase partitioning is again uniform, with an added Poissonian component, with a total $\Delta\psi = 20°$ corresponding to the actual micro-bunch duration expressed as phase interval for Linac [11]. In Figure 5, we report the aforementioned electron distribution (Figure 5a) together with the corresponding power spectrum (Figure 5b) calculated with Equation (10). The total power, integrated over the whole bandwidth, results in $P_{TOT} \sim 55$ W.

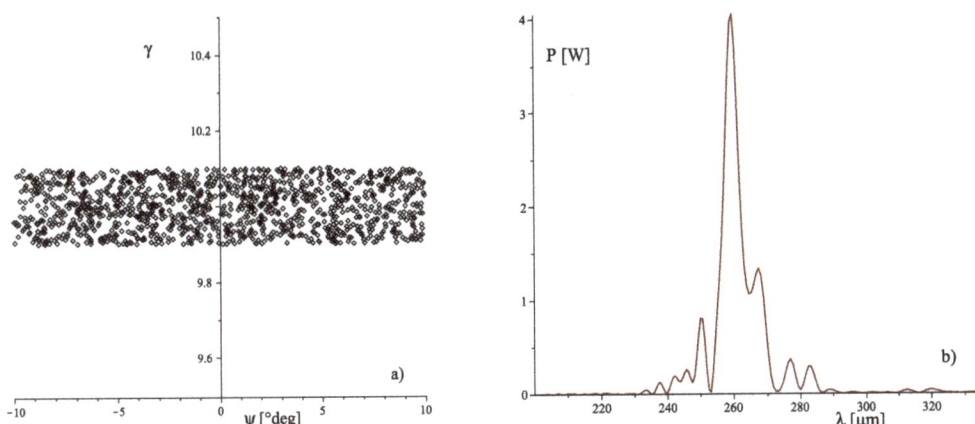

Figure 5. Emission by undulator–radiator: not the modulated case: (**a**) phase-space; and (**b**) power spectrum.

As anticipated, a similar calculation can be performed for the electron distribution of Figure 5a), to which the energy modulation $\Delta \gamma_j$ of Equation (9) is added for each electron of the distribution with its actual phase ψ_j and energy (through the velocity $\beta_{e,j}$). The amplitude of the electric field is the one evaluated at the end of Section 3 from the saturated intracavity radiation power $E_{0z} \sim 1.8 \times 10^7$ [V/m]. In Figure 6, we report the energy modulated electron distribution (Figure 6a) together with the corresponding power spectrum (Figure 6b), again calculated by means of Equation (10). As can be clearly seen, the emission is strongly increased by orders of magnitude due to the modulation introduced which, moreover, is not clearly distinguishable when looking at Figures 5a and 6a. It is further worth underlining how the total bandwidth is slightly reduced with respect to the unmodulated case. The total power, integrated over the whole bandwidth, now results as $P_{TOT} \sim 1.28 \times 10^7$ W.

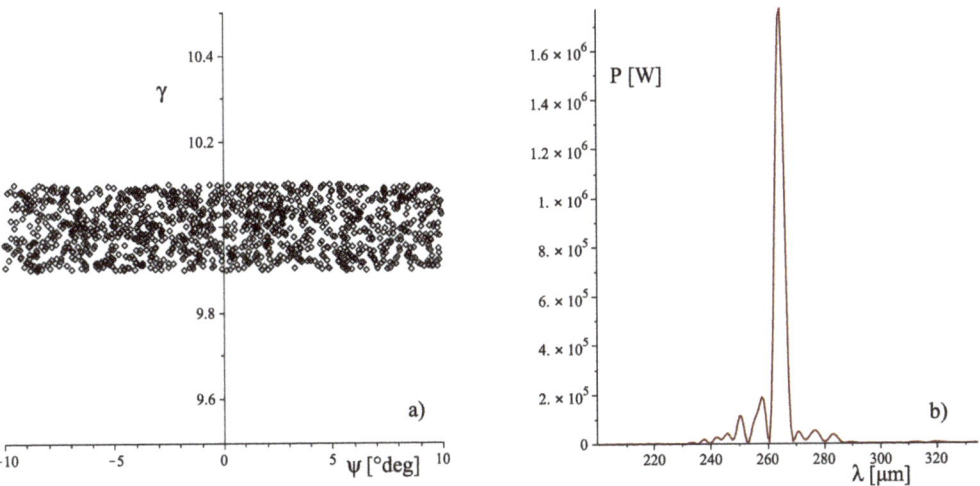

Figure 6. Emission by undulator–radiator: modulated case: (**a**) phase-space; and (**b**) power spectrum.

We may now ask whether there is any optimisation procedure to further increase the power radiated by the undulator. The most relevant tool is the distance between the Cerenkov electromagnetic resonator and the entrance of the magnetic undulator. This is because the energy modulation acquired by the electrons in the cavity transforms into a velocity modulation, and consequently bunches before entering the undulator interaction region. This "drift space" allows a ballistic process that correlates the velocity variation of each electron, with its position, and therefore phase, in the bunch. In Equation (11), we report the phase term that should be inserted in the set of Equation (10) that takes into account the phase variation, after the velocity modulation expressed by $(v_z)_j$ and for a specific drift space L_{Drift}. The index "j" indicates the specific electron and v_{ref} is the velocity of the "reference electron":

$$\left(\Psi_{Drift}\right)_j = \omega_{RF} L_{Drift} \left(\frac{1}{(v_z)_j} - \frac{1}{v_{ref}}\right) + \psi_j \tag{11}$$

Considering a series of values for L_{Drift} ranging from 0 to 3.5 metres, the power spectrum was calculated and reported in Figure 7. As can be appreciated, the peak power, starting from a specific value, tends to reduce, while increasing L_{Drift}, and the spectrum itself tends to broaden with a couple of peaks appearing. A further increase in the modulator radiator distance produces a spectral band reduction and a peak power increase up to the final value.

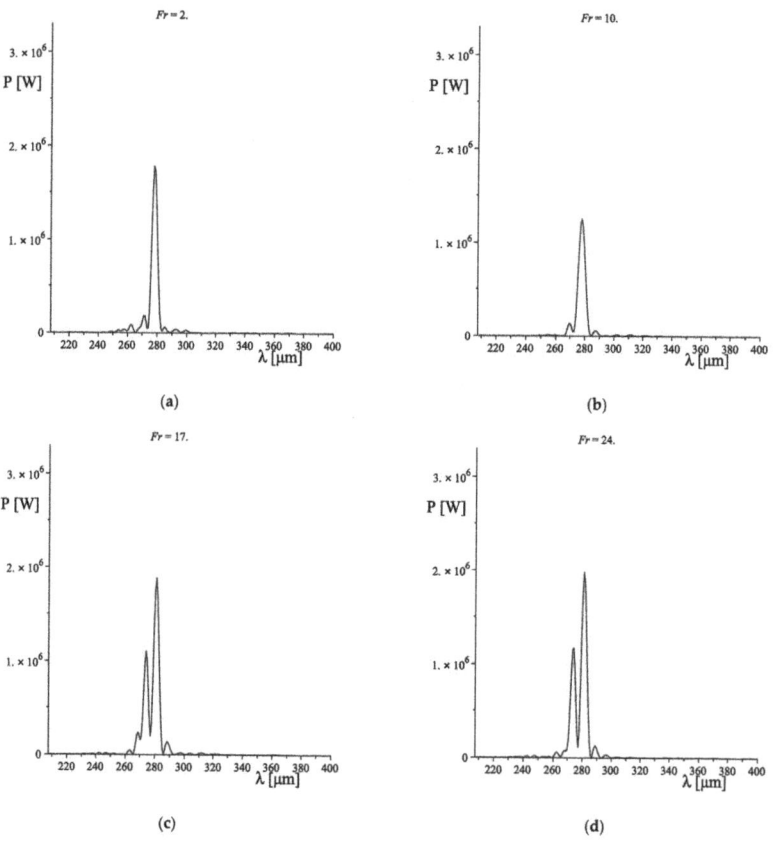

Figure 7. Cont.

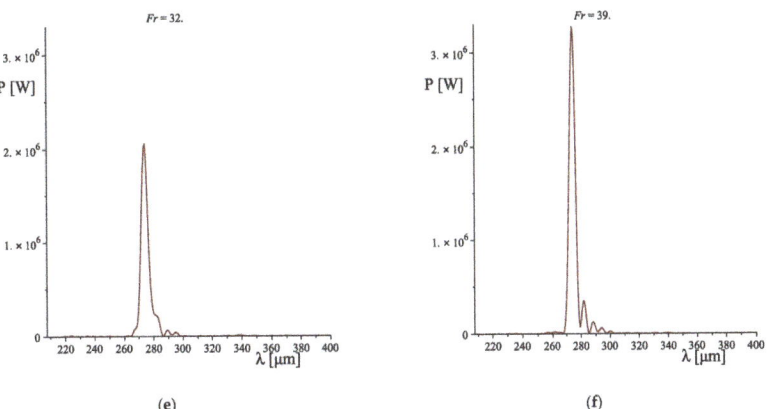

Figure 7. Power spectrum for different drift-space values: (**a**) L_{Drift} = 0.18 m; (**b**) L_{Drift} = 0.90 m; (**c**) L_{Drift} = 1.52 m; (**d**) L_{Drift} = 2.15 m; (**e**) L_{Drift} = 2.87 m; and (**f**) L_{Drift} = 3.50 m.

5. Conclusions

The example reported to date indicates how a hybrid scheme for free electron devices can be effective for the power enhancement of the electromagnetic radiation generated. This two-elements scheme, based on an oscillator, in which intracavity radiation acts as an energy modulator, and a magnetic undulator as a radiator, is a versatile arrangement because the oscillator section can be chosen among a series of different devices. As anticipated, together with the Cerenkov device, other sources can be taken into account; among which the Smith–Purcell is an interesting choice because it offers characteristics that lay between that of a Cerenkov FEL (being a slow-wave device) and an undulator FEL (wavelength scales inversely with the electron energy, as can be seen in Equation (12)). The synchronic condition, in fact, results to be [10,28]:

$$\lambda_{SP} = \frac{\Lambda}{|n_{so}|}\left(\frac{1}{\beta_e} - \cos\theta\right) \qquad (12)$$

where Λ represents the grating period, n_{so} indicates the grating spectral order and θ is the angle between the electron beam direction (parallel to the grating surface) and the observer. A new parameter, in the Smith–Purcell-based FEL, is evident from Equation (12) and is the angle θ that offers a wide and continuous range of spectral tunability [28] that can be exploited, keeping fixed other parameters like the electron energy and the grating geometry. This characteristic increases the flexibility of the hybrid scheme FEL because it easily allows to obtaining the condition $\lambda_U = \lambda_{SP}/n$, where $n = 1, 2, \ldots$, because the $\cos\theta$ term can be used to obtain the maximum wavelength extension:

$$\lambda_{SP}^{(+)} = \frac{\Lambda}{|n_{so}|}\frac{1}{\beta_e} \Rightarrow \lambda_{SP}^{(-)} = \frac{\Lambda}{|n_{so}|}\left(\frac{1-\beta_e}{\beta_e}\right).$$

The harmonic number n is, therefore, a pivotal parameter for extending the spectral emission of such a coherent source [5–7], that with a proper combination of all the parameters involved, for both the oscillator and the radiator, prove to be a promising and versatile device, with the additional feature of compactness.

Funding: This research received no external funding.

Institutional Review Board Statement: Not applicable.

Informed Consent Statement: Not applicable.

Data Availability Statement: Not applicable.

Conflicts of Interest: The authors declare no conflict of interest.

References

1. Pantell, R.H.; Soncini, G.; Puthoff, H.E. Stimulated photon-electron scattering. *IEEE J. Quantum Electron.* **1968**, *QE-4*, 905–907. [CrossRef]
2. Deacon, D.A.G.; Elias, L.R.; Madey, J.M.J.; Ramian, G.J.; Schwettman, H.A.; Smith, T.I. First Operation of a Free-Electron Laser. *Phys. Rev. Lett.* **1977**, *38*, 892–894. [CrossRef]
3. van Amersfoort, P.W.; Bakker, R.J.; Bekkers, J.B.; Best, R.W.B.; van Buuren, R.; Delmee, P.F.M.; Faatz, B.; van der Geer, C.A.J.; Jaroszynski, D.A.; Manintveld, P.; et al. First lasing with FELIX. *Nucl. Instr. Meth.* **1992**, *A318*, 42–46. [CrossRef]
4. Milton, S.V.; Gluskin, E.; Arnold, N.D.; Benson, C.; Berg, W.; Biedron, S.G.; Borland, M.; Chae, Y.C.; Dejus, R.J.; Den Hartog, P.K.; et al. Exponential gain and saturation of a self-amplified spontaneous emission free-electron laser. *Science* **2001**, *292*, 2037–2040. [CrossRef] [PubMed]
5. Bonifacio, R.; De Salvo Souza, L.; Pierini, P.; Scharlemann, E.T. Generation of XUV Light by Resonant Frequency Tripling in a two Wiggler FEL Amplifier. *Nucl. Instr. Meth.* **1990**, *A296*, 787–790. [CrossRef]
6. Dattoli, G.; Doria, A.; Giannessi, L.; Ottaviani, P.L. Bunching and exotic undulator configurations in SASE FELs. *Nucl. Instr. Meth.* **2003**, *A507*, 388–391. [CrossRef]
7. Ciocci, F.; Dattoli, G.; De Angelis, A.; Faatz, B.; Garosi, F.; Giannessi, L.; Ottaviani, P.L.; Torre, A. Design Considerations on a High-Power VUV FEL. *IEEE J. Quantum Electron.* **1995**, *QE-31*, 1242–1252. [CrossRef]
8. Asgekar, V.; Dattoli, G. Hybrid free electron laser devices. *J. Appl. Phys.* **2007**, *101*, 063111-1–063111-4. [CrossRef]
9. Ciocci, F.; Dattoli, G.; Doria, A.; Schettini, G.; Torre, A.; Walsh, J.E. Spontaneous Emission in Cerenkov FEL Devices: A Preliminary Theoretical Analysis. *Il Nuovo Cimento* **1988**, *10D*, 1–20. [CrossRef]
10. Urata, J.; Goldstein, M.; Kimmitt, M.F.; Naumov, A.; Platt, C.; Walsh, J.E. Superradiant Smith-Purcell Emission. *Phys. Rev. Lett.* **1998**, *80*, 516–519. [CrossRef]
11. Dattoli, G.; Doria, A.; Sabia, E.; Artioli, M. *Charged Beam Dynamics, Particle Accelerators and Free Electron Lasers*, 1st ed.; IOP Publishing Ltd.: Bristol, UK, 2017.
12. Roberts, S.; Coon, D.D. Far-Infrared Properties of Quartz and Sapphire. *J. Opt. Soc. Am.* **1962**, *52*, 1023–1029. [CrossRef]
13. Collin, R.E. *Foundations of Microwave Engineering*; McGraw-Hill: Singapore, 1966.
14. Walsh, J.E. Stimulated Cerenkov Radiation. *Adv. Electron. Electron Phys.* **1982**, *58*, 271–310.
15. Dattoli, G.; Doria, A.; Gallerano, G.P.; Renieri, A.; Schettini, G.; Torre, A. A Single-Particle Calculation of the FEL-Cerenkov Gain. *Il Nuovo Cim.* **1988**, *101B*, 79–84. [CrossRef]
16. Ciocci, F.; Dattoli, G.; Doria, A.; Gallerano, G.P.; Schettini, G.; Torre, A. Spontaneous Emission in a Double Dielectric Slab for Cerenkov Free-Electron-Laser Operation. *Phys. Rev. A* **1987**, *36*, 207–210. [CrossRef] [PubMed]
17. Dattoli, G. Logistic function and evolution of free-electron-laser oscillators. *J. Appl. Phys.* **1998**, *84*, 2393–2398. [CrossRef]
18. Andrews, H.L.; Brau, C.A. Three-dimensional theory of the Cerenkov free-electron laser. *J. Appl. Phys.* **2007**, *101*, 104904-1–104904-6. [CrossRef]
19. Rigrod, W.W. Gain Saturation and Output Power of Optical Masers. *J. Appl. Phys.* **1963**, *34*, 2602–2603. [CrossRef]
20. Herman, A.H. Theory of mode locking with a fast saturable absorber. *J. Appl. Phys.* **1975**, *46*, 3049–3058.
21. Dattoli, G.; Cabrini, S.; Giannessi, L. Simple model of gain saturation in free-electron lasers. *Phys. Rev. A* **1991**, *44*, 8433–8434. [CrossRef]
22. Dattoli, G.; Giannessi, L.; Ottaviani, P.L.; Carpanese, M. A simple model of gain saturation in high gain single pass free electron lasers. *Nucl. Instr. Meth.* **1997**, *A393*, 133–136. [CrossRef]
23. Dattoli, G.; Doria, A.; Gallerano, G.P.; Schettini, G.; Torre, A.; Walsh, J.E. Pulse Propagation Theory for the Cerenkov Free-Electron Laser. *Il Nuovo Cim.* **1989**, *103B*, 281–289. [CrossRef]
24. Wangler, T.P. *Introduction to Linear Accelerator Theory*; LAUR-93-805; Los Alamos National Laboratory: Washington, DC, USA, 1993.
25. Doria, A.; Gallerano, G.P.; Giovenale, E.; Letardi, S.; Messina, G.; Ronsivalle, C. Enhancement of Coherent Emission by Energy-Phase Correlation in a Bunched Electron Beam. *Phys. Rev. Lett.* **1998**, *80*, 2841–2844, and references therein. [CrossRef]
26. Doria, A.; Gallerano, G.P.; Giovenale, E. Novel Schemes for Compact FELs in the THz Region. *Condens. Matter* **2019**, *4*, 90. [CrossRef]
27. Bahrdt, J. Shaping Photon Beams with Undulators and Wigglers. In *Synchrotron Light Sources Free Electron Lasers*; Springer: Berlin/Heidelberg, Germany, 2016; pp. 751–819.
28. Doucas, G.; Kimmitt, M.F.; Doria, A.; Gallerano, G.P.; Giovenale, E.; Messina, G.; Andrews, H.L.; Brownell, J.H. Determination of longitudinal bunch shape by means of coherent Smith-Purcell radiation. *Phys. Rev. Accel. Beams* **2002**, *5*, 072802-1–072802-8. [CrossRef]

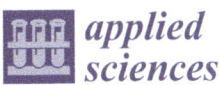

Review

Three-Dimensional, Time-Dependent Analysis of High- and Low-*Q* Free-Electron Laser Oscillators

Peter J. M. van der Slot [1,*,†] and Henry P. Freund [2,3,†]

1. Laser Physics and Nonlinear Optics, Mesa$^+$ Institute for Nanotechnology, Department of Science and Technology, University of Twente, 7544NE Enschede, The Netherlands
2. Department of Electrical and Computer Engineering, University of New Mexico, Albuquerque, NM 87131, USA; freundh0523@gmail.com
3. NOVA Physical Science and Simulations, Vienna, VA 22182, USA
* Correspondence: p.j.m.vanderslot@utwente.nl
† These authors contributed equally to this work.

Abstract: Free-electron lasers (FELs) have been designed to operate over virtually the entire electromagnetic spectrum, from microwaves through to X-rays, and in a variety of configurations, including amplifiers and oscillators. Oscillators can operate in both the low and high gain regime and are typically used to improve the spatial and temporal coherence of the light generated. We will discuss various FEL oscillators, ranging from systems with high-quality resonators combined with low-gain undulators, to systems with a low-quality resonator combined with a high-gain undulator line. The FEL gain code MINERVA and wavefront propagation code OPC are used to model the FEL interaction within the undulator and the propagation in the remainder of the oscillator, respectively. We will not only include experimental data for the various systems for comparison when available, but also present, for selected cases, how the two codes can be used to study the effect of mirror aberrations and thermal mirror deformation on FEL performance.

Keywords: free-electron laser; oscillator; regenerative amplifier

1. Introduction

Free-electron laser (FEL) oscillators (FELO) have been part of the overall research activity since the beginnings of the field. An FEL oscillator consists of an undulator placed within an optical resonator, also known as an optical cavity, that typically consists of two spherical mirrors separated by a distance L_{cav}. Note that the undulator is not necessarily centered within the optical resonator. Furthermore, an electron beam is directed into the cavity through the undulator, and out of the cavity, as is schematically shown in Figure 1, which is taken from Reference [1]. The optical pulse generated by the electrons streaming through the undulator is extracted from the cavity either by a partially reflective (i.e., transmissive) mirror or through a hole in the mirror. Observe that multiple optical pulses may be contained within the resonator depending upon the repetition rate of the electron bunches and the roundtrip time for the optical pulses to circulate through the resonator. We also note that, when the growth of the optical field exponentiates in a single pass through the undulator, i.e., in case of a high-gain FEL [2], a large fraction of the light can be extracted from the resonator.

The first FEL oscillator driven by a relativistic electron beam was realized in 1977 [3], shortly after the coherent amplification of radiation of the same wavelength was experimentally demonstrated [4]. Coherent undulator radiation was first demonstrated using the so-called Ubitron, which was configured both as amplifier and oscillator, and which is nowadays considered to be the first (non-relativistic) FEL [5]. In the early days of FEL development, the technology available to generate high-quality, high-brightness electron beams, that are necessary for efficient FEL operation, was relatively primitive by today's standards. At that time, the limited available gain, which in part may be due to space restrictions, favoured oscillator configurations to bring the laser into saturation and provide fully coherent output, as mirrors were readily available all the way from the visible to well into the microwave spectral range. Although we limit ourselves here to infrared wavelengths or shorter, exciting FEL research also takes place at longer wavelengths.

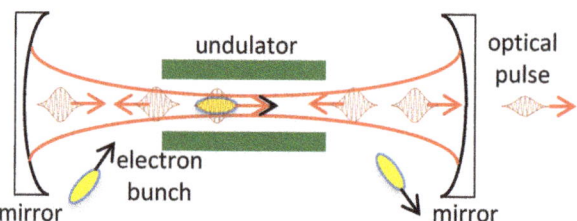

Figure 1. Schematic representation of a typical layout for an FEL oscillator. The electron beam consisting of electron pulses is guided through the undulator and around the mirrors. The optical pulse that is amplified within the undulator is recirculating within the resonator and extracted through one of the mirrors. Reproduced with permission from [1]. Copyright Springer, 2018.

The unique properties of FEL oscillators, in particular to fill the spectral gap for coherent light sources in the visible to microwave spectral range, resulted quickly in the establishment of several facilities for applied research. The characteristics of user facilities using FEL oscillators depends, in part, on the accelerator technology used, which includes electrostatic acceleration [6–9], energy recovery linear accelerators (linacs) [10–15], non-recovery linacs [16–30], microtrons [31,32] and synchrotrons [33–37]. Research performed at these user facilities includes, amongst others, biological and material science [38]. A more complete overview of the various FEL oscillators, together with the main system parameters, can be found in Ref. [39].

As mentioned, the optical properties of FEL oscillators are in part determined by the electron accelerator used. For example, electrostatic accelerators can only accelerate electrons up to a kinetic energy of a few MeV and, consequently, the spectral range is limited to microwave and THz frequencies [39]. The much higher electron energies of storage rings allow the FEL oscillators to operate in the visible down to the deep UV wavelengths [39], while RF linacs can, in principle, accelerate electrons to still higher energies, from a few MeV up to tens of GeV, allowing FELs to cover a large fraction of the electromagnetic spectrum, from microwaves all the way down to hard X-rays [39].

Furthermore, electrostatic accelerators are capable of long to continuous wave electron pulses, that can result in single longitudinal mode oscillation, with a relative linewidth of about 10^{-8} over a time of 5 µs, which was set by the voltage droop present in the accelerator [6] at the time of measurement. On the other hand, the short duration of, and spread in, electron energy for the electron pulses produced by RF linacs typically leads to a relative linewidth of the order of 10^{-4} to 10^{-2} [13,29,40–53], unless additional spectral filtering is used. For example, using the Vernier effect of a double cavity resonator to reduce the number of intra-cavity longitudinal modes and subsequent external filtering, an RF-linac-based FEL oscillator was able to provide a single longitudinal mode [54]. FEL oscillators based on storage rings provide a lower relative linewidth within the range 10^{-5} to 5×10^{-4} [34,55–63], due to the higher electron beam quality of storage rings.

Finally, the average and peak power are, to a large extent, determined by the accelerator technology. Superconducting energy recovery linacs are the primary drivers for high average power FEL oscillators [64–70]; however, other types of FEL oscillators have used various techniques to increase the output pulse energy including, but not limited to, optical klystrons [34,36,48,57,58,60,63,71–76], cavity dumping [77–81], pulse stacking in an external cavity [82–84], electron beam energy ramping [85,86] or dynamic cavity desynchronization [87–92]. Tapering of the undulator [93–95] has also been used to improve the peak power in the pulse [96–100], however, tapering of the undulator in FEL oscillators leads to complicated dynamics and a strong dependence on system parameters [101–104].

The wavelength tuning of FEL oscillators is typically obtained by selecting a set of electron beam energies and varying the undulator gap. Operation at other wavelength ranges is possible through harmonic generation [105–107] and such harmonics were quickly observed [40]. Lasing on the third harmonic was first demonstrated using the Standford MARK-III FEL oscillator [108], quickly followed by others [43,48,58,61,97,109–121]. The simultaneous generation of multiple wavelengths may be beneficial for certain applications. The fixed relation between the fundamental and its harmonics can be overcome using different undulators in a single optical cavity [19,122–125], two undulators driven by a single electron beam at a single beam energy, but each having its own optical resonator [126] or having different beam energies [127,128] to allow operation at two independently chosen wavelengths.

FEL oscillators share many characteristics with amplifier systems, however, there are also many differences. For example, slippage between the optical and electron pulse, in combination with cavity desynchronization, will effect the FEL oscillator dynamics. Here, a cavity is considered synchronized when it is tuned to a length where the roundtrip time for the optical pulse matches an integer multiple of the time separating two subsequent electron pulses. Maxima in the gain and extraction efficiency are found for different cavity desynchronizations. In particular, dynamic cavity desynchronization [87] can be used to first set a cavity length corresponding to maximum gain for a quick initial growth of the optical pulse energy and then switched to a cavity length for maximum extraction efficiency that is obtained at small cavity desynchronization. The latter is typically also associated with the generation of short optical pulses [19,88,92,129–134]. For short pulse FEL oscillators, i.e., where the root-mean-square (rms) width of the electron bunch is smaller than the total slippage distance, the oscillator is operating in the superradiant regime [132,134–142]. An analytic theory for this regime predicts a scaling of the optical pulse energy E_L with the bunch charge q as $E_L \propto q^{3/2}$ and a scaling of the temporal width τ_L of the optical pulse as $\tau_L \propto q^{-1/2}$ [138], which has been experimentally confirmed [139], although higher extraction efficiencies have also been observed for a perfectly synchronized cavity length, where the analytic theory breaks down [92,132]. Furthermore, short pulse FEL oscillators operating in the large-slippage regime also show a stable oscillation in the macropulse power, known as limit-cycle oscillations, for certain cavity lengths detuned from perfect synchronization, which has been observed both experimentally [102,137,143–146] and in numerical simulations [136,138,147–149].

Techniques well known from laser physics have also been applied to FEL oscillators, either experimentally or in a conceptual study, such as injection seeding [150–155] and mode locking [133,151,152,156]. On the other hand, the unique nature of the gain process in FELs allows for the micro-structuring of the gain medium [157–159] to enhance the gain, which is not readily available for ordinary lasers. One important application of this technique is to transfer coherence from a low-frequency optical beam to a higher frequency optical beam. This process is known as high-gain harmonic generation (HGHG) [160]. This technique has been successfully used to generate fully coherent light at soft X-ray frequencies [161]. Alternative methods currently investigated, in particular to reach even shorter wavelengths, and rely on Bragg reflections from atomic layers using appropriated crystals [162].

The drive to higher gain per unit length and to shorter wavelengths has pushed accelerator development; in particular, research into photo-cathode based electron sources [163,164] that typically produce higher quality electron beams has contributed to today's state-of-the-art accelerator technology. The availability of electron beams with improved beam quality has driven FEL development over the years, especially the capability to generate shorter wavelengths. Due to a lack of suitable mirrors, initial focus was on FELs relying on self-amplified spontaneous emission (SASE), with a proof-of-principle experiment at 530 nm [165], followed by demonstrations at shorter wavelengths [166]. To overcome poor temporal coherence, HGHG is used to provide completely coherent output pulses down to 4-nm wavelength [167], while for even smaller wavelengths, FEL oscillators using the above-mentioned Bragg mirrors are considered [162].

Along with increasingly sophisticated FEL oscillator designs and experiments, analytical theories [101,138,168–171] have been developed for an initial assessment of oscillator performance. An initial theoretical description of the FEL gain was quantum mechanical in nature [172,173], however, it was quickly demonstrated that the gain could be described using classical theory [174]. Furthermore, the more complete simulation codes have also become adept at treating increasingly complicated designs and include both steady-state and time-dependent simulations in one- and three-dimensions.

In the remainder of this paper, we will focus on the simulation of a few different FEL oscillators. To model these oscillators, we have selected the FEL gain code MINERVA, which models the light amplification within the undulator line, and the optical wavefront propagation code OPC, which models the light propagation in the remainder of the resonator. The mathematical formulations of these codes are presented in Section 2. Subsequently, we present some considerations on resonators relevant for FEL oscillators in Section 3. We continue with a discussion on a low-gain/high-Q oscillators, taking the Infrared Demo and Infrared Upgrade experiments performed at the Thomas Jefferson National National Accelerator Facility (JLab) as examples. Both are discussed in Section 4. We compare this with a high-gain/low-Q oscillator, also known as a regenerative amplifier (RAFEL), also operating in the infrared, and investigate the performance of such a system in the soft X-ray spectral range. These systems are described in Section 5. We conclude with a summary and discussion in Section 6.

2. Numerical Formulation

Simulations of FEL oscillators have appeared in the literature by including optical propagation algorithms to existing FEL simulation codes, as well as self-contained FEL oscillator codes [103,149,175–182]. In this paper, we describe the use of an existing FEL simulation code to treat the interaction within the undulators and to link that to a code specifically designed to propagate the optical field through various resonator configurations. Such optics codes are sufficiently general to be able to treat a variety of resonator designs, and many may have been originally created to deal with other types of lasers. In this simulation environment, the FEL code hands off the optical field at the resonator exit to the optics code, which then propagates the field around the resonator and back to the undulator entrance, after which it is handed off to the FEL code for another pass through the undulator.

Among the earliest applications of this method was to simulations of the IR-Demo [64,65], as described in Section 4.1, and the 10-kW Upgrade experiments at JLab [183], which employed the MEDUSA FEL code [184] and OPC [185] and successfully reproduced many of the essential features of the experiment. OPC has also been interfaced with the GENESIS FEL code [186] and the PUFFIN FEL code [187] to study VUV FEL oscillators [188,189]. In this paper, we discuss the linkage of the MINERVA simulation code with OPC.

As will be described below, while MINERVA represents the optical field as a superposition of Gaussian modes with two independent polarization directions, OPC propagates the field on a grid. This necessitates the mapping of the Gaussian modes in MINERVA at the undulator exit to the grid supported by OPC, and the decomposition of the optical field in OPC at the undulator entrance back into Gaussian modes for both polarization components.

2.1. The MINERVA Simulation Code

MINERVA is a time-dependent, three-dimensional simulation code that models the interaction between electrons and a co-propagating optical field through an undulator line, which may include strong-focusing quadrupoles and/or dipole chicanes [1,190–192]. The optical fields are described using a superposition of Gauss-Hermite modes, using two independent polarization directions taken to be in the x- and y-directions with the z-direction taken along the axis of the undulator line. The Gauss–Hermite modes constitute a complete set, and together with the two independent polarizations, are able to describe the generation of arbitrary polarizations that might arise for any given undulator geometry. The vector potential representing the optical field in terms of the Gauss–Hermite modes is given by

$$\delta \mathbf{A}(\mathbf{x},t) = \hat{\mathbf{e}}_x \sum_{\substack{l,n=0 \\ h=1}}^{\infty} e_{l,n,h}^{(x)}(\mathbf{x},t) \left(\delta A_{l,n,h}^{(1,x)}(z,t) \sin(\varphi_h^{(x)}(\mathbf{x},t)) + \delta A_{l,n,h}^{(2,x)}(z,t) \cos(\varphi_h^{(x)}(\mathbf{x},t)) \right) + $$
$$\hat{\mathbf{e}}_y \sum_{\substack{l,n=0 \\ h=1}}^{\infty} e_{l,n,h}^{(y)}(\mathbf{x},t) \left(\delta A_{l,n,h}^{(1,y)}(z,t) \sin(\varphi_h^{(y)}(\mathbf{x},t)) + \delta A_{l,n,h}^{(2,y)}(z,t) \cos(\varphi_h^{(y)}(\mathbf{x},t)) \right), \quad (1)$$

where (l,n) are the transverse mode numbers, h is the harmonic number and $\delta A_{l,n,h}$ are the mode amplitudes. Furthermore, $\hat{\mathbf{e}}_j$ is a unit vector in the j-direction, $j = x, y$ and

$$e_{l,n,h}^{(j)}(\mathbf{x},t) = \frac{w_{0,h}^{(j)}}{w_h^{(j)}(z-z_0,t)} e^{-r^2/(w_h^{(j)}(z-z_0,t))^2} H_l(\zeta_x^{(j)}(x,z,t)) H_n(\zeta_y^{(j)}(y,z,t)) \quad (2)$$

are the transverse eigenfunctions for polarization direction j $r = \sqrt{x^2 + y^2}$, H_l and H_n are the Hermite polynomials of order l and n, respectively, $\zeta_x^{(j)}(x,z,t) = \sqrt{2}x/w_h^{(j)}(z-z_0,t)$, $\zeta_y^{(j)}(y,z,t) = \sqrt{2}y/w_h^{(j)}(z-z_0,t)$ and $w_{0,h}^{(j)}$ and $w^{(j)}(z-z_0,t)$ are the beam radii in the waist at $z = z_0$ and at location z along the optical axis. Note, $e_{l,n,h}^{(j)}$ and $w^{(j)}$ are dependent on time through the source dependent expansion (SDE) [193], as different parts of the optical pulse will experience different gain. Finally, the optical phases $\varphi_h^{(j)}(\mathbf{x},t)$ are given by

$$\varphi_h^{(j)}(\mathbf{x},t) = h(k_0 z - \omega_0 t) + \alpha_h^{(j)}(z,t) \left(\frac{r}{w_h^{(j)}(z-z_0,t)} \right)^2, \quad (3)$$

where $k_0 = \omega_0/c$ is the vacuum wavenumber belonging to the carrier frequency ω_0, c is the speed of light in vacuo and $\alpha_h^{(j)}(z,t)$ is the curvature of the wavefront for harmonic h. In this formulation, we assume that the mode amplitudes, curvature of the phase fronts and radii of the modes are slowly varying functions of z and t. The total optical power is given by

$$P(z,t) = \sum_{\substack{l,n=0 \\ h=1}}^{\infty} P_{l,n,h}(z,t) = \frac{m_e^2 c^5}{8e^2} k_0^2 \sum_{\substack{l,n=0 \\ h=1}}^{\infty} 2^{l+n-1} l! n! \sum_{j=x,y} (w_{0,h}^{(j)})^2 \left((\delta a_{l,n,h}^{(1,j)}(z,t))^2 + (\delta a_{l,n,h}^{(2,j)}(z,t))^2 \right), \quad (4)$$

where $\delta a_{l,n,h}^{(i,j)}(z,t) = e \delta A_{l,n,h}^{(i,j)}(z,t)/m_e c^2$ are the components of the normalized mode amplitudes, $i = 1, 2$, $j = x, y$ and m_e is the electron rest mass.

The optical fields are driven by accelerated electrons, as they co-propagate through the magnetic fields that are placed along the transport line. Of main interest here is the amplification of the optical field by the electrons within the undulators that can be placed in arbitrary configuration along the electron beam transport line. Within the slowly varying phase and amplitude approximation, the evolution of the normalized mode amplitudes $\delta a_{l,n,h}^{(i,j)}(z,t)$ is given by

$$\frac{d}{dz} \begin{pmatrix} \delta a_{l,n,h}^{(1,j)}(z,t) \\ \delta a_{l,n,h}^{(2,j)}(z,t) \end{pmatrix} + K_{l,n,h}^{(j)}(z) \begin{pmatrix} \delta a_{l,n,h}^{(2,j)}(z,t) \\ -\delta a_{l,n,h}^{(1,j)}(z,t) \end{pmatrix} = \begin{pmatrix} S_{l,n,h}^{(1,j)}(z,t) \\ S_{l,n,h}^{(2,j)}(z,t) \end{pmatrix}, \quad (5)$$

where d/dz is the convective derivative and $K^{(j)}_{l,n,h}(z,t)$ is given by

$$K^{(j)}_{l,n,h}(z,t) = (1+l+n)\left[\frac{\alpha^{(j)}_h(z,t)}{w^{(j)}_h(z,t)}\frac{dw^{(j)}_h(z,t)}{dz} - \frac{1}{2}\frac{d\alpha^{(j)}_h(z,t)}{dz} - \frac{1+(\alpha^{(j)}_h(z,t))^2}{k_0(w^{(j)}_h(z,t))^2}\right]. \quad (6)$$

The source terms $S^{(i,j)}_{l,n,h}(z,t)$ in Equation (5) are given by

$$\begin{pmatrix}S^{(1,j)}_{l,n,h}(z,t)\\S^{(2,j)}_{l,n,h}(z,t)\end{pmatrix} = \frac{1}{\pi}\frac{\omega_b^2}{k_0c^2}\frac{1}{2^{l+n-1}}\frac{1}{l!n!}\frac{1}{(w^{(j)}_{0,h})^2}\left\langle e^{(j)}_{l,n,h}(\mathbf{x})\frac{v_j(z,t)}{|v_z(z,t)|}\begin{pmatrix}-\cos(\varphi^{(j)}_h(z,t))\\\sin(\varphi^{(j)}_h(z,t))\end{pmatrix}\right\rangle, \quad (7)$$

where ω_b is the nominal plasma frequency, v_j is the component of the electron velocity in direction j, v_z is the longitudinal velocity component and $\langle\langle\ldots\rangle\rangle$ is an average over the electron distribution given by

$$\langle\langle\ldots\rangle\rangle = \int_0^{2\pi}\frac{d\psi_0}{2\pi}\int_1^\infty\frac{d\gamma_0}{\sqrt{\pi/2}\Delta\gamma}\frac{e^{-(\gamma_0-\gamma_{\mathrm{avg}})^2/2\Delta\gamma^2}}{1+\mathrm{erf}(\gamma_{\mathrm{avg}}/\sqrt{2}\Delta\gamma)}\iint\frac{dx_0dy_0}{2\pi\sigma_r^2}\iint\frac{dp_{x0}dp_{y0}}{2\pi\sigma_p^2}e^{-r^2/2\sigma_r^2}e^{-p_{\perp 0}^2/2\sigma_p^2}(\ldots). \quad (8)$$

In Equation (8), γ_{avg} and $\Delta\gamma$ are the relativistic factors corresponding to the initial average electron energy and energy spread, and σ_r and σ_p describe the width of the initial distribution function in transverse and momentum phase space, respectively.

The particle distribution described by Equation (8) is supplemented in the simulation code MINERVA, with methods to import 6-dimensional particle distributions which may be obtained from various sources, such as electron beam transport models, and this allows full start-to-end simulation capabilities.

To minimize the number of modes required to accurately describe the amplified optical field within the undulators, the so-called source dependent expansion [193] is used. Within this approximation, the spot size and curvature of the eigenmodes for each of the polarization directions $j = x, y$ are allowed to evolve according to

$$\frac{dw^{(j)}_h(z,t)}{dz} = \frac{2\alpha^{(j)}_h(z,t)}{hk_0 w^{(j)}_h(z,t)} - w^{(j)}_h(z,t)Y^{(j)}_h(z,t) \quad (9)$$

and

$$\frac{1}{2}\frac{d\alpha^{(j)}_h(z,t)}{dz} = \frac{1+(\alpha^{(j)}_h(z,t))^2}{hk_0(w^{(j)}_h(z,t))^2} - X^{(j)}_h(z,t) - \alpha^{(j)}_h(z,t)Y^{(j)}_h(z,t), \quad (10)$$

where

$$X^{(j)}_h(z,t) = \frac{2}{(\delta a^{(j)}_{0,0,h}(z,t))^2}\left[\left(S^{(1,j)}_{2,0,h}(z,t)+S^{(1,j)}_{0,2,h}(z,t)\right)\delta a^{(1,j)}_{0,0,h}(z,t) - \left(S^{(2,j)}_{2,0,h}(z,t)+S^{(2,j)}_{0,2,h}(z,t)\right)\delta a^{(2,j)}_{0,0,h}(z,t)\right] \quad (11)$$

and

$$Y^{(j)}_h(z,t) = -\frac{2}{(\delta a^{(j)}_{0,0,h}(z,t))^2}\left[\left(S^{(1,j)}_{2,0,h}(z,t)+S^{(1,j)}_{0,2,h}(z,t)\right)\delta a^{(1,j)}_{0,0,h}(z,t) + \left(S^{(2,j)}_{2,0,h}(z,t)+S^{(2,j)}_{0,2,h}(z,t)\right)\delta a^{(2,j)}_{0,0,h}(z,t)\right]. \quad (12)$$

Furthermore, in Equations (11) and (12), $(a_{0,0,h}^{(j)}(z,t))^2 = (a_{0,0,h}^{(1,j)}(z,t))^2 + (a_{0,0,h}^{(2,j)}(z,t))^2$. Note that SDE (Equations (9)–(12)) recovers vacuum diffraction when no electron beam is present $[X_h^{(j)}(z,t) = Y_h^{(j)}(z,t) \equiv 0]$.

The source terms in Equation (5) depend on the evolution of the electron coordinates and velocities that are given by the Newton–Lorentz equations

$$\frac{dx}{dz} = \frac{v_x}{v_z}, \tag{13}$$

$$\frac{dy}{dz} = \frac{v_y}{v_z}, \tag{14}$$

$$\frac{d\mathbf{p}}{dz} = -\frac{e}{v_z}\left[\delta\mathbf{E} + \frac{\mathbf{v}}{c} \times (\mathbf{B} + \delta\mathbf{B})\right], \tag{15}$$

and the evolution of the ponderomotive phase ψ given by

$$\frac{d\psi}{dz} = k + k_u - \frac{\omega}{v_z}. \tag{16}$$

Using the Coulomb gauge, the optical fields $\delta\mathbf{E} = -\frac{1}{c}\frac{\partial \delta\mathbf{A}}{\partial t}$ and $\delta\mathbf{B} = \nabla \times \delta\mathbf{A}$ are derived from the optical vector potential given by Equation (1), while $\mathbf{B}$ is the static magnetic field produced by the magnetic elements along the electron transport line. The model presented here ignores space-charge effects, however, this can be easily incorporated [1].

The dynamical equations for the particles and fields are integrated simultaneously using a 4th order Runge–Kutta algorithm. Hence, the number of equations in the simulation is $N_{\text{equations}} = N_{\text{slices}}[6N_{\text{particles}} + 4(N_{\text{modes}} + N_{\text{harmonics}})]$, where N_{slices} is the number of slices in the simulation, and $N_{\text{particles}}$ is the number of particles in each slice, N_{modes} is the total number of modes in the fundamental and all the harmonics, and $N_{\text{harmonics}}$ is the number of harmonics. The Runge-Kutta algorithm allows the step size to change so optimized step sizes can be used in each magnetic element or in the drift spaces while this imposes no limitation on the placement of components along the electron beam path.

The formulation self-consistently tracks the generation of the optical field with arbitrary polarizations depending on the undulator configuration. The polarization state of the output light, therefore, can be determined by calculation of the Stokes parameters [194]. Measurements of the polarization in FELs have been characterized by the Stokes parameters [195,196].

Magnetic field elements, such as undulators, quadrupoles and dipoles, can be placed in arbitrary sequences to specify a variety of different transport lines, and the gap lengths between different undulators can be varied as well. Field configurations can be set up for single or multiple undulator segments and can contain quadrupoles placed between the segments or be superimposed on the lattice to create a FODO lattice. Magnetic elements can also be dipole chicanes to model optical klystron, high-gain harmonic generation (HGHG) or phase shifters. See Section 2.2 for analytical models for the various static magnetic field elements.

2.2. Analytical Models for Static Magnetic Fields

The various types of undulators are modeled using three-dimensional analytical representations. Two models are available for the planar undulator, representing a flat-pole face and a parabolic-pole face with weak two-plane focusing, respectively. The flat-pole-face undulator with the magnetic field oscillating in the y-plane is described by

$$\mathbf{B}_u(\mathbf{x}) = B_u(z)\left[\left(\sin(k_u z) - \frac{\cos(k_u z)}{k_u B_u(z)}\frac{dB_u}{dz}\right)\hat{\mathbf{e}}_y \cosh(k_u y) + \hat{\mathbf{e}}_z \sinh(k_u y)\cos(k_u z)\right], \tag{17}$$

where B_u is the amplitude of the undulator field, $k_u = 2\pi/\lambda_u$, λ_u is the undulator period and $B_u(z)$ describes the entrance and exits taper at the ends of an undulator segment. The field described in Equation (17) is both curl- and divergence-free when the amplitude is constant. The analytic entrance and exit taper function $B_u(z)$ is given by

$$B_u(z) = \begin{cases} B_{u0}\sin^2\left(\frac{k_u z}{4N_{tr}}\right) & 0 \leq z \leq N_{tr}\lambda_u \\ B_{u0} & N_{tr}\lambda_u \leq z \leq L_{tr}, \\ B_{u0}\cos^2\left(\frac{k_u(L_{tr}-z)}{4N_{tr}}\right) & L_{tr} \leq z \leq L_u \end{cases} \quad (18)$$

where B_{u0} is the undulator amplitude in the homogeneous part of the undulator, L_w is the length of the undulator segment, N_{tr} is the number of undulator periods in the transition region and $L_{tr} = L_w - N_{tr}\lambda_u$ is the location of the start of the exit taper. The field in the taper regions has zero divergence, and the z-component of the curl also vanishes. The transverse components of the curl do not vanish, but are of the order of $1/(k_u B_u(z))dB_u/dz$, which is usually small.

A parabolic-pole-face undulator with the magnetic field orientation in the y-plane and weak focusing in the x- and y-planes is described by the analytical model

$$\mathbf{B}_u(\mathbf{x}) = B_u(z)\left[\left(\cos(k_u z) - \frac{\sin(k_u z)}{k_u B_u(z)}\frac{dB_u}{dz}\right)\hat{\mathbf{e}}_\perp(x,y) - \sqrt{2}\hat{\mathbf{e}}_z\cosh\left(\frac{k_u x}{\sqrt{2}}\right)\sinh\left(\frac{k_u y}{\sqrt{2}}\right)\sin(k_u z)\right], \quad (19)$$

where

$$\hat{\mathbf{e}}_\perp(x,y) = \hat{\mathbf{e}}_x\sinh\left(\frac{k_u x}{\sqrt{2}}\right)\sinh\left(\frac{k_u y}{\sqrt{2}}\right) + \hat{\mathbf{e}}_y\cosh\left(\frac{k_u x}{\sqrt{2}}\right)\cosh\left(\frac{k_u y}{\sqrt{2}}\right) \quad (20)$$

and the taper function $B_u(z)$ is again given by Equation (18). As in the case of the flat-pole-face model, Equation (19) is divergence free and the z-component of the curl also vanishes. Both, the flat-pole-face and parabolic-pole-face ideally produce linearly polarized light.

Circular polarized light is produced by helical undulators that are described by

$$\mathbf{B}_u(\mathbf{x}) = 2B_u(z)\left[\left(\cos(\chi) - \frac{\sin(\chi)}{k_u B_u(z)}\frac{dB_u}{dz}\right)I_1'(k_u r)\hat{\mathbf{e}}_r - \left(\sin(\chi) - \frac{\cos(\chi)}{k_u B_u(z)}\frac{dB_u}{dz}\right)\frac{I_1(k_u r)}{k_u r}\hat{\mathbf{e}}_\theta + I_1(k_u r)\sin(\chi)\hat{\mathbf{e}}_z\right] \quad (21)$$

in cylindrical coordinates r, θ, z, where $\chi = k_u z - \theta$, I_1 is the regular Bessel function of the first kind, the prime (′) indicates the derivative of the function with respect to its argument and $B_u(z)$ is again given by Equation (18).

Finally, a magnetic field with varying degrees of ellipticity is produced by an APPLE-II undulator, which can be approximated by a superposition of two flat-pole-face undulators that are oriented perpendicularly to each other, and one of which can be displaced with respect to the other along the axis of symmetry. As such, the field is represented by

$$\mathbf{B}_u(\mathbf{x}) = B_u(z)\left[\left(\sin(k_u z + \phi) - \frac{\cos(k_u z + \phi)}{k_u B_u(z)}\frac{dB_u}{dz}\right)\cosh(k_u x)\hat{\mathbf{e}}_x + \left(\sin(k_u z) - \frac{\cos(k_u z)}{k_u B_u(z)}\frac{dB_u}{dz}\right)\cosh(k_u y)\hat{\mathbf{e}}_y + (\sinh(k_u x)\cos(k_u z + \phi) + \sinh(k_u y)\cos(k_u z))\hat{\mathbf{e}}_z\right], \quad (22)$$

where ϕ, $0 \leq \phi \leq \pi$, represents the phase shift between the two linear undulators and as before, $B_u(z)$ is given by Equation (18). This model is valid near the axis the axis of symmetry. The ellipticity, u_e of the APPLE-II undulator is given by

$$u_e = \frac{1 - |\cos(\phi)|}{1 + |\cos(\phi)|}. \quad (23)$$

We note that the APPLE-II undulator configured as linear undulator has $u_e = 0$, while $u_e = 1$ for a helical configuration.

The remaining static magnetic field models are used to describe quadrupole magnets, using

$$\mathbf{B}_Q(z) = B_{Q0}(z)(y\hat{\mathbf{e}}_x + x\hat{\mathbf{e}}_y), \tag{24}$$

where $B_{Q0}(z)$ is the constant field gradient over some range $z_1 \leq z \leq z_2$, and dipole magnets using a field model that is described by a constant field oriented perpendicularly to the axis of symmetry over some range $z_3 \leq z \leq z_4$. Both, the field models for quadrupole and dipole magnets, have hard-edge field transitions and are curl- and divergence-free over the range where these are defined.

2.3. Performance of the MINERVA FEL Code

To illustrate the performance of the MINERVA FEL code, we briefly compare the predictions of this code with experimental data from two SASE FEL experiments. We consider the "Sorgente Pulsata ed Amplificata di Radiazione Coerente" (SPARC) experiment, a SASE FEL located at ENEA Frascati [197], and the Linac Coherent Light Source (LCLS), which is a SASE FEL at the Stanford Linear Accelerator Center [198].

2.3.1. The SPARC SASE FEL

The experimental parameters of SPARC [197] are as follows. The electron beam energy was 151.9 MeV, with a bunch charge of 450 pC, and a bunch width of 12.67 ps. The peak current was approximately 53 A for a parabolic temporal bunch profile. The x- and y-emittances were 2.5 mm-mrad and 2.9 mm-mrad respectively, and the rms energy spread was 0.02 percent. There were six undulators, each of which were 77 periods in length, with a period of 2.8 cm and an amplitude of 7.88 kG. Each undulator was modeled using Equation (17) with one period for the entrance up-taper and another for the exit down-taper. Furthermore, in the simulation, eight undulators were used to show saturation of the system. The gap between the undulators was 0.4 m in length and the quadrupoles (0.053 m in length with a field gradient of 0.9 kG/cm), forming a strong focusing lattice were located 0.105 m downstream from the exit of the previous undulator. Note that the quadrupole orientations were fixed and did not alternate. The electron beam was matched into the undulator/focusing lattice. The resonance occurred at a wavelength of 491.5 nm. In the experiment, the pulse energies were measured in the gaps between the undulator segments.

A comparison of the pulse energy as found in the simulation (blue line) and from the experiment (red markers) is shown in Figure 2, where the simulation result is averaged over 20 simulation runs with different noise seeds. This yields convergence to better than 5 percent. Energy conservation in the simulation is maintained to within better than one part in 10^4. Each marker represents a single measurement that is repeated several times, while the error bar indicates the error in the measurement. The experimental data are courtesy of L. Giannessi. Agreement between the simulation and the measured performance is excellent.

A comparison between the evolution of the relative linewidth as determined from simulation (blue line) and by measurement (red markers, data courtesy of L. Giannessi) is shown in Figure 3. Agreement between the simulation and the measured linewidth is within about 35 percent after 15 m. As shown, the predicted linewidths are in substantial agreement with the measurements.

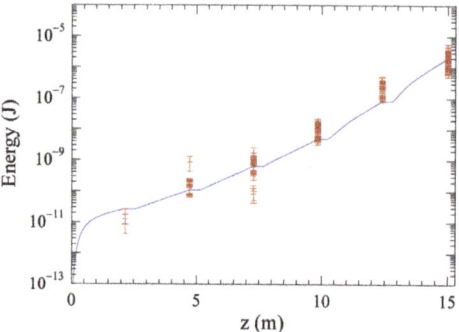

Figure 2. Simulated (blue line) and measured (red crosses) pulse energy as a function of the propagation distance z for the SPARC experiment. The different points correspond to individual measurements and the error bar indicates the error in each of the measurements. The simulation result is an average over 20 noise realizations.

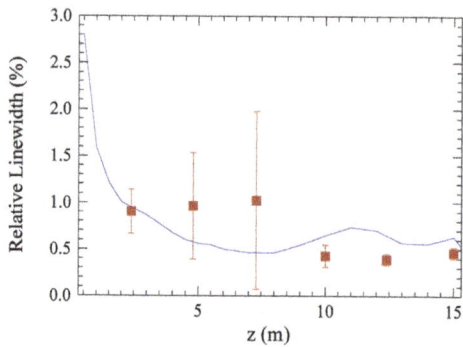

Figure 3. Simulated (blue line) and measured (red data points) relative linewidth as a function of the propagation distance z for the SPARC experiment. The error bar indicates the error in the measurement. The simulation result is, on average, over 20 noise realizations.

2.3.2. The LCLS SASE FEL

To illustrate the performance of MINERVA at much shorter wavelengths, we also briefly compare with experimental data from LCLS [198], which is a SASE FEL user facility that became operational in 2009, operating at a 1.5 Å wavelength.

To operate at 1.5 Å, LCLS employs a 13.64 GeV/250 pC electron beam with a flat-top temporal pulse shape of 83 fs duration. The normalized emittance (x and y) is 0.4 mm-mrad and the rms energy spread is 0.01 percent. The undulator line consisted of 33 segments with a period of 3.0 cm and a length of 113 periods. In the simulation, each segment is modeled using Equation (17), with one period each in entry and exit tapers. A mild down-taper in field amplitude of -0.0016 kG/segment starting with the first segment (with an amplitude of 12.4947 kG and $K_{rms} = 2.4748$) and continuing from segment to segment was used. This is the so-called gain taper. The electron beam was matched into a FODO lattice consisting of 32 quadrupoles, each with a field gradient of 4.054 kG/cm and a length of 7.4 cm. Each quadrupole was placed a distance of 3.96 cm downstream from the end of the preceding undulator segment, and the gap lengths between the undulators followed a repetitive sequence of short (0.48 m)-short (0.48 m)-long (0.908 m).

The LCLS produces pulses of about 1.89 mJ at the end of the undulator line [198], and saturation is found after about 65–75 m along the undulator line. A comparison between the measured pulse energies (red circles), as obtained by giving the electrons a kick to disrupt the FEL process, and the simulation (blue) is shown in Figure 4. The experimental data are courtesy of P. Emma and H.-D. Nuhn at SLAC, and the simulation results represent an average over an ensemble of 25 runs performed with different noise seeds. As shown in Figure 4, the simulations are in good agreement with the measurements in the exponential growth region with close agreement for the gain length. The simulation exhibits saturation at the same distance as the experiment in the range of 65–75 m at a pulse energy of 1.5 mJ. After saturation, in view of the gain taper, the pulse energy grows more slowly to about 2.02 mJ at the end of the undulator line, which is approximately 8 percent higher than the observed pulse energy.

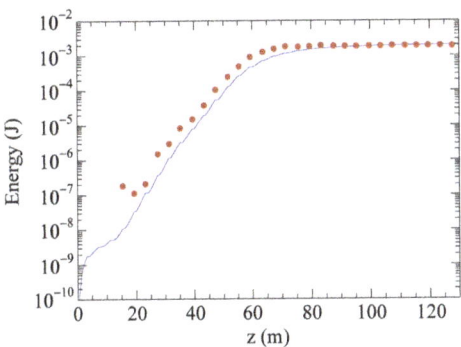

Figure 4. Simulated (blue line) and measured (red circles) optical pulse energy as a function of the propagation distance z for the LCLS experiment. The simulation result is on average over 25 noise realizations.

The agreement between simulation and experiment for the pulse energy is poorer during the early stages of the interaction. This may be due to a variety of reasons. On the experimental side, as the pulse energy grows by 5 to 6 orders of magnitude from the initial shot noise to saturation, it is difficult to calibrate the detectors for the low pulse energies at the early stages of the interaction. Moreover, while kicking the electrons provides a fast measurement method, it is accompanied by a larger background signal and the possibility of restarting the FEL process downstream the undulator line when the kick is performed at the beginning of the undulator line [198]. On the simulation side, there may be some inaccuracies in the shot noise algorithm or the finite number of optical modes used that underestimates the initial noise level.

2.4. The Optical Propagation Code OPC

When modeling FEL oscillators, the electron–light interaction within the undulator segments needs to be modeled, as well as the propagation of the light through the remainder of the oscillator. The light propagators internal to FEL gain codes, including that in MINERVA, are typically not very efficient when considering free-space propagation over large distances and interaction with various optical elements.

The wavefront propagator [185,199] is based upon the scalar paraxial Helmholtz equation [200]

$$\frac{\partial^2 u}{\partial x^2} + \frac{\partial^2 u}{\partial y^2} - 2ik_0 \frac{\partial u}{\partial z} = 0, \qquad (25)$$

where u is the complex scalar wave amplitude that describes the transverse profile of a time-harmonic optical beam, $k_0 = 2\pi/\lambda_0$, and λ_0 is the free-space wavelength. By applying a two-dimensional spatial Fourier transform, Equation (25) transforms into

$$(k_x^2 + k_y^2)\tilde{u} - 2ik_0 \frac{\partial \tilde{u}}{\partial z} = 0, \qquad (26)$$

where

$$\tilde{u}(k_x,k_y,z) \equiv \int_{-\infty}^{\infty}\int_{-\infty}^{\infty} dxdy\, u(x,y,z)e^{-i(k_xx+k_yy)} \tag{27}$$

is the two-dimensional Fourier transform of $u(x,y,z)$. Given a known profile $u_0(x,y) = u(x,y,0)$ at $z = 0$, e.g., at the exit of the undulator line, the analytical solution in reciprocal space to Equation (26) is given by

$$\tilde{u}(k_x,k_y,z) = \tilde{u}_0(k_x,k_y)e^{iz\lambda_0(k_x^2+k_y^2)/\pi}. \tag{28}$$

The solution in normal space at location z is found by the inverse spatial Fourier transform of Equation (28),

$$u(x,y,z) \equiv \frac{1}{4\pi^2}\int_{-\infty}^{\infty}\int_{-\infty}^{\infty} dk_x dk_y\, \tilde{u}(k_x,k_y,z)e^{i(k_xx+k_yy)}). \tag{29}$$

This wavefront propagation is known as spectral propagation and is very suitable for propagation over short and large distances. However, when propagating over long distances, care has to be taken that the complete optical field remains contained within the transverse domain of the two-dimensional spatial Fourier transform (Equation (27)), e.g., as a result of a fast Fourier transform implementation, to avoid artificial reflections from the edges of this domain.

By substituting Equation (28) into Equation (29), using the initial profile $u_0(x,y)$ and Equation (27), changing the order of integration and performing the integration over k_x and k_y, we obtain the Fresnel diffraction integral [201]

$$u(x,y,z) = -\frac{i}{\lambda_0 z}\int_{-\infty}^{\infty}\int_{-\infty}^{\infty} d\xi d\eta\, u_0(\xi,\eta)e^{i\pi[(x-\xi)^2+(y-\eta)^2]/\lambda_0 z}. \tag{30}$$

Note that the Fresnel diffraction integral can be derived using various methods, including the free-space Green's function [202], or by applying the paraxial approximation to the spherical wavelets in Huygens' integral [200]. It can also be shown that propagation through a cascaded set of paraxial optical components described by an overall ray-optical ABCD matrix can be described by a single Huygens' integral, given by [200]

$$u(x,y,z) = e^{-ik_0 z}\int_{-\infty}^{\infty}\int_{-\infty}^{\infty} d\xi d\eta\, K(x,y,\xi,\eta)u_0(\xi,\eta), \tag{31}$$

where Huygens' kernel K is given by

$$K(x,y,\xi,\eta) \equiv \frac{i}{\lambda_0\sqrt{B_xB_y}}e^{-i\frac{\pi}{B_x\lambda_0}(A_x\xi^2-2\xi x+D_xx^2)}e^{-i\frac{\pi}{B_y\lambda_0}(A_y\eta^2-2\eta y+D_yy^2)}, \tag{32}$$

and A_i, B_i, C_i and D_i are the components of the system ABCD matrix for $i = x,y$. The ABCD matrix can describe real or complex orthogonal paraxial optical systems that may contain astigmatism [200]. Note, in the presence of apertures, the optical field must be propagated from aperture to aperture, since apertures cannot be included in the ABCD matrix.

An efficient calculation of the integrals appearing in the spectral propagation method and Fresnel's diffraction integrals relies on fast Fourier transforms. By applying a transformation to Equation (31), it can be put into a form that also allows the use of fast Fourier transforms to efficiently evaluate the integrals. We define $M_x = a_2/a_1$, where a_1 and a_2 are measures for the size of the optical field, such that the optical field becomes negligible for $|x| \geq a_{1,2}$ at the input and output plane, respectively. Similarly, $M_y = a_3/a_4$ where a_3 and a_4 are measures for the size of the optical field, such that the optical field becomes negligible for $|y| \geq a_{3,4}$ in the input and output plane, respectively. Using the transformation $x' = a_1 x, \xi' = a_2 \xi, y' = a_3 y, \eta' = a_4 \eta$,

$$v_0(\xi', \eta') = \sqrt{a_1 a_3} u_0(\xi, \eta) e^{-i\pi \frac{(A_x - M_x)\xi^2}{B_x \lambda_0}} e^{-i\pi \frac{(A_y - M_y)\eta^2}{B_y \lambda_0}}, \tag{33}$$

and

$$v(x', y') = \sqrt{a_2 a_4} u(x, y) e^{i\pi \frac{(D_x - M_x^{-1})x^2}{B_x \lambda_0}} e^{i\pi \frac{(D_y - M_y^{-1})y^2}{B_y \lambda_0}}. \tag{34}$$

Equation (31) can be transformed into

$$v(x', y') = i\sqrt{N_{c,x} N_{c,y}} \int_{-1}^{1} \int_{-1}^{1} d\xi' d\eta' \, K(x', y', \xi', \eta') v_0(\xi', \eta') \tag{35}$$

with the kernel K given by

$$K(x', y', \xi', \eta') = e^{i\pi N_{c,x}(x' - \xi')^2} e^{i\pi N_{c,y}(y' - \eta')^2}. \tag{36}$$

In Equations (35), $N_{c,x}$ and $N_{c,y}$ are equivalent collimated Fresnel numbers [200] defined as

$$N_{c,x} = \frac{M_x a_1^2}{B_x \lambda_0}, \quad N_{c,y} = \frac{M_y a_3^2}{B_y \lambda_0}. \tag{37}$$

We shall refer to Equation (35) as the modified Fresnel diffraction integral, and this integral can also be efficiently evaluated using fast Fourier transforms, with the added benefit that independent magnification factors in the x- and y-directions can be applied in going from the input to the output plane. This means that the output plane can grow or shrink in size with the optical beam when it expands or contracts in propagating from the input to the output plane that are defined by the system ABCD matrix used in the propagation.

2.4.1. Optical Elements

To allow the modeling of FEL oscillators, the optical field needs to interact with various types of optical elements, such as lenses, mirrors or diaphragms. Diaphragms are implemented as hard edge apertures that reduce the optical field to zero outside the aperture. Various apodization functions are available that can be applied to the edge of the aperture. Lenses and mirrors are implemented as elements that apply a phase shift to the optical field. This is done by multiplying the optical field by $e^{-iq(x,y)}$, where $q(x,y)$ is the local phase shift in the transverse plane. For example, a thin lens is modeled as $q(x,y) = k_0(x^2 + y^2)/2f$ with f as the focal strength of the lens. Mirrors are modeled as thin lenses using $f = R/2$, where R is the radius of curvature of the mirror. More complicated optical elements as thick lenses or a combination of lenses can be implemented by determining the overall ABCD matrix and using the modified Fresnel diffraction integral (Equation 35). OPC also allows for more complicated phase masks that can be created using Zernike polynomials [194]. These can be used to implement not only various types of mirror and lens aberrations, but also mirror distortion resulting from thermal loading [203,204] (see Section 2.4.2 for more detail). In the latter case, OPC can set a scaling factor for the aberrations depending on the (average) optical power loading of the mirror.

Typically, it is assumed that the FEL gain bandwidth is sufficiently small that dispersive effects within the optical elements can be neglected. However, this is not the case when crystal Bragg mirrors are used, e.g., to model oscillator configurations at X-ray wavelengths. For such mirrors, the angle of reflection and mirror loss strongly depend on the type of crystal used, its orientation and the X-ray photon energy [205]. To properly model the reflection of Bragg mirrors, the incident optical field needs to be Fourier transformed into the frequency domain to handle the different photon energies in the optical field, and a two-dimensional spatial Fourier transform of the incident field is needed to deal with the various angles of incidence on the mirror.

Several optical elements can be combined to form a more complex optical component, e.g., by combining a mirror with a diaphragm element, extraction of radiation from a resonator through a hole in one of the mirrors can be modeled. Another example is to use an external finite element program to simulate mirror surface distortion due to thermal loading of the mirror. This surface distortion can then be converted to a phase mask, the amplitude of which can be dynamically scaled at each roundtrip to model mirror distortion during the start-up of the oscillator.

Finally, the collection of wavefront propagators together with the optical components and interfaces with several FEL gain codes is known as the optical propagation code (OPC). As OPC is specifically designed to work several FEL gain codes to model FEL oscillators, some of the optical components allow for the forking of the optical propagation path. For example, at the mirror used for coupling the light out of the resonator, the tracking of the light within the resonator can temporarily be suspended to propagate the light outside the resonator to some diagnostic point where several optical properties of the light can be obtained. Afterwards, the propagation of the light within the resonator can be continued. This allows simultaneous monitoring of the light properties at some external diagnostic point, as well as the build-up of the light within the resonator.

2.4.2. Modeling Mirrors

The default optical components used by OPC are ideal thin lenses and spherical mirrors. However, by using amplitude and phase masks, additional optical components can be added, in particular more realistic lenses and mirrors. Here, we limit ourselves to phase masks that are generated using the circle polynomials $R_n^{|m|}$ of Zernike [194]. These polynomials are used to generate a phase difference $d\theta$ defined on a transverse plane that is applied to the optical field as

$$d\theta = D_{mn} R_n^{|m|}(\rho) \times \begin{cases} \cos(m\phi) & m \leq 0 \\ \sin(m\phi) & m < 0 \end{cases}, \tag{38}$$

where ρ is a scaled radial distance, $\rho = \sqrt{x^2 + y^2}/\rho_c$ with ρ_c some characteristic length scale, ϕ is the angle $\tan^{-1}(y/x)$ and D_{mn} is the amplitude of the polynomial. The indices m, n describe the type of aberration, for example, $m = 0$ and $n = 4$ correspond to spherical aberration and $m = 1$ and $n = 3$ to coma [194]. Therefore, adding a phase mask and applying it at the location of a lens of mirror adds the associated aberrations to create a more realistic model of the component.

It is also possible to use these Zernike polynomials to generate new optical components. For example, adding the polynomials $m, n = 2, 2$ with $m, n = 0, 2$ with appropriate amplitudes generates a cylindrical lens of a certain focal strength. This can be used to correctly model the performance of a spherical mirror with a non-zero angle of incidence, e.g., when used in a ring resonator, to model for the different foci in tangential and sagittal direction.

Another application is to use the Zernike polynomials to model mirror surface distortions, in particular, due to thermal loading of the mirror. Here, we assume that round mirror is uniformly cooled at its circumference and that the heat loading is axi-symmetric. A finite element program can be used to calculate the steady state deviation $\delta z(r/r_0)$, where r_0 is some characteristic length, that results from the heat generation in the mirror due to some absorbed power P_{abs}. A fit using $R_n^0(r/r_0)$ Zernike polynomials with n taken even is then used to determine the amplitudes to be used in generating the phase mask. To convert the mirror distortion δz into a localized change in phase for the optical field, we set

$$d\theta(r/r_0) = -\frac{4\pi \delta z(r/r_0)}{\lambda}, \tag{39}$$

where the minus sign is required to comply with the phase advance used in OPC and the phase change is proportional to twice the mirror displacement. It is reasonable to assume that a stable transverse field distribution is established after starting from noise when the intracavity optical starts to heat the mirror. Therefore, the phase distortion due to mirror heating can be obtained by scaling Equation (39) with a factor $P_i(t)\tau/(P_{abs}T_{rep})$ with P_{abs} the absorbed power used to calculate δz, P_i the instantaneous absorbed power, τ the duration of the optical pulse and T_{rep} the repetition time for the optical pulses.

3. Some Considerations for Optical Resonators Used in Free-Electron Lasers

Most optical resonators used in laser oscillators consist of two spherical mirrors separated by a distance L_{cav}, as schematically shown in Figure 1. When the radius of curvature R_c of the mirrors is equal, the resonator is called concentric when $L_{cav} = 2R_c$ and confocal when $L_{cav} = R_c$. Other configurations with an unequal radii of curvature of different distances between the mirrors are known as generalized resonators.

Most of the low-gain FEL oscillators employ stable concentric resonators to ensure that the optical pulse train does not "walk" out of the cavity. Consider a generalized resonator with a cavity length L_{cav}, as shown in Figure 5, which shows the radii of curvature, $R_{c,i}(i = 1, 2)$, for the two mirrors, as well as the distances z_i from the mode waist to each of the mirrors. The transverse optical modes of the cold resonator, i.e., without a gain medium (electron beam) present, can be described as either Gauss–Hermite cf. Equations (1)–(3) or Gauss–Laguerre modes.

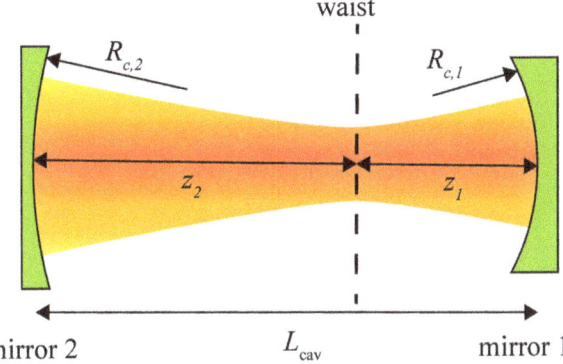

Figure 5. Schematic representation of a generalized two-mirror resonator, defining some of its parameters.

Defining

$$g_i = 1 - \frac{L_{cav}}{R_{c,i}} \qquad (40)$$

then the Rayleigh range z_R for the Gaussian eigenmodes in the cavity is given by

$$z_R = L_{cav}\sqrt{\frac{g_1 g_2(1 - g_1 g_2)}{g_1 + g_2 - 2g_1 g_2}} \qquad (41)$$

Since the Rayleigh range must be positive, we must have $0 \leq g_1 g_2 \leq 1$, which is the condition for resonator stability [200]. This means that Gaussian beams can only be eigenmodes of stable resonators. The stability condition implies that

$$L_{cav} < R_1 + R_2. \qquad (42)$$

We also note that the waist of the Gaussian mode is at a distance

$$z_1 = L_{\text{cav}} \frac{g_2(1 - g_1)}{g_1 + g_2 - 2g_1 g_2} \tag{43}$$

from mirror 1 and at a distance $z_2 = L_{\text{cav}} - z_1$ from mirror 2. Note that the sign convention used for the ray-optic ABCD formalism [200] applies here as well, meaning that $R_c > 0$ for a concave mirror and $R_c < 0$ for a convex mirror and that the distances z_i have a sign.

The Gauss–Hermite transverse modes as described by Equations (1)–(3) are eigenmodes of an empty generalized resonator with a particular Rayleigh range and location of the waist defined by the resonator. Whenever the resonator contains internal apertures clipping the optical field, partial waveguiding, or if the light is extracted via a hole, a single transverse Gaussian mode can no longer be an eigenmode of the resonator. The Fox–Li method [206] can be used to find the eigenmodes of such resonators [207].

The resonant frequencies, or longitudinal modes, of the resonator are those frequencies for which the total roundtrip phase is an integer multiple of 2π. As a result, the resonant frequencies differ for the different transverse optical modes [200]. The frequency spacing between two subsequent resonances of the same transverse mode is known as the free-spectral range $\Delta\nu_{\text{FSR}}$. FEL resonators typically have a $\Delta\nu_{\text{FSR}}$ that is much smaller than the gain bandwidth, due to the large mirror separation used. Consequently, most FEL oscillators are operating on multiple longitudinal modes.

As shown in Figure 1, the resonator may contain more than one optical pulse if the roundtrip time in the resonator is larger than the time between subsequent electron bunches. The resonator design must ensure synchronism between the optical pulses and the electron bunches and optimal performance is typically found near the synchronous or zero-detuning cavity length, where the incoming electron bunch coincides with the returning optical pulse train. This zero-detuning cavity length, L_0, is given by

$$\frac{M}{f_{\text{rep}}} = \frac{2L_0 - L_u}{c} + \frac{L_u}{v_g}, \tag{44}$$

where M is the number of simultaneous electron bunches in the optical cavity, f_{rep} is the repetition rate of the electron bunches, L_u is the undulator length and v_g is the group velocity of the light within the undulator. Solving for L_0 gives

$$L_0 = \frac{cM}{2f_{\text{rep}}} - \frac{L_u}{2} \frac{c}{v_g} \left(1 - \frac{v_g}{c}\right), \tag{45}$$

which reduces to the well-known expression

$$L_0 = \frac{cM}{2f_{\text{rep}}}, \tag{46}$$

for low gain oscillators where $v_g \approx c$. As will be discussed in the Section 5 on high-gain/low-Q oscillators, exponential gain in the undulator results in a reduction in the group velocity, which has the effect of shortening the zero-detuning cavity length compared to that for low-gain/high-Q oscillators (Equation (46)).

In general, the dynamics in an oscillator are set by the interplay between the instantaneous gain and loss, where in a free-electron laser, the gain is provided by the electrons streaming through the undulator and loss is due to out-coupling of the radiation and other loss mechanisms that may be present within the resonator. The total loss of the resonator determines the quality factor Q of the resonator [200]. To obtain laser oscillation, the roundtrip small-signal gain has to be higher than the loss per roundtrip. The so-called threshold gain is the roundtrip small-signal gain needed to just balance the loss per roundtrip. When the light builds up inside the resonator, the gain is reduced and a stationary state is obtained when the saturated gain equals the loss per roundtrip. Note that this is the same condition as for threshold, i.e., the saturated gain is equal to the threshold gain. If we denote the output power on the *n*th pass as P_n, then the power after the (*n*+1)th pass is $P_{n+1} = (1-L)(1+G)P_n$. Equilibrium is characterized by $P_{n+1} = P_n$; at which point, $G = L/(1-L)$.

In FELs, where the bunch charge/peak current is relatively small and the gain cannot reach the exponential regime in a single pass through the undulator, the resonator Q must be high enough that the oscillator can lase. In such cases, most of the energy extracted from the electrons remains circulating in the resonator and a small fraction of the power is out-coupled. This implies that the loss, which is often dominated by the fraction of radiation that is coupled out of the resonator, but also includes losses at the mirrors or within the resonator, can impose difficulties if mirror absorption is large enough to result in excessive heating or degradation of the reflectivity. In such cases, the mirrors must be cooled or otherwise protected. For example, storage ring FELs have a low small-signal gain and thus require high-quality mirrors that are susceptible to the higher-harmonics generated. Short-wavelength X-ray FEL oscillators also have a low small-signal gain and the available X-ray mirror technology is pushed to its limits to produce mirrors with sufficiently low loss. High average power operation may require the cryogenic cooling of the mirrors to prevent mirror distortion due to thermal loading.

The efficiency of a low-gain/high-Q oscillator is predicted to be $\eta = 1/2.4N_u$ [1], where N_u denotes the number of uniform periods in the undulator; hence, high efficiency requires relatively short undulators. Because of this, oscillator design is a balance between having a sufficiently long undulator for the gain to exceed the losses, set by the quality Q of the resonator, but not so long that the efficiency is negatively impacted.

4. Low-Gain/High-Q Oscillators

In this section, we describe simulations of two low-gain/high-Q infrared FEL oscillator experiments conducted at JLab: the IR-Demo [50,64,65] and the 10-kW Upgrade [11]. Both of these experiments were conceived as demonstrations for high average power infrared FELs based on energy recovery linacs.

4.1. The IR-Demo Experiment at JLab

The IR Demo experiment [50,64,65] was based on a superconducting energy recovery linac at JLab that produced 0.4 (±0.1) ps rms electron bunches, with energies of about 38 MeV bunch charges of 60 pC (60 A peak current) at a repetition rate of 18.7 MHz corresponding to an average current of 1.2 mA. The transverse emittance of the bunches was 7.5(±1.5) mm-mrad (rms) and the rms energy spread was about 0.25 percent. The experiment uses a 42-period flat-pole-face planar undulator with a period of 2.7 cm and an on-axis amplitude of 5.56 kG, yielding an undulator strength parameter of $K_{rms} = 0.99$. Therefore, the simulation model uses Equation (17) to model the undulator with one period entry and exit tapers. The resonant wavelength was 4.8 µm and a concentric resonator was used with a optical cavity length of about 8 m [208]. The radii of curvature of the mirrors were 4.045 m with a cold cavity Rayleigh range of 40 cm. Transmissive out-coupling through the downstream mirror was used and had a transmittance of approximately 10 percent. The outer radius of the mirrors was 2.54 cm. OPC uses the modified Fresnel propagator (Equation (35)) to handle the divergence and convergence of the optical beam inside the resonator using a fixed number of grid points.

Simulations of this experiment were conducted with MEDUSA/OPC. MEDUSA [184] and MINERVA both employ Gaussian representations for the optical field and integrate the three-dimensional Lorentz force equations for the electron trajectories without performing an average over the wiggle-motion. However, MEDUSA is the more primitive code and MINERVA contains many additions and incorporates superior algorithms not present in MEDUSA. Nevertheless, in cases where the two codes have been compared, their predictions for FEL performance are in agreement to within about 10 percent.

The evolution of the output energy found in simulation versus pass is shown in Figure 6 for a cavity length near the peak of the detuning curve of 8.01049 m. Observe that saturation is found after about 70 passes at a pulse energy of 0.17 mJ, corresponding to an average power of about 318 W, at a repetition rate of 18.7 MHz. This represents an average efficiency of about 0.70 percent, which is close to the theoretically predicted efficiency of about 1.0 percent for an undulator with 40 uniform periods.

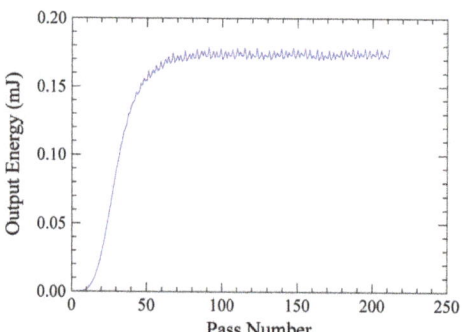

Figure 6. Simulated pulse energy as a function of roundtrip number n at a near optimal cavity detuning of $L_{cav} = 8.01049$ m for the IR Demo experiment. Remaining parameters as described in the text.

The average power found in simulation near the peak in the detuning curve is consistent with the observation of 311 W during CW operation of the IR Demo [50,64,65]. This is also shown in Figure 7, which shows the detuning curves found in simulation (blue) and during pulsed operation of the IR Demo (green). The average power during CW operation is indicated by the dashed line. Observe that the zero-detuning point in the simulation is shifted by about 5 μm from that observed in the experiment. This may be due to an uncertainty in the cavity length measurement by up to 10 μm. The full width of the detuning curve is found to be within about 30–35 μm.

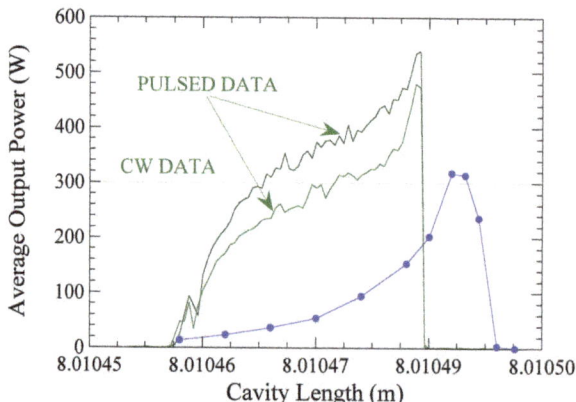

Figure 7. Tuning curve for the IR Demo experiment including measurements from CW and pulsed runs (green) and from simulation (blue). Other parameters as described in the text.

Higher bunch charges were used in the pulsed runs than in the CW runs in the IR Demo. Lower bunch charges were used in the CW runs in order to reduce distortion due to mirror heating. Indeed, mirror distortion made it difficult to obtain a detuning curve during CW operation. Mirror heating was not a serious problem in the pulsed runs. When the gain to loss ratio is small, as in the CW runs and in the simulation, it is expected that the tuning curve for a low-gain/high-Q oscillator will display a peak at the zero detuning point, followed by a rapid decline as the cavity length decreases, and this is what is found in simulation. However, when the gain-to-loss ratio increases, then the detuning curve will exhibit a shoulder, as indicated in the detuning curves for the pulsed runs. This shoulder will be much more prominent in the RAFEL simulations discussed below.

4.2. The 10-kW Upgrade Experiment at JLab

This experiment represented an upgrade to the original IR-Demo experiment [65] and numerous elements represent upgrades. For example, the accelerating modules were upgraded to achieve higher energy, bunch charge, and average current. Effort was also made to reduce/mitigate the beam breakup instability in view of the higher average current. The original undulator was replaced to achieve high gain and resonance at a shorter wavelength. In order to handle the higher power, the resonator was lengthened to reduce the mirror loading and cryogenic, edge-cooling was used for the mirrors. As a result, the kinetic energy was increased to 115 MeV, while the energy spread of 0.3 percent remained approximately the same. The charge of the electron bunch was almost doubled to 115 pC with a pulse length of 390 fs. The normalized emittance of 9 mm-mrad in the wiggle plane and 7 mm-mrad in the plane orthogonal to the wiggle plane was similar as in the IR demo experiment, and the maximum repetition rate of 74.85 MHz for the electron bunches remained unchanged. Note, that although the IR-Demo experiment was capable of running at 74.85 MHz, the results reported in Section 4.1 corresponded to operation at 17.85 MHz. To operate at somewhat shorter wavelengths, the planar undulator, which is modeled in the simulation using Equation (19) with one period up- and down-taper, had a longer period of 5.5 cm, a total of 30 periods, and a peak on-axis magnetic field of 3.75 kG. The electron beam was focused into the undulator with the focus at the center of the undulator. The concentric resonator was also updated [209] and had a length of about 32 m with a cold-cavity Rayleigh length of 0.75 m. The total loss in the resonator was 21 percent with about 18 percent out-coupled per pass from the downstream mirror. For these settings, the wavelength was 1.6 µm.

In simulating this experiment, the number of particles in MINERVA was 5832 per slice, while the separation between slices was 5.4 fs. The number of optical modes was dynamically adjusted each roundtrip to accommodate the evolution of the optical field inside the resonator. OPC uses, again, the modified Fresnel propagator (Equation (35)) to handle the divergence and convergence of the optical beam inside the resonator.

The length of the optical cavity must be selected so that the returning optical pulse is in synchronism with the electron bunches. The roundtrip time for the optical pulses in the cavity is $\tau_r = 2L_{cav}/c$ and the separation between electron bunches is $\tau_{sep} = 1/f_{rep}$, where L_{cav} is the cavity length and f_{rep} is the electron bunch repetition rate. Perfect synchronism (referred to as zero-detuning) is obtained when $\tau_r = M\tau_{sep}$, which leads to Equation (46). Here, M is the number of optical pulses in the cavity. In this case, there were 16 optical pulses in the cavity and the zero-detuning length is L_0 = 32.041946079 m. The cavity detuning curve obtained from simulations is shown in Figure 8 as a function of the difference between the cavity length L_{cav} and the zero-detuning length. With a maximum pulse energy of 0.194 mJ and a repetition rate of 74.85 MHz, we find that the maximum output power of 14.52 kW occurs for a positive detuning of 2 µm and is close to the measured value of 14.3 ± 0.72 kW [69]. As a result, the predicted extraction efficiency is about 1.4 percent, which is close to the theoretical value of η = 1.7 percent. We remark that the previous simulation of this experiment with MEDUSA/OPC [183] yielded an average output power of 12.3 kW, and the present formulation is in better agreement with the experiment than in the earlier simulation. As in the previous simulation [183], the roughly triangular shape of the detuning curve is also in agreement with the experimental observation.

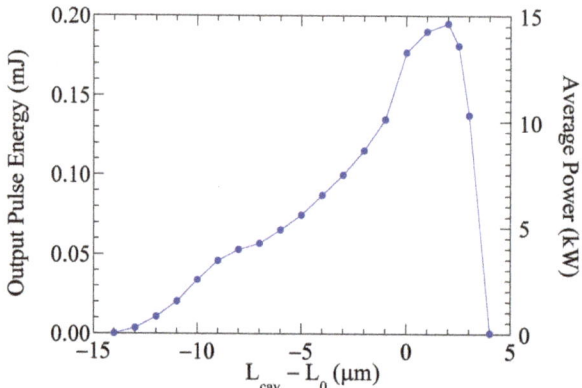

Figure 8. Tuning curve for the IR upgrade experiment. Simulation parameters as described in the text.

The temporal profiles of the optical pulse at the undulator entrance and exit as well as that of the electron bunch current are shown in Figure 9 for the zero-detuning cavity length after pass 100, which corresponds to a stable, saturated steady-state. Observe that the electron bunch is centered in the time window, which has a duration of 1.4 ps. This is at zero-detuning, as indicated by the fact that the incoming optical pulse at the undulator entrance is in close synchronism with the electron bunch. It is also evident that the center of the optical pulse advances by about 0.16 ps, as it propagates through the undulator, and this is in good agreement with the theoretical slippage estimate of $N_u \lambda / c$ for a low-gain FEL, where N_u is the number of periods in the undulator. Finally, it should be remarked that this is in the steady-state regime where the losses in the resonator and the out-coupling are compensated by the gain in the undulator.

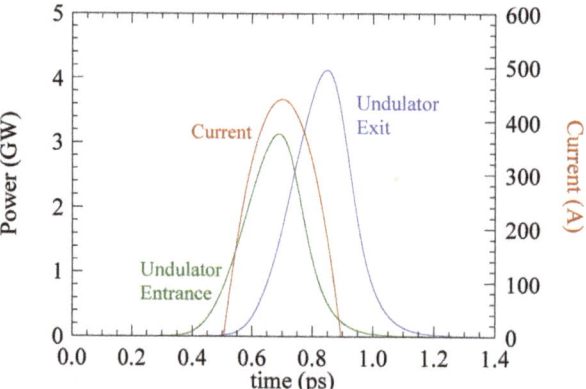

Figure 9. Temporal profiles of the power in the optical pulse after 100 passes at the undulator entrance (green) and exit (blue), as well as the current in the electron bunch (right axis, red) for the IR upgrade experiment. The cavity length is $L_{cav} = 32.041946079$ m and other parameters, as described in the text.

5. High-Gain/Low-Q Oscillators

An alternate approach to oscillator design is to use a high-gain undulator where the radiation grows exponentially on a single pass through the undulator [2]. Because the gain is high, the permissible resonator loss can be relatively high; hence, a large fraction of the power can be coupled out of the resonator. This type of oscillator has been referred to as a regenerative amplifier FEL (RAFEL), and the concept has been experimentally demonstrated at the Los Alamos National Laboratory [210]. Hence, a RAFEL may also be thought of as a low-Q oscillator and has advantages, both for (1) high power designs, since the mirror loading can be kept below mirror deformation or damage thresholds, and (2) for VUV and X-ray oscillators.

RAFELs differ from low-gain oscillators in a number of ways. One difference is that, as shown in Madey's theorem [211], a low-gain oscillator exhibits no gain directly on the resonance. In contrast, the growth rate in the exponential gain regime has a peak on-resonance, and this is reflected in the wavelengths excited in a RAFEL. A second difference is the overall efficiency. The saturation efficiency, η, of a low-gain oscillator is $\eta = 1/2.4N_u$, where N_u is the number of periods in the undulator. Since the radiation exponentiates in each pass through the undulator in the RAFEL, the efficiency is given by that found in the high-gain Compton regime, where $\eta = \rho$ where ρ is the Pierce parameter. A third difference is in the linewidth, which scales inversely with N_u in a low-gain oscillator, but which is given by the linewidth of the exponential interaction in the high-gain Compton regime. A fourth difference is in the longitudinal and transverse mode structure, which is determined largely by the resonator properties in a low-gain oscillator. In a RAFEL, by contrast, the exponential gain leads to saturation in a very small number of passes through the resonator, and the mode structure is largely governed by the interaction in the undulator. A fifth difference is in the effect of slippage. Slippage in a low-gain oscillator scales with N_u. However, the high-gain in a RAFEL results in a reduction in the group velocity, such that slippage scales with $N_u/3$. However, one point of similarity that the RAFEL shares with low-gain oscillators, is the presence of limit-cycle oscillations.

In this section, we discuss simulations of an infrared RAFEL with the intention of illustrating many of the general properties of a RAFEL and how it compares both to low-gain/high-Q oscillators and SASE FELs [212] and simulations of an X-ray RAFEL concept, making use of hole out-coupling [213]. We note that the infrared RAFEL simulations were performed with MEDUSA/OPC, while the X-ray RAFEL simulations were performed with MINERVA/OPC.

5.1. An Infrared RAFEL

The electron beam, undulator, and resonator parameters are summarized in Table 1. Observe that the temporal profile of the electron bunch is parabolic with a full width of 1.2 ps, and that the undulator is a two-plane-focusing (i.e., parabolic pole face) design. Consequently, Equation (17) is used to model the undulator with the first and last periods tapered up and down to model the injection and ejection of the beam. Since there is exponential growth and, hence, the optical guiding of the radiation, we use a matched beam in the undulator. The resonator is concentric with the power coupled out through a 5.0 mm hole in the downstream mirror, which provides for a typical average out-coupling of about 97 percent. Given the repetition rate, f_rep, the nominal zero-detuning cavity length, L_0, is 6.85239904 m when $M = 4$ and assuming $v_g = c$ (see Equation (46)). The temporal window is an important numerical consideration, and must be chosen to be large enough to accommodate the maximum cavity detuning length that is consistent with pass-to-pass amplification so that the optical pulse remains within the time window for all the usable choices of cavity length. In practice, for this example, we choose a temporal window of 4.0 ps and include 182 temporal slices, which corresponds to the inclusion of one temporal slice every three wavelengths. OPC uses the modified Fresnel propagator (Equation (35)) to handle the divergence and convergence of the optical beam inside the resonator, using a grid with a fixed number of grid points.

Table 1. Electron beam, undulator and resonator parameters for the IR RAFEL.

Electron Beam			
Energy	55	MeV	
Charge	800	pC	
Bunch duration	1.2	ps	parabolic
Repetition rate	87.5	MHz	
Normalized emittance	15	mm-mrad	
Energy spread	0.25%		
Matched beam radius	392	μm	
Undulator			two-plane focusing
Period	2.4	cm	
Magnitude	6.5–7.0	kG	
K_{rms}	1.03–1.11		
Length	$100\lambda_u$		98 uniform
Resonator			Concentric
Wavelength	2.2	μm	
Length	6.852	m	
Radii of curvature	3.5	m	
Rayleigh range	0.5	m	
Hole radius	5.0	mm	
Out-coupling	97%		

We first consider the single-pass gain because this will affect the performance of the RAFEL. Since the undulator is long enough to achieve exponential growth, we show the gain length, L_G, found in simulation versus the undulator field strength in Figure 10. The optimal (i.e., minimal) gain length of 0.176 m occurs for an on-axis undulator field strength of about 6.7 kG, which corresponds to an rms undulator strength parameter of K_{rms} = 1.06. This is in good agreement with the prediction based on the parameterization of the interaction by Ming Xie [214].

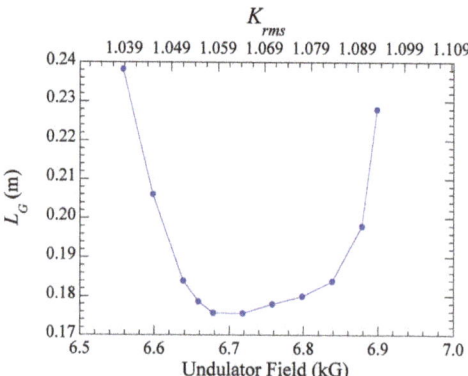

Figure 10. Gain length L_G versus on-axis undulator field amplitude B_u for the IR RAFEL. Other parameters as in Table 1.

It should be noted that the well-known resonance condition $\lambda = \lambda_u(1 + K_{rms}^2)/2\gamma^2$ predicts an undulator field of about 6.81 kG ($K_{rms} = 1.08$) at a 2.2 μm wavelength. This shift in the resonance is due to three-dimensional effects and is in disagreement with the shift in the resonance associated with low-gain oscillators. The gain length has implications over the permissible range of K_{rms} for which the RAFEL will operate (i.e., over which there is pass-to-pass amplification). Since the RAFEL will saturate when the gain balances the loss, and the loss for the resonator is about 97 percent, this implies that the RAFEL will operate as long as the single-pass gain exceeds about 3200–3300 percent. In order to identify this range more closely, we perform multi-pass simulations and take the average gain over the first 10 passes. We take an average because there are fluctuations in the gain on a pass-to-pass basis (i.e., limit-cycle like oscillations), which will be discussed in more detail below. The average gain is shown as a function of the on-axis undulator field under the assumption of a cavity length of 8.65238 in Figure 11. This represents a cavity detuning with respect to the zero-detuning length of $\Delta L_{cav} = -8\lambda$. It is clear from Figure 11 that the gain is relatively constant over the range of about 6.65–6.85 kG (K_{rms} = 1.054–1.085) and falls off rapidly as the field diverges outside this range, which is consistent with the behavior of the gain length shown in Figure 10. The cutoff for a gain of about 3300 percent occurs for field levels of about 6.518 kG (K_{rms} = 1.03) at the low end and 6.878 kG (K_{rms} = 1.09) at the high end, and we do not expect the RAFEL to function outside of this range of undulator fields.

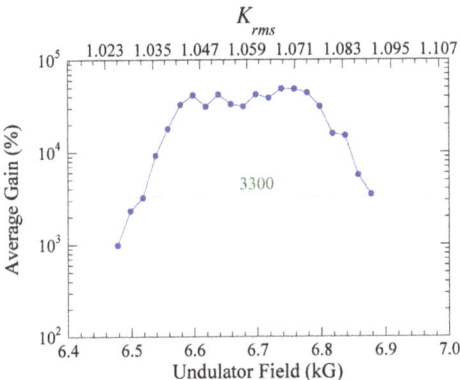

Figure 11. Average gain produced by the IR RAFEL over the first 10 passes versus the undulator field B_u for a cavity length of L_{cav} = 8.62538144 m ($\Delta L_{cav} = -8\lambda$). Other parameters as in Table 1.

In order to demonstrate how the saturation efficiency of a RAFEL differs from that of a low-gain oscillator, it is instructive to compare the RAFEL with an equivalent SASE FEL. The performance of the RAFEL is shown in Figure 12, where we plot the average pulse energy (blue circles) in the steady-state as a function of the on-axis undulator field for the same cavity detuning ($\Delta L_{cav} = -8\lambda$), as used for Figure 11. The error bars characterize the limit-cycle oscillations. The RAFEL reaches its peak pulse energy for an undulator field of 6.678 kG (K_{rms} = 1.058) and falls to zero outside the range predicted in Figure 10. We also plot the equivalent SASE saturated pulse energy (red triangles). In order to deal with the statistical fluctuations inherent in the SASE output, a large number of runs were made with different shot noise distributions, and found the average (red triangles) and standard deviations (error bars). Note that the SASE results represent the pulse energies over whatever length of undulator is required to reach saturation. Observe that (1) the RAFEL configuration saturates with a higher pulse energy than the SASE configuration, (2) the fluctuations in the RAFEL in the steady-state regime are comparable in magnitude to the statistical fluctuations found in SASE, however, the fluctuations of the RAFEL are deterministic in nature, and (3) the FWHM of the tuning range in K_{rms} is comparable for both the RAFEL and SASE configurations.

The RAFEL saturates with about a 0.28 mJ pulse energy, which corresponds to an extraction efficiency of about 0.64 percent. This compares well with the empirical formula [214] that predicts a saturation efficiency of about 0.76 percent. In contrast, the saturation efficiency of a low-gain oscillator is predicted to be $\eta = 1/(2.4 N_u) = 0.43\%$.

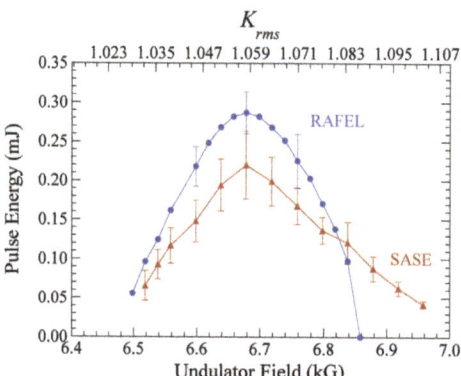

Figure 12. Output pulse energy for the IR RAFEL (blue circles) and an equivalent SASE FEL (red triangles) as a function of the undulator field strength B_u. The cavity detuning for the IR RAFEL is $\Delta L_{cav} = -8\lambda$, while the other simulation parameters are given in Table 1. The error bars indicate energy fluctuations due to limit-cycle-like oscillations for the RAFEL and pulse-to-pulse rms energy fluctuations in case of SASE.

The spectral linewidth of the RAFEL also differs from that of a low-gain oscillator. The full width of the spectrum for a typical low-gain oscillator is given by $\Delta\omega/\omega = 1/N_u = 0.01$ for the example under consideration. This can be translated into a tuning range over the undulator field, as follows

$$\left|\frac{\Delta B_u}{B_u}\right| = \frac{1 + K_{rms}^2}{K_{rms}^2}\left|\frac{\Delta\omega}{\omega}\right|. \tag{47}$$

This implies a full width tuning range of $\Delta B_u = 0.063$ kG ($\Delta K_{rms} = 0.001$), which is narrower than what we find in the simulation. The relative SASE linewidth is given by $(\Delta\omega/\omega)_{rms} = \rho$ [215] where ρ denotes the Pierce parameter. Here, $\rho = 0.0097$ and $(\Delta\omega/\omega)_{rms} = 0.0097$. Converting this to a tuning range in the undulator field and going from the rms width to a FWHM tuning range, we obtain $(\Delta B_u/B_u)_{FWHM} = 0.022$, which compares well with the simulation results that give $(\Delta B_u/B_u)_{FWHM} = 0.019$. Hence, the RAFEL behaves more like a SASE FEL than a typical low-gain oscillator in regards to the spectral linewidth.

Another way in which the RAFEL differs from a low-gain oscillator is in the cavity detuning. In a low-gain FEL oscillator, the zero-detuning length is obtained by assuming that the group velocity v_g equals the speed of light in vacuo c throughout the resonator. However, v_g is reduced in a RAFEL by the interaction in the undulator, and results in smaller synchronous cavity length. This makes the cavity detuning dependent on the gain of the FEL. The change in group velocity also affects slippage. In a low-gain oscillator, the group velocity reduction is small and the slippage is one wavelength per undulator period; hence, the slippage distance is $l_{slip} = N_u\lambda$. However, the slippage per undulator period is reduced in a high-gain RAFEL, or in any FEL where there is exponential growth because they have medium decreases, in both the phase and group velocities. The reduced phase velocity results in the optical guiding of the radiation, while the reduced group velocity results in less slippage. It has been shown that $l_{slip} = N_u\lambda/3$ at the resonant wavelength [216]. For the example under consideration, this yields $l_{slip} = 72$ µm, which is much less than the slippage length of 220 µm if the RAFEL behaved as a low-gain oscillator.

In order to estimate the effect of this on the detuning length, we note that the zero-detuning length is found by equating the roundtrip time of the radiation through the cavity with the spacing between electron bunches ($1/f_{rep}$), cf. Equation (45). As a result, in the high gain regime where $v_g = c/(1 + 1/3\gamma_\parallel^2)$, the difference in synchronous cavity length ΔL_0 for a high-gain RAFEL and a low-gain FEL oscillator is given by Equation (45) as

$$\Delta L_0 = \frac{L_u}{6\gamma^2}(1 + K_{\text{rms}}^2) = -\frac{N_u \lambda}{3}. \tag{48}$$

This is comparable to what is found in the simulation.

The detuning curve found in the simulation is shown in Figure 13, where we plot the output pulse energy versus cavity detuning for an undulator field of 6.658 kG (K_{rms} = 1.055). Here, we define the cavity detuning relative to the nominal zero detuning length (Equation (46) with $M = 1$), so that $\Delta L_{\text{cav}} = L_{\text{cav}} - L_0$. As shown in Figure 13, we find a full width detuning range of about 50–110 µm and an FWHM detuning range of about 40 µm, which are in reasonable agreement with the estimate based on the one-dimensional analysis of slippage.

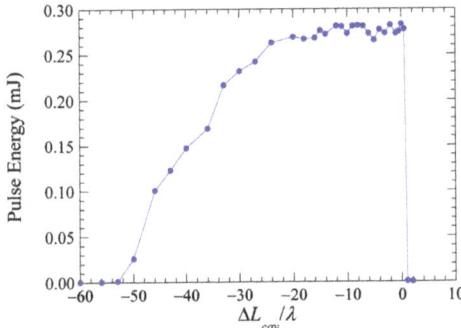

Figure 13. Cavity detuning curve of the IR RAFEL for an on-axis undulator field of $B_u = 6.658$ kG (K_{rms} = 1.055), while the other parameters are given in Table 1.

The temporal evolution of the pulse energy is shown for an undulator field of 6.658 kG (K_{rms} = 1.055) in Figure 14, where we plot the pulse energy versus pass number through the undulator for the choice of several cavity detunings that samples the complete detuning curve. It is clear that significant fluctuations are found over a large range of detunings and that both the magnitude and period of the fluctuations decrease as the magnitude of the detuning increases, although the magnitude of the fluctuations decreases as well near the zero-detuning length.

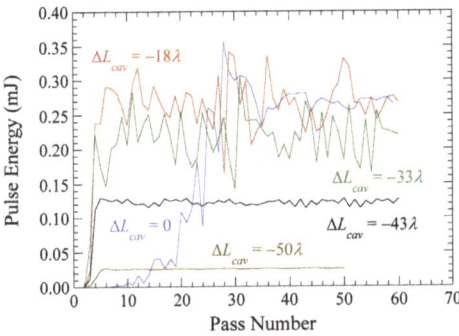

Figure 14. Temporal evolution of the pulse energy for cavity detunings of $\Delta L_{\text{cav}} = 0$, $-18\lambda, -33\lambda, -43\lambda$ and -50λ. The on-axis undulator field is $B_u = 6.658$ kG (K_{rms} = 1.055), while the other parameters are given in Table 1.

The fluctuations seen in simulation can be rapid and irregular. There are two possible explanations for this. One is that due to the high gain and high out-coupling, small changes in the mode structure from pass to pass can result in relatively large changes in the gain and, hence, the pulse energy. These "small" changes can include variations in the transverse mode structure (both in terms of the modal decomposition and spot size), and the temporal pulse shape. The second explanation, related to the first, is that since we have employed hole out-coupling, these relatively small changes in the transverse mode structure at the mirror can give rise to large differences in the out-coupling of the optical mode. It is not surprising, therefore, that the magnitude of the fluctuations varies depending on the cavity detuning. In Figure 15, we show the variation in the rms magnitude of the fluctuations in the out-coupled pulse energy as a function of the cavity detuning. It is clear from Figure 15 that the fluctuation level is relatively constant, at about the 0.03 mJ level over most of the detuning range, but with rapid declines at the end of the detuning range. Furthermore, the oscillation period is of the order of a few passes through the resonator.

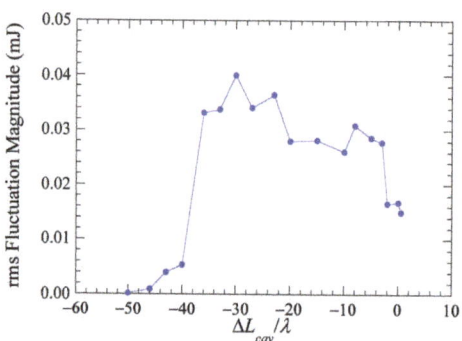

Figure 15. Standard deviation of the optical pulse energy as a function of cavity detuning $\Delta L_{cav}/\lambda$ for a undulator field strength of B_u = 6.658 kG (K_{rms} = 1.055), while the other parameters are given in Table 1.

Fluctuations/oscillations have been observed in low-gain oscillators and are referred to as limit-cycle oscillations. The observation of limit-cycle behavior in the low-gain FELIX FEL oscillator corresponds to an oscillation period of [143]

$$\Delta \tau = -\tau_{slip} \frac{L_{cav}}{\Delta L_{cav}}, \tag{49}$$

where $\tau_{slip} = l_{slip}/c$ is the slippage time. For the case of FELIX, L_{cav} = 6 m, λ = 40 µm, and N_u = 38, and the cavity detuning ranges over about 160 µm. As a result, τ_{slip} = 5.1 ps and τ_r (=$2L_{cav}/c$) = 40 ns is the nominal roundtrip time; hence, this implies that the limit cycle oscillation occurs over a period of about 3 µs or 75 passes for a cavity detuning of −100 µm.

In contrast, if we apply the slippage time for the high gain RAFEL under consideration

$$\Delta \tau = -\frac{N_u \lambda}{3 \Delta L_{cav}} \frac{L_{cav}}{c} = -\frac{\tau_r}{2} \frac{N_u \lambda}{3 \Delta L_{cav}}. \tag{50}$$

As such, we expect the oscillation period to occur on the scale of a small number of passes for the indicated cavity detuning range. This is indeed what is observed in Figure 14. For example, the oscillations occur approximately every 2–4 passes for $\Delta L_{cav}/\lambda$ = −8, which is consistent with Equation (50). However, there is not a great deal of variation with detuning possible when the oscillations occur on such a fast time scale, and we must take Equations (49) and (50) as approximate measures of the oscillation period. Still, the observed oscillation period is well described by the formula for the oscillation period for limit-cycle oscillations found in low-gain oscillators when the appropriate slippage is taken into account. For a high-gain RAFEL, the much lower slippage results in very short oscillation periods.

The limit-cycle-like oscillations in the RAFEL are correlated with the fluctuations/oscillations in the transverse mode structure. The transverse mode structure in a low-gain oscillator is largely (but not completely) determined by the mode structure in the cold cavity, since the optical guiding of the radiation in the undulator is weak. This is not the case in a RAFEL where the mode is guided through the undulator. As a result, the mode structure that forms as the RAFEL saturates differs substantially from the cold cavity modes, and our choice of a Rayleigh range of 0.5 m serves mainly to determine the radii of curvature of the mirrors. Since the radiation is guided in the undulator, the spot size at the undulator exit may be smaller than it would be in the cold cavity, which means that the Rayleigh range of the radiation as it exits the undulator is smaller than it would be in the cold cavity. This implies, in turn, that the optical mode will expand more rapidly as it propagates to the downstream mirror. Alternatively, decomposing the smaller spot size at the undulator exit in cold cavity modes, necessarily leads to higher order transverse modes in the optical field. After propagating to the outcoupler, the superposition of these modes determine the fraction of the optical field coupled out through the hole, and, similarly, after propagation to the undulator entrance, the superposition sets the field profile at undulator entrance. Small variations in the exponential growth rate, e.g., due to changing coupling of the electrons to the optical field at the undulator entrance, lead to relatively larger effects on the optical guiding of the radiation. This in turn changes the spot size at the undulator exit and, hence, the energy coupled out of the resonator and the spot size at the undulator entrance.

The oscillation in mode size has also been observed in simulation of low-gain oscillators [183] where the magnitude of the oscillation depends on the amount of optical guiding, which may vary between the FEL gain codes used [204]. Furthermore, it is found that mirror aberrations, e.g., spherical aberration, also effect the variation in optical mode size observed from pass to pass [204].

This is illustrated in Figure 16, where we plot the pass-to-pass variation in the width of the optical mode on the downstream and upstream mirrors for $B_u = 6.585$ kG ($K_{rms} = 1.043$) and $\Delta L_{cav} = -8\lambda$. It is clear that both the spot size and the fluctuations of the spot size on the upstream mirror are greater than those on the downstream mirror, due to the optical properties of the resonator. At saturation, the location of the smallest optical beam size moves over the axis of the undulator and this changes the optical magnification. Consequently, the size of the optical field at both mirrors as well as at the entrance of the undulator changes from pass to pass, as can be observed in Figure 16.

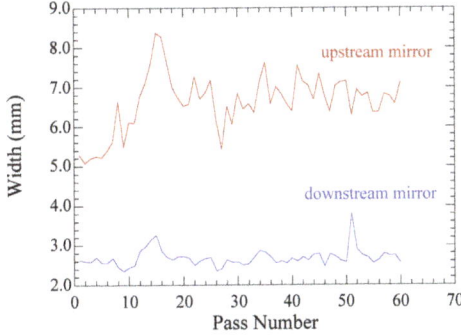

Figure 16. Variation in the width (rms diameter) of the optical beam incident on the upstream mirror (red) and downstream mirror (blue) as a function of the number of passes for a cavity detuning of $\Delta L_{cav} = -8\lambda$ and an undulator field strength of $B_u = 6.658$ kG ($K_{rms} = 1.055$). The other parameters are given in Table 1.

The transverse mode structure is not only a result of optical guiding; it is also affected by the hole out-coupling. Consider the case of B_u = 6.658 kG (K_{rms} = 1.055) and $\Delta L_{cav} = -18\lambda$. The cross-section of the field delivered to the undulator entrance on pass 60 is shown in Figure 17, where we plot the normalized power in the x-direction (i.e., the wiggle plane). Observe that the bulk of the power is at the edge of the optical field, but there is a spike at the center that seeds the subsequent pass through the undulator. Despite the multiple peaks in the cross section at the undulator entrance, the strength of the interaction in the undulator yields a near-Gaussian mode peaked on-axis at the undulator exit, as shown in Figure 18a. What has happened is that the interaction with the electron beam, which has a diameter of about 0.784 mm, essentially amplifies and guides the central peak shown in Figure 17, while the power in the wings falls outside the electron beam and is not amplified. This near-Gaussian mode then propagates to the downstream mirror, during which it expands by about a factor of three, as shown in Figure 18b, where the FWHM is about 3.9 mm in width. The FWHM of the modal superposition at the undulator exit is about 1.2 mm.

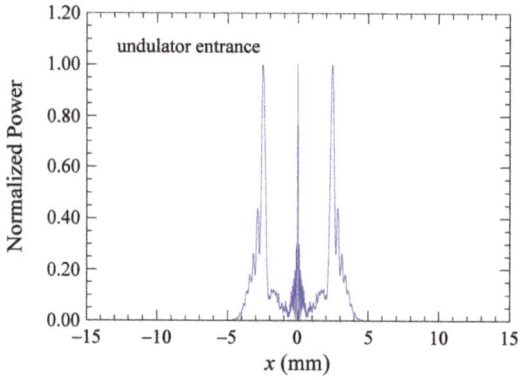

Figure 17. Cross-section of the optical field at the undulator entrance on pass 60 for a cavity detuning $\Delta L_{cav} = -18\lambda$ and an undulator field strength of B_u = 6.658 kG (K_{rms} = 1.055). The other parameters are given in Table 1.

Ignoring the hole in the out-coupling mirror, the waist (0.59 mm) of the fundamental cold cavity mode is designed to be about $\sqrt{2}$ times the matched electron beam radius in the undulator. The FWHM of the fundamental cold cavity mode at the undulator exit and downstream mirror are 1.84 and 4.82 mm, respectively. We thus observe that the optical mode in the RAFEL expands faster from the undulator exit to the downstream mirror than the fundamental cold cavity mode (factor 3.25 and 2.62 respectively). That the RAFEL mode size is still smaller at the downstream mirror is the result of a balance between the faster expansion and smaller spot size of the RAFEL optical mode at the undulator exit compared to the cold cavity mode. The smaller spot size at the undulator exit is due to gain guiding as described above. Both the smaller spot size at the undulator exit and faster expansion of the RAFEL optical beam again indicate that at the undulator exit, the optical field consists of fundamental and higher order cold-cavity modes. Note, a fundamental Gaussian beam having a waist at the undulator exit with the same size as the RAFEL optical beam would have a Rayleigh range of 1.49 m. Finally, the cross section of the mode incident on the upstream mirror is shown in Figure 18c. After reflection from the upstream mirror and propagation through the resonator to the undulator entrance, this field results in a modal pattern similar to that shown in Figure 17.

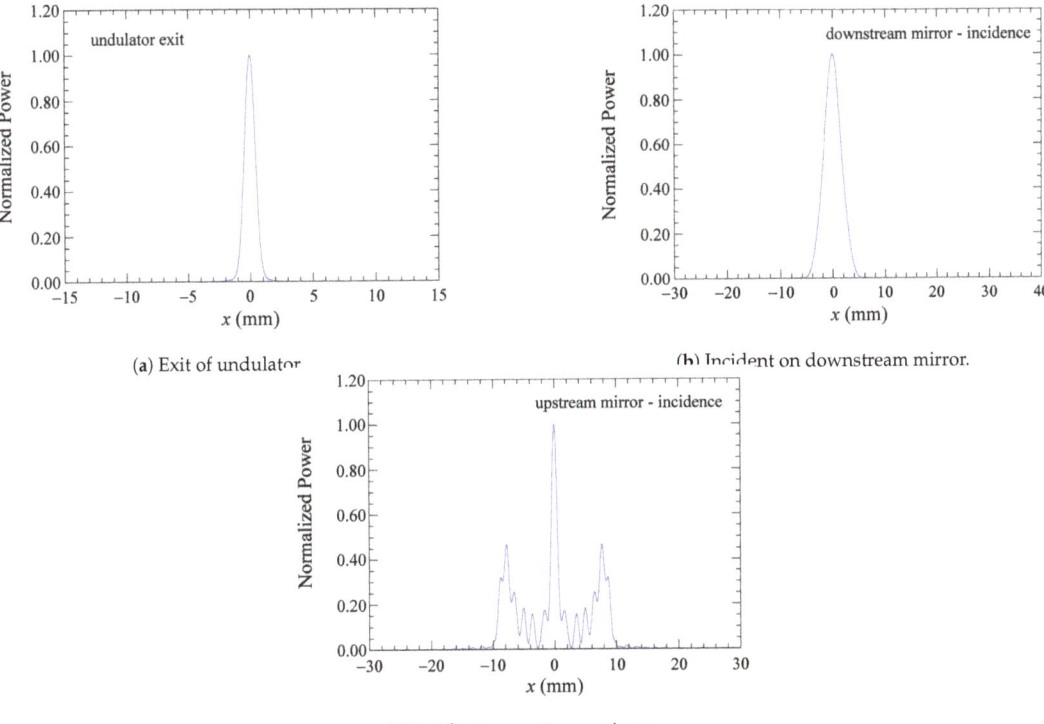

Figure 18. Cross-section of the optical field at various location on pass 60 for a cavity detuning $\Delta L_{cav} = -18\lambda$ and an undulator field strength of $B_u = 6.658$ kG ($K_{rms} = 1.055$). The other parameters are given in Table 1.

Now consider the formation of temporal coherence. Since the RAFEL starts from shot noise on the beam, the initial growth of the mode starts from spiky noise and, just as in a SASE FEL, develops coherence as it propagates through the undulator. However, the undulator is not long enough to reach saturation on a single pass, so that the evolution to temporal coherence is expected to develop over multiple passes. In Figure 19, we plot the temporal pulse shapes found on the first pass (a) at z = 0.5 m (blue) and 1.0 m (red), and (b) at z = 2.0 m (blue) and 2.4 m (red), the latter being at the undulator exit, for an on-axis undulator field amplitude $B_u = 6.658$ kG ($K_{rms} = 1.055$). Figure 19 shows the full simulation time window, and it should be noted that the electron beam is centered in the time window with a full (parabolic) width of 1.2 ps. The pulse shows many spikes at 0.5 m, but that it has coalesced into about 5 spikes after 1.0 m. The development of temporal coherence continues, until at the undulator exit at 2.4 m, only two spikes remain.

The multi-pass development of temporal coherence after the first pass depends strongly on the cavity detuning. The temporal pulse shapes on the 60th pass at the undulator exit for $B_u = 6.658$ kG ($K_{rms} = 1.055$) and for cavity detunings of $\Delta L_{cav} = 0, -8\lambda, -18\lambda$ and -43λ are shown in Figure 20. As demonstrated previously, the synchronized cavity length for a RAFEL is shorter than the synchronized cavity length of a low-gain FEL oscillator. Therefore, as we have used the speed of light in vacuo, instead of the actual group velocity to define the cavity detuning, we note that $\Delta L_{cav} = 0$ actually corresponds to a cavity length that is larger than the synchronized length for the high-gain RAFEL. Consequently, the returning optical pulse will lag behind the center of the electron bunch. The pulse will be amplified as it propagates through the undulator, but as shown in Figure 19, the two spikes formed over the first pass remain. This behavior is also found for small detunings, as shown in Figure 20b for $\Delta L_{cav} = -8\lambda$.

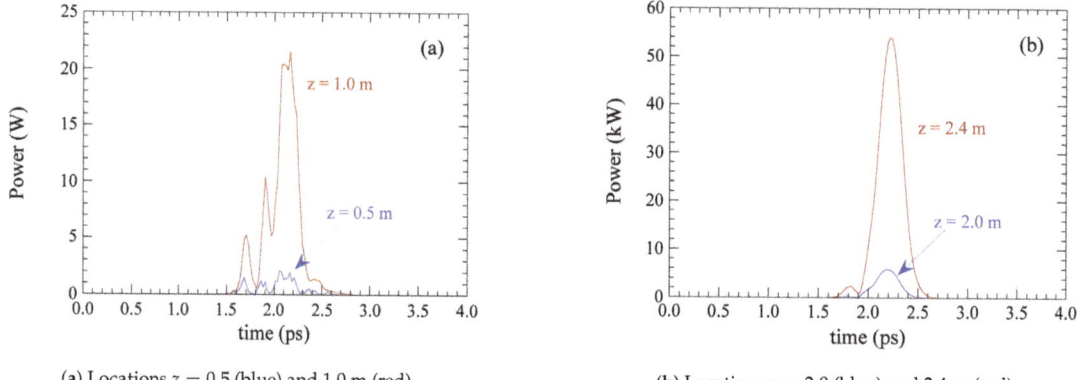

(a) Locations $z = 0.5$ (blue) and 1.0 m (red).

(b) Locations $z = 2.0$ (blue) and 2.4 m (red).

Figure 19. Temporal pulse shape at various locations along the undulator for the first pass when using a cavity detuning $\Delta L_{cav} = -18\lambda$ and an undulator field strength of $B_u = 6.658$ kG ($K_{rms} = 1.055$). The other parameters are given in Table 1.

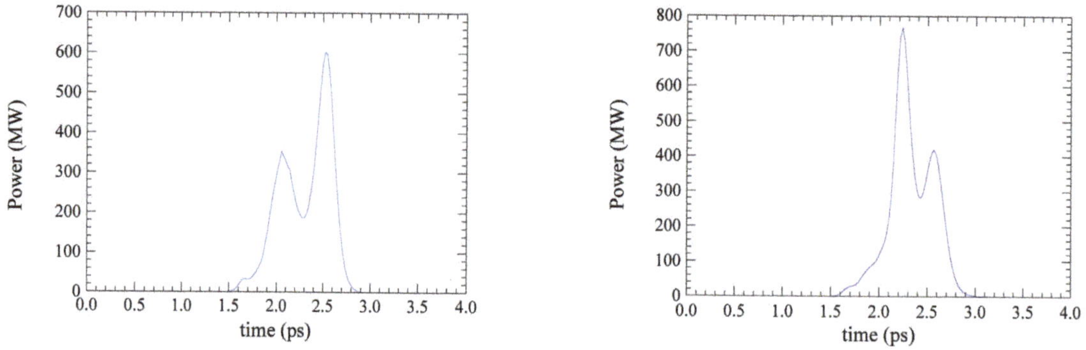

(a) $\Delta L_{cav} = 0$

(b) $\Delta L_{cav} = -8\lambda$

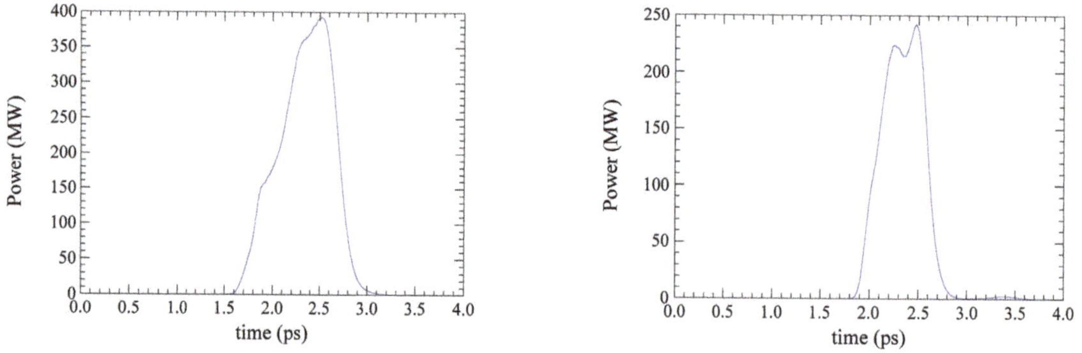

(c) $\Delta L_{cav} = -18\lambda$

(d) $\Delta L_{cav} = -43\lambda$

Figure 20. Temporal pulse shape at the exit of the undulator after 60 passes, and for various cavity detunings. The undulator field strength is $B_u = 6.658$ kG ($K_{rms} = 1.055$). The other parameters are given in Table 1.

If the detuning is closer to the center of the detuning range, then the synchronism between the returning optical pulse and the electrons is a better match, and the multiple spikes are "washed out". This is shown in Figure 20c, where $\Delta L_{cav} = -18\lambda$ and we see that a broader pulse has formed. As the cavity length is decreased further, the optical pulse arrives increasingly near the head of the electron bunch. In this case, there is not enough gain to wash out the multi-spike character of the signal. This is shown in Figure 20d for $\Delta L_{cav} = -43\lambda$, where the total power (or pulse energy is much reduced).

5.2. An X-ray RAFEL

The impetus driving research into X-ray free-electron laser oscillators (XFELOs) and RAFELs is the character of SASE emission. Since there are no seed lasers available at X-ray wavelengths, fourth generation FEL light sources [198,217–221] at these wavelengths are based on SASE over a single pass through a long undulator line. While pulse energies of the order of 2 mJ have been achieved at Ångstrom to sub-Ångstrom wavelengths, with the potential to reach multi-TW peak powers [222–227], SASE exhibits shot-to-shot fluctuations in the output spectra and power of about 10–20 percent. For many applications, these fluctuations are undesirable, and efforts are underway to find alternatives.

The utility of an XFELO has been under study for a decade [162,228–233], making use of resonators based upon Bragg scattering from atomic layers within diamond crystals [234–238]. The development of these crystals is a major breakthrough in the path toward an XFELO. Estimates indicate that using a superconducting RF linac producing 8 GeV electrons at a 1 MHz repetition rate is capable of producing 10^{10} photons per pulse at a 0.86 Å wavelength, with a FWHM bandwidth of about 2.1×10^{-7}. This design is consistent with the LCLS-II High Energy Upgrade [239]. As a consequence, an XFELO on a facility, such as the LCLS-II and LCLS-II-HE, is expected to result in a decrease in SASE fluctuations in the power and spectrum, and to narrow the spectral linewidth.

As with the majority of FELOs to date, the aforementioned XFELOs use low gain/high-Q resonators with transmissive out-coupling through thin diamond crystals [229]. Potential difficulties with low-gain/high-Q resonators derive from sensitivities to electron beam properties, mirror loading and alignments. In addition, transmissive out-coupling with high intra-cavity power can result in mirror damage. While experiments show that diamond crystals can sustain relatively high thermal and radiation loads [238], transmissive out-coupling cannot be easily achieved at the photon energies of interest here. Because of this, X-ray RAFELs [213,240,241] using a variety of out-coupling schemes are receiving a great deal of attention, and we consider a RAFEL design using a pinhole in one of the mirrors [210,213,240] here.

Optics propagation codes such as OPC must treat reflections from the diamond crystal Bragg mirrors, where the mirror losses and angles of reflection depend on the crystal orientation/geometry and the X-ray photon energy. X-ray Bragg mirrors typically have a very narrow reflection bandwidth and a narrow angle of acceptance [205]. For the X-ray RAFEL, and for computational efficiency, a temporal Fourier transform is applied at the beginning of the optical path, when the optical field is passed from MINERVA to OPC and the propagation is performed in the wavelength domain, i.e., each wavelength is independently propagated through the resonator using the modified Fresnel propagator (Equation (35)). The inverse Fourier transform is calculated at the end of the optical path, before the field is handed back to MINERVA. As the optical field inside the cavity is typically not collimated, a spatial Fourier transform in the transverse coordinates is calculated for each of the wavelengths when a Bragg mirror is encountered. Each combination of transverse and longitudinal wavenumber corresponds to a certain photon energy and angle of incidence on the Bragg mirror, and these parameters are used to calculate the complex reflection and transmission coefficients of the Bragg mirror [205]. After applying the appropriate parameter to the optical field, depending on whether it is reflected or transmitted, the inverse spatial Fourier transform is calculated and the field is propagated to the next optical element along the path until the end is reached.

Here, we consider a six-crystal, tunable, compact cavity [236], as illustrated in Figure 21, which shows both a top and a side view. The crystals are arranged in a non-coplanar (3-D) scattering geometry. There are two backscattering units comprising three crystals (C_1, C_2, and C_3) on one side of the undulator and three crystals (C_4, C_5, and C_6) on the other side. Collimating and focusing elements are shown as CRL1,2, which could be grazing incidence mirrors, but are represented in Figure 21 by another possible alternative—compound refractive lenses [242,243]. In each backscattering unit, three successive Bragg reflections take place from three individual crystals to reverse the direction of the beam from the undulator. Assuming that all the crystals and Bragg reflections are the same, the Bragg angles can be chosen within the range $30° < \theta < 90°$; however, Bragg angles close to $\theta = 45°$ should be avoided to ensure high reflectivity for both linear polarization components, as the reflection plane orientations for each crystal change. The cavity allows for tuning the photon energy in a large spectral range by synchronously changing all Bragg angles. In addition, to ensure constant time of flight, the distance L (which brackets the undulator), and the distance between crystals, as characterized by H, have to be changed with θ. The lateral size G is kept constant as the resonator is tuned.

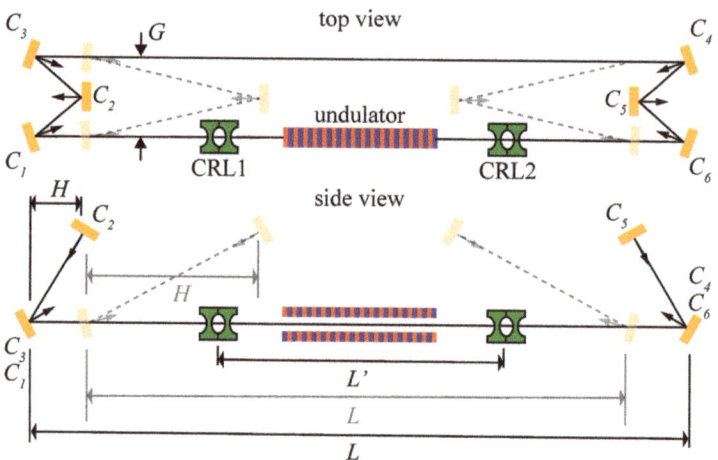

Figure 21. Schematic view of a 6-mirror ring resonator for an X-ray FEL oscillator using plane Bragg mirrors $C_1 \ldots C_6$ and compound refractive lenses, CRL1 and CRL2 for focusing. After [236].

Because the C_1C_6 and C_3C_4 lines are fixed, intracavity radiation can be out-coupled simultaneously for several users at different places in the cavity, although we only consider out-coupling through C_6 at the present time. Out-coupling through crystals C_3 and C_6 are most favourable, since the direction of the out-coupled beams do not change with photon energy, but out-coupling for more users through crystals C_1 and C_4 is also possible. Such multi-user capability is in stark contrast with present SASE beamlines, which support one user at a time. We consider that the electron beam propagates from left to right through the undulator and the out-coupling is accomplished through a pinhole in the first downstream mirror (C_6).

Consider the LCLS-II beamline [239] with the HXR undulator corresponding to an electron energy of 4.0 GeV, a bunch charge in the range of 10–30 pC with an rms bunch duration (length) at the undulator of 2–173 fs (0.6–52 µm) and a repetition rate of 1 MHz. The peak current at the undulator is 1000 A, with a normalized emittance of 0.2–0.7 mm-mrad, and an rms energy spread of about 125–1500 keV. The HXR undulator [239] is a plane-polarized, hybrid permanent magnet undulator with a variable gap, a period of 2.6 cm, and a peak field of 10 kG. Each HXR undulator has 130 periods. In the simulation, each undulator is modeled using Equation (17) and we consider that the first and last period describe an entry/exit taper. There is a total of 32 segments that can be installed. The break sections between the undulators are 1.0 m in length and contain steering, focusing and diagnostic elements, although we only consider the focusing quadrupoles in the simulation, which we position in the center of the breaks. The quadrupoles are assumed to be 7.4 cm in length with a field gradient of 1.71 kG/cm.

A fundamental resonance at 3.05 keV (=4.07 Å) implies an undulator field of 5.61 kG. We assume that the electron beam has a normalized emittance of 0.45 mm-mrad and a relative energy spread of 1.25×10^{-4}, corresponding to the nominal design specification for LCLS-II. This yields a Pierce parameter of $\rho = 5.4 \times 10^{-4}$. In order to match this beam into the undulator/FODO line, the initial beam size in the $x(y)$-direction is 37.87 (31.99) µm with Twiss $\alpha_x = 1.205$ ($\alpha_y = -0.8656$). Note that this yields Twiss $\beta_x = 24.9$ m and $\beta_y = 17.80$ m.

The resonator dimensions were fixed by means of estimates of the gain using the Ming Xie parameterization [214], and MINERVA simulations indicated that about 40–60 m of undulator would be required to operate as a RAFEL. As such, the distance, L, between the two mirrors framing the undulator was chosen to be 130 m, which is also the distance separating the two mirrors on the back side of the resonator (elements C_3 and C_4). In studying the cavity tuning via time-dependent simulations, these two distances are allowed to vary while holding fixed the configurations of the backscattering units. The compound refractive lenses, which are modeled as thin lenses by OPC, are placed symmetrically around the undulator and are designed to place the optical focus at the center of the undulator in vacuo. In this study, the focal length is approximately 94.5 m.

In order to out-couple the X-rays through a transmissive mirror at the wavelength of interest, the diamond crystal would need to be impractically thin (about 5 µm); hence, we consider out-coupling through a hole in the first downstream mirror (C_6). We consider all the mirrors to be 100 µm thick. Due to the high computational requirements of time-dependent simulations, we begin with an optimization of the RAFEL with respect to the hole radius and the undulator length using steady-state (i.e., time-independent) simulations.

The choice of hole radius is important, because if the hole is too small then the bulk of the power remains within the resonator while if the hole is too large then the losses become too great and the RAFEL cannot lase. The results for the optimization of the hole radius indicate that the optimum hole radius is 135 µm, which allows for 90 percent out-coupling, where we fixed the undulator line to consist of 11 HXR undulator segments. This is shown in Figure 22, where we plot the output power as a function of pass number for the optimum hole radius and the variation in the saturated power with the hole radius (inset).

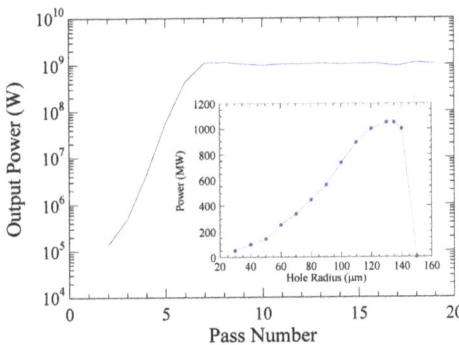

Figure 22. Output power versus number of passes through the resonator for a whole radius of 135 µm. The inset shows the output power as a function of hole radius. Other simulation parameters are described in the text.

A local optimization on the undulator length for a hole radius of 135 µm is shown in Figure 23, where we plot the peak recirculating power (left axis) and the average output power (right axis). The error bars in the figure indicate the level of pass-to-pass fluctuations in the power which is generally smaller than the level of shot-to-shot fluctuations in SASE. Note that while this represents steady-state simulations, the average power is calculated under the assumption of an electron bunch with a flat-top temporal profile having a duration of 24 fs which yields a duty factor of 2.4×10^{-8}. Each point in the figure refers to a given number of HXR undulators ranging from 9–13 segments. It is evident from the figure that the optimum length is 47.18 m, corresponding to 11 segments.

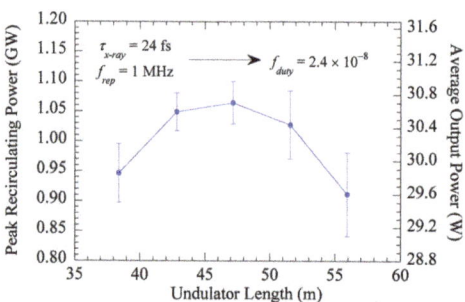

Figure 23. Recirculating output power versus length of the undulator L_u for a hole radius of 135 µm. Other simulation parameters as described in the text.

Time-dependent simulations were performed under the assumption of electron bunches with a flat-top temporal profile having a full width duration of 24 fs and a peak current of 1000 A. This corresponds to a bunch charge of 24 pC. The detuning curve defining what cavity lengths are synchronized with the repetition rate of the electrons is shown in Figure 24. For simplicity, we take the synchronous cavity length L_0 as $L_0 = c/f_{rep}$ (cf. Equation (46)), where a single optical pulse is assumed to be inside the cavity and the effect of gain on the group velocity is ignored. Here $L_0 = 299.7924580$ m. The range of cavity lengths with overlap between the optical pulse and an electron pulse with a length of about 7.2 µm is given by $L_0 - 7.2$ µm $< L_{cav} < L_0 + 7.2$ µm, where L_{cav} is taken here to be the total roundtrip length of the cavity.

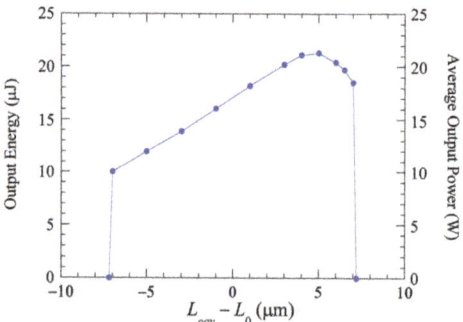

Figure 24. Output energy as a function of the cavity detuning $\Delta L_{cav} = L_{cav} - L_0$ for a hole radius of 135 µm. The simulation parameters are as described in the text.

The evolution of the output energy at the fundamental and the 3rd harmonic, and the spectral linewidth of the fundamental, vs. pass is shown in Figure 25 for a detuning of 5 µm, which is close to the peak in the detuning curve (Figure 24). While it is not evident in the figure, the rms fluctuation in the energy from pass to pass is of the order of about 3 percent, which is lower than the shot-to-shot fluctuations expected from SASE. At least as important as the output power is that the linewidth contracts substantially during the exponential growth phase and remains constant through saturation. Starting with a linewidth of about 3.7×10^{-4} after the first pass corresponding to SASE, the linewidth contracts to about 6.0×10^{-5} at saturation. The SASE linewidth after the first pass through the undulator is slightly smaller than the predicted linewidth based on 1-D theory [240], which is approximately 4.5×10^{-4}. Hence, the RAFEL is expected to have both high average power and a stable narrow linewidth, which is to a large extent determined by the spectral filtering of the Bragg mirrors.

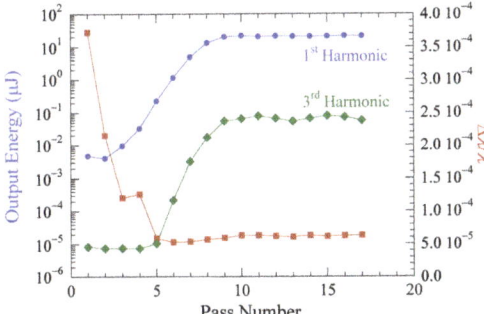

Figure 25. Evolution of the fundamental pulse energy (blue, left) and the 3rd harmonic (green, left), as well as the relative linewidth (red, right) when the cavity detuning is $\Delta L_{cav} = 5$ µm and for an electron beam energy spread $\Delta E_b/E_b = 1.25 \times 10^{-4}$. Other parameters as described in the text.

The 3rd harmonic grows parasitically from high powers/pulse energies at the fundamental in a single pass through the undulator [184] and has been shown to reach output intensities of 0.1 percent that of the fundamental in a variety of FEL configurations, and this is what we find in the RAFEL simulations. As shown in Figure 25, the 3rd harmonic intensity remains small until the fundamental pulse energy reaches about 1 µJ after which it grows rapidly and saturates after about 12 passes. This is close to the point at which the fundamental saturates as well. The saturated pulse energies at the 3rd harmonic reach about 0.067 µJ. Given a repetition rate of 1 MHz, this corresponds to a long-term average power of 67 mW.

The reduction in the linewidth after saturation shown in Figure 25 indicates that a substantial level of longitudinal coherence has been achieved in the saturated regime. The RAFEL starts from shot noise on the beam during the first pass through the undulator, and longitudinal coherence develops over the subsequent passes. Hence, we expect that the temporal profile of the optical field will exhibit the typical spiky structure associated with SASE at the undulator exit after the first pass and this is indeed depicted in Figure 26a which shows the temporal profile at the undulator exit after the first pass. The number of spikes expected, N_{spikes}, is given approximately by $N_{spikes} = l_b/(2\pi l_c)$, where l_b is the rms bunch length and l_c is the coherence length. For the present case, $l_b = 7.2$ µm and $l_c = 60$ nm; hence, we expect that $N_{spikes} = 19$. We observe about 14 spikes in Figure 26a which is in reasonable agreement with the expectation. Note that the time axis encompasses the time window used in the simulation. As indicated in Figure 25, the linewidth after the first pass is of the order of 4.3×10^{-4} which is relatively broad and corresponds to the interaction due to SASE. This is reflected in the output spectrum from the undulator after the first pass, which is shown in Figure 26b.

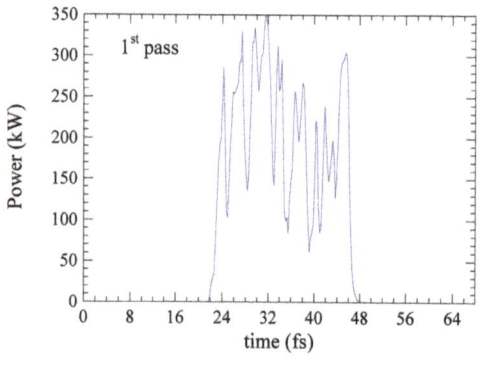
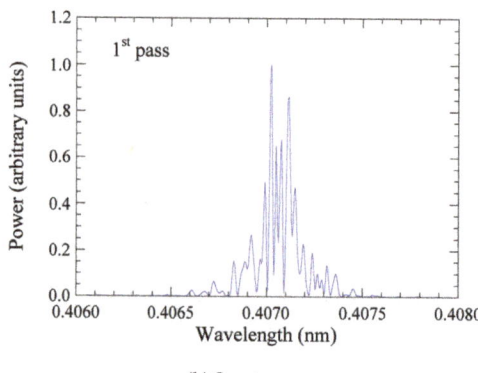

(a) Temporal profile

(b) Spectrum

Figure 26. Temporal pulse shape and spectrum of the optical pulse at the exit of the undulator for the first pass. Other parameters as described in the text.

The spectral narrowing that is associated with the development of longitudinal coherence as the interaction approaches saturation results in a smoothing of the temporal profile. This is illustrated in Figure 27a, where we plot the temporal profiles of the optical field at the undulator exit corresponding to passes 12–16, which are after saturation, has been achieved (left axis). As shown in the figure, the temporal pulse shapes from pass-to-pass are relatively stable and exhibit a smooth plateau with a width of about 23–24 fs, which corresponds to, and overlaps, the flat-top profile of the electron bunches, which is shown on the right axis. Significantly, the smoothness of the profiles corresponds with the narrow linewidth and contrasts sharply with the SASE output after the first pass through the undulator (see Figure 26b). Both the pass-to-pass stability and smoothness of the output pulses contrast markedly with the large shot-to-shot fluctuations and the spikiness expected from the output pulses in pure SASE.

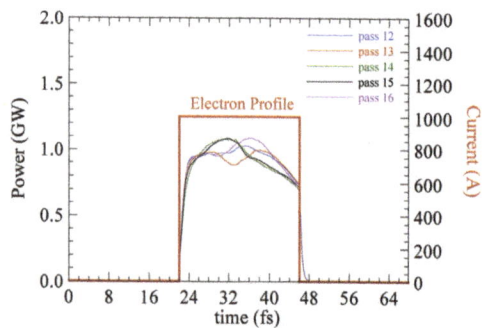
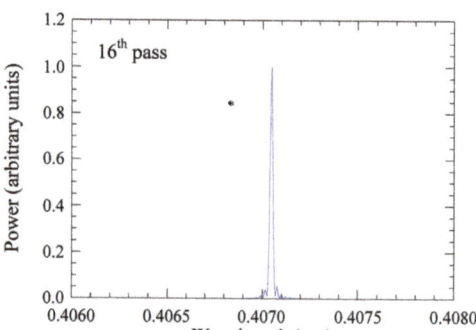

(a) Temporal profile for the optical pulse after different number of passes and current pulse (red).

(b) Spectrum at the exit of the undulator after 16 passes

Figure 27. Temporal pulse shape for the electron bunch and optical pulse after different number of passes and the spectrum at pass number 16 of the optical pulse at the exit of the undulator. Other parameters as described in the text.

The narrow relative linewidth in this regime of about 7.3×10^{-5} at the undulator exit, as shown in Figure 27b after pass 16, as well as the smooth temporal profiles shown in Figure 27a, are associated with longitudinal coherence after saturation is achieved.

6. Summary and Conclusions

The development of both low-gain/high-Q and high-gain/low-Q oscillators is an active and ongoing area of research into FEL sources over virtually the entire electromagnetic spectrum [30,86,91,92,241,244–248]. Both types of FEL oscillators have their own merits. For example, high-gain/low-Q are typically better suited for higher peak power operation, due to a reduced mirror loading [203] and higher extraction efficiency, as found in Section 5. On the other hand, properties like gain bandwidth, and stability of the output, are closer to SASE FELs than low-gain/high-Q FEL oscillators. However, we have not yet explored the full range of feedback, and increasing the feedback may shift the performance in this respect closer to that of low-gain/high-Q oscillators.

As we have described in this paper, great progress has been made in our ability to simulate both the interaction through the undulator and in multi-pass configurations through the undulator and the resonator. This was demonstrated in Section 4 by the excellent agreement found between the simulations and the IR Demo and 10-kW Upgrade experiments at JLab, after which the simulations of both an infrared and an X-ray RAFEL were described in Section 5.

The combination of a three-dimensional, time-dependent FEL simulation code with an optics propagation code provides enormous flexibility in being able to study a wide range of undulator and optical resonator configurations. In particular, the use of a general FEL code such as MINERVA allows the simulation of variable polarization (Section 2.1) governed by the choice of undulator geometries (Section 2.2) and ultra-short electron bunches [249] down to the neighborhood of the cooperation length in the undulators, which defines the limit of applicability of the slowly varying amplitude and phase approximation. The use of OPC permits the simulation of arbitrary optical resonators, including thermal heating and distortion as well as Bragg reflections.

In summary, the numerical algorithms that have been implemented for the simulation of FEL oscillators are now sufficiently mature to serve as reliable design tools for virtually any conceivable undulator and oscillator configuration.

Author Contributions: Both authors contributed equally to conceptualization, methodology, software, validation, analysis, writing—original draft preparation, writing—review and editing, and visualization. All authors have read and agreed to the published version of the manuscript.

Funding: The work described was supported over the course of time by multiple contracts with the U.S. Office of Naval Research, the Department of Defense Joint Technology Office, and the Department of Energy.

Data Availability Statement: Data is available from the authors on request.

Acknowledgments: The authors would like to thank numerous staff members at JLab for many helpful discussions about the IR Demo and 10-kW Upgrade experiments. We would also like to thank Heinz-Dieter Nuhn and Paul Emma for providing assistance with understanding the data from the LCLS and thank Luca Giannessi for assistance concerning the SPARC data. The work described was supported over the course of time by multiple contracts with the U.S. Office of Naval Research, the Department of Defense High Energy Laser Joint Technology Office, and the Department of Energy.

Conflicts of Interest: The authors declare no conflict of interest. Furthermore, the funders had no role in the design of the study; in the collection, analyses, or interpretation of data; in the writing of the manuscript, or in the decision to publish the results.

Abbreviations

The following abbreviations are used in this manuscript:

BPM	beam position monitor
CRL	compound refractive lens
CW	continuous wave
FEL	free-electron laser

FELO	free-electron laser oscillator
FODO	focusing and defocusing
FWHM	full width at half maximum
HGHG	high gain harmonic generation
IR	infrared
JLab	Thomas Jefferson National Accelerator Facility
LCLS	linac coherent light source
linac	linear accelerator
RAFEL	regenerative amplifier free-electron laser
RF	radio frequency
rms	root mean square
SASE	self-amplified spontaneous emission
SDE	source dependent expansion
SPARC	sorgente pulsata ed amplificata di radiazione coerente
VUV	vacuum ultraviolet
XFELO	X-ray free-electron laser

References

1. Freund, H.P.; Antonsen, T.M., Jr. *Principles of Free Electron Lasers*, 3rd ed.; Springer: Cham, Switzerland, 2018.
2. Moore, G.T. The high-gain regime of the free electron laser. *Nucl. Instrum. Methods Phys. Res. Sect. A Accel. Spectrometers Detect. Assoc. Equip.* **1985**, *239*, 19–28. [CrossRef]
3. Deacon, D.A.G.; Elias, L.R.; Madey, J.M.J.; Ramian, G.J.; Schwettman, H.A.; Smith, T.I. First operation of a free-electron laser. *Phys. Rev. Lett.* **1977**, *38*, 892–894. [CrossRef]
4. Elias, L.R.; Fairbank, W.M.; Madey, J.M.J.; Schwettman, H.A.; Smith, T.I. Observation of stimulated emission of radiation by relativistic electrons in a spatially periodic transverse magnetic field. *Phys. Rev. Lett.* **1976**, *36*, 717–720. [CrossRef]
5. Phillips, R.M. History of the Ubitron. *Nucl. Instrum. Methods Phys. Res. Sect. A Accel. Spectrometers Detect. Assoc. Equip.* **1988**, *272*, 1–9. [CrossRef]
6. Elias, L.R.; Ramian, G.; Hu, J.; Amir, A. Observation of single-mode operation in a free-electron laser. *Phys. Rev. Lett.* **1986**, *57*, 424–427. [CrossRef]
7. Ramian, G. The new UCSB free-electron lasers. *Nucl. Instrum. Methods Phys. Res. Sect. A Accel. Spectrometers Detect. Assoc. Equip.* **1992**, *318*, 225–229. [CrossRef]
8. Gover, A.; Faingersh, A.; Eliran, A.; Volshonok, M.; Kleinman, H.; Wolowelsky, S.; Yakover, Y.; Kapilevich, B.; Lasser, Y.; Seidov, Z.; et al. Radiation measurements in the new tandem accelerator FEL. *Nucl. Instrum. Methods Phys. Res. Sect. A Accel. Spectrometers Detect. Assoc. Equip.* **2004**, *528*, 23–27. [CrossRef]
9. Gover, A.; Pinhasi, Y. Electrostatic-accelerator free-electron lasers. In *Electrostatic Accelerators: Fundamentals and Applications*; Springer: Berlin/Heidelberg, Germany, 2005; pp. 378–390. [CrossRef]
10. Minehara, E.J.; Sawamura, M.; Nagai, R.; Kikuzawa, N.; Sugimoto, M.; Hajima, R.; Shizuma, T.; Yamauchi, T.; Nishimori, N. JAERI superconducting RF linac-based free-electron laser-facility. *Nucl. Instrum. Methods Phys. Res. Sect. A Accel. Spectrometers Detect. Assoc. Equip.* **2000**, *445*, 183–186. [CrossRef]
11. Neil, G.R.; Behre, C.; Benson, S.V.; Bevins, M.; Biallas, G.; Boyce, J.; Coleman, J.; Dillon-Townes, L.A.; Douglas, D.; Dylla, H.F.; et al. The JLab high power ERL light source. *Nucl. Instrum. Methods Phys. Res. Sect. A Accel. Spectrometers Detect. Assoc. Equip.* **2006**, *557*, 9–15. [CrossRef]
12. Thomas, A.W.; Williams, G.P. The free electron laser at Jefferson Lab: The technology and the science. *Proc. IEEE* **2007**, *95*, 1679–1682. [CrossRef]
13. Thompson, N.R.; Clarke, J.A.; Craig, T.; Dunning, D.J.; Kolosov, O.V.; Moss, A.; Saveliev, Y.M.; Surman, M.; Tovee, P.D.; Weightman, P. Status of the Alice IR-FEL: From ERL demonstrator to user facility. In *Proceedings of the 37th International Free Electron Laser Conference*, JACoW Publishing: Daejeon, Korea, 2015; pp. 379–383. [CrossRef]
14. Vinokurov, N.A.; Arbuzov, V.S.; Chernov, K.N.; Davidyuk, I.V.; Dementyev, E.N.; Dovzhenko, B.A.; Getmanov, Y.V.; Knyazev, B.A.; Kolobanov, E.I.; Kondakov, A.A.; et al. Novosibirsk high-power THz FEL facility. In *Proceedings of the 2016 International Conference Laser Optics (LO)*; IEEE: Piscataway, NJ, USA, 2016; pp. R10–R14. [CrossRef]
15. Shevchenko, O.A.; Melnikov, A.R.; Tararyshkin, S.V.; Getmanov, Y.V.; Seredyakov, S.S.; Bykov, E.V.; Kubarev, V.V.; Fedin, M.V.; Veber, S.L. Electronic modulation of THz radiation at NovoFEL: technical aspects and possible applications. *Materials* **2019**, *12*, 3063. [CrossRef]
16. Smith, T.I.; Frisch, J.C.; Rohatgi, R.; Schwettman, H.A.; Swent, R.L. Status of the SCA-FEL. *Nucl. Instrum. Methods Phys. Res. Sect. A Accel. Spectrometers Detect. Assoc. Equip.* **1990**, *296*, 33–36. [CrossRef]
17. van der Wiel, M.J.; van Amersfoort, P.W.; Team, F. FELIX: from laser to user facility. *Nucl. Instrum. Methods Phys. Res. Sect. A Accel. Spectrometers Detect. Assoc. Equip.* **1993**, *331*, ABS30–ABS33. [CrossRef]

18. Tomimasu, T.; Saeki, K.; Miyauchi, Y.; Oshita, E.; Okuma, S.; Wakita, K.; Kobayashi, A.; Suzuki, T.; Zako, A.; Nishihara, S.; et al. The FELI FEL facilities—Challenges at simultaneous FEL beam sharing systems and UV-range FELs. *Nucl. Instrum. Methods Phys. Res. Sect. A Accel. Spectrometers Detect. Assoc. Equip.* **1996**, *375*, 626–631. [CrossRef]
19. Ortega, J.M. The CLIO infrared FEL facility. *Synchrotron Radiat. News* **1996**, *9*, 20–33. [CrossRef]
20. Ortega, J.M. Operation and extension to far-infrared of the CLIO FEL facility. *Jpn. J. Appl. Phys.* **2002**, *41*, 20–28. [CrossRef]
21. Schwettman, H.A.; Smith, T.I.; Swent, R.L. The Stanford picosecond FEL center. *Nucl. Instrum. Methods Phys. Res. Sect. A Accel. Spectrometers Detect. Assoc. Equip.* **1996**, *375*, 662–663. [CrossRef]
22. Horiike, H.; Tsubouchi, N.; Awazu, K.; Asakawa, M.; Heya, M. Status of the Institute of Free-Electron Laser, Osaka university. *Jpn. J. Appl. Phys.* **2002**, *41*, 10–14. [CrossRef]
23. Tanaka, T.; Hayakawa, K.; Hayakawa, Y.; Sato, I.; Science, Q. Guiding optics system for LEBRA FEL user facility. In *Proceedings of the 26th International Free Electron Laser Conference*; JACoW Publishing: Trieste, Italy, 2004; pp. 427–430.
24. van der Zande, W.J.; Jongma, R.T.; van der Meer, L.; Redlich, B. FELIX facility: Free electron laser light sources from 0.2 to 75 THz. In *Proceedings of the 2013 38th International Conference on Infrared, Millimeter, and Terahertz Waves (IRMMW-THz)*; IEEE: Piscataway, NJ, USA, 2013; pp. 1–2. [CrossRef]
25. Schöllkopf, W.; Gewinner, S.; Junkes, H.; Paarmann, A.; von Helden, G.; Bluem, H.; Todd, A.M.M. The new IR and THz FEL facility at the Fritz Haber Institute in Berlin. In *Proceedings of the SPIE Proceedings Volume 9512—Advances in X-ray Free-Electron Lasers Instrumentation III*; Biedron, S.G., Ed.; SPIE: Prague, Czech Republic, 2015; 95121L. [CrossRef]
26. Zen, H.; Suphakul, S.; Kii, T.; Masuda, K.; Ohgaki, H. Present status and perspectives of long wavelength free electron lasers at Kyoto university. *Phys. Procedia* **2016**, *84*, 47–53. [CrossRef]
27. Klopf, J.M.; Zvyagin, S.; Helm, M.; Kehr, S.C.; Lehnert, U.; Michel, P.; Pashkin, A.; Schneider, H.; Seide, W.; Winnerl, S. FELBE—upgrades and status of the IR/THz FEL user facility at HZDR. In *Proceedings of the 2018 43rd International Conference on Infrared, Millimeter, and Terahertz Waves (IRMMW-THz)*; IEEE: Piscataway, NJ, USA, 2018; pp. 1–2. [CrossRef]
28. Li, M.; Yang, X.; Xu, Z.; Wu, D.; Wang, H.; Xiao, D.; Shu, X.; Lu, X.; Huang, W.; Dou, Y. China's First Tera-Hertz Free Electron Laser Oscillator. In *Proceedings of the 2018 International Conference on Microwave and Millimeter Wave Technology (ICMMT)*; IEEE: Chengdu, China, 2018; pp. 1–3. [CrossRef]
29. Schöllkopf, W.; Gewinner, S.; Todd, A.M.M.; Colson, W.B.; de Pas, M.; Dowell, D.; Gottschalk, S.C.; Junkes, H.; Rathke, J.W.; Schultheiss, T.J.; et al. The FHI FEL upgrade design. In *Proceedings of the 39th International Free-Electron Laser Conference*; JACoW Publishing: Geneva, Switzerland, 2019; pp. 52–55. [CrossRef]
30. Zhao, Z.; Li, H.; Jia, Q.; He, Z.; Zhu, Y. Proposal of an operation mode of FELiChEM for generating high-power ultra-short infrared FEL pulses. *Nucl. Instrum. Methods Phys. Res. Sect. A Accel. Spectrometers Detect. Assoc. Equip.* **2020**, *984*, 164634. [CrossRef]
31. Gallerano, G.P.; Doria, A.; Giovenale, E.; Renieri, A. Compact free electron lasers: From Cerenkov to waveguide free electron lasers. *Infrared Phys. Technol.* **1999**, *40*, 161–174. [CrossRef]
32. Jeong, Y.U.; Kazakevitch, G.M.; Lee, B.C.; Park, S.H.; Cha, H.J. Laboratory-scale wide-band FIR user facility based on a compact FEL. *Nucl. Instrum. Methods Phys. Res. Sect. A Accel. Spectrometers Detect. Assoc. Equip.* **2004**, *528*, 88–91. [CrossRef]
33. Hara, T.; Couprie, M.E.; Garzella, D.; Nahon, L.; Marsi, M.; Bakker, R.; Billardon, M. Progress of the Super-ACO storage ring free electron laser in the UV as a source for users. *J. Electron Spectrosc. Relat. Phenom.* **1996**, *80*, 317–320. [CrossRef]
34. Litvinenko, V.N.; Burnham, B.; Park, S.H.; Wu, Y.; Cataldo, R.; Emamian, M.; Faircloth, J.; Goetz, S.; Hower, N.; Madey, J.M.J.; et al. First UV/visible lasing with the OK-4/Duke storage ring FEL. *Nucl. Instrum. Methods Phys. Res. Sect. A Accel. Spectrometers Detect. Assoc. Equip.* **1998**, *407*, 8–15. [CrossRef]
35. Hosaka, M.; Katoh, M.; Mochihashi, A.; Shimada, M.; Takashima, Y.; Hara, T. High power deep UV lasing on the UVSOR-II storage ring FEL. In *Proceedings of the 28th International Free Electron Laser Conference*; JACoW Publishing: Berlin, Germany, 2006; pp. 368–370.
36. Wu, Y.K.; Vinokurov, N.A.; Mikhailov, S.; Li, J.; Popov, V. High-gain lasing and polarization switch with a distributed optical-klystron free-electron laser. *Phys. Rev. Lett.* **2006**, *96*, 224801. [CrossRef]
37. Wu, Y.K. Accelerator physics research and light source development programs at Duke university. In *Proceedings of the 2007 IEEE Particle Accelerator Conference (PAC)*; IEEE: Piscataway, NJ, USA, 2007; pp. 1215–1217. [CrossRef]
38. Edwards, G.S.; Allen, S.J.; Haglund, R.F.; Nemanich, R.J.; Redlich, B.; Simon, J.D.; Yang, W.C. Applications of free-electron lasers in the biological and material sciences. *Photochem. Photobiol.* **2007**, *81*, 711–735. [CrossRef]
39. Neyman, P.J.; Colson, W.B.; Gottshalk, S.C.; Todd, A.M.M. Free electron lasers in 2017. In *Proceedings of the 38th International Free-Electron Laser Conference*; JACoW Publishing: Sante Fe, NM, USA, 2017; pp. 204–209. [CrossRef]
40. Newnam, B.; Warren, R.; Sheffield, R.; Stein, W.; Lynch, M.; Fraser, J.; Goldstein, J.; Sollid, J.; Swann, T.; Watson, J.; et al. Optical performance of the Los Alamos free-electron laser. *IEEE J. Quantum Electron.* **1985**, *21*, 867–881. [CrossRef]
41. Bamford, D.J.; Deacon, D.A.G. Measurement of the coherent harmonics emitted in the Mark III free electron laser. *Nucl. Instrum. Methods Phys. Res. Sect. A Accel. Spectrometers Detect. Assoc. Equip.* **1989**, *285*, 23–30. [CrossRef]
42. O'Shea, P.G.; Bender, S.C.; Carlsten, B.E.; Early, J.W.; Feldman, D.W.; Lumpkin, A.H.; Feldman, R.; Goldstein, J.C.; McKenna, K.; Martineau, R.; et al. Performance of the APEX free-electron laser at Los Alamos National Laboratory. *Nucl. Instrum. Methods Phys. Res. Sect. A Accel. Spectrometers Detect. Assoc. Equip.* **1993**, *331*, 62–68. [CrossRef]

43. Prazeres, R.; Berset, J.M.; Glotin, F.; Jaroszynski, D.A.; Ortega, J.M. Optical performance of the CLIO infrared FEL. *Nucl. Instrum. Methods Phys. Res. Sect. A Accel. Spectrometers Detect. Assoc. Equip.* **1993**, *331*, 15–19. [CrossRef]
44. van der Meer, A.F.G.; Bakker, R.J.; van der Geer, C.A.; Oepts, D.; van Amersfoort, P.W.; Gillespie, W.A.; Martin, P.F.; Saxon, G. Optimization of the FELIX accelerator with respect to laser performance. *Nucl. Instrum. Methods Phys. Res. Sect. A Accel. Spectrometers Detect. Assoc. Equip.* **1993**, *331*, 282–286. [CrossRef]
45. O'Shea, P.G.; Bender, S.C.; Byrd, D.A.; Early, J.W.; Feldman, D.W.; Fortgang, C.M.; Goldstein, J.C.; Newnam, B.E.; Sheffield, R.L.; Warren, R.W.; et al. Demonstration of ultraviolet lasing with a low energy electron beam. *Nucl. Instrum. Methods Phys. Res. Sect. A Accel. Spectrometers Detect. Assoc. Equip.* **1994**, *341*, 7–11. [CrossRef]
46. Nguyen, D.C.; Gierman, S.M.; Goldstein, J.C.; Kinross-Wright, J.M.; Kong, S.H.; Plato, J.G.; Russell, S.J.; Sheffield, R.L.; Sigler, F.E.; Sherwood, B.A.; et al. Recent progress of the compact AFEL at Los Alamos. *Nucl. Instrum. Methods Phys. Res. Sect. A Accel. Spectrometers Detect. Assoc. Equip.* **1995**, *358*, 27–30. [CrossRef]
47. Xie, J.; Zhuang, J.; Huang, Y.; Li, Y.; Lin, S.; Ying, R.; Zhong, Y.; Zhang, L.; Wu, G.; Zhang, Y.; et al. The saturation of the Beijing FEL. *Nucl. Instrum. Methods Phys. Res. Sect. A Accel. Spectrometers Detect. Assoc. Equip.* **1995**, *358*, 256–259. [CrossRef]
48. Berryman, K.W.; Smith, T.I. First lasing, capabilities, and flexibility of FIREFLY. *Nucl. Instrum. Methods Phys. Res. Sect. A Accel. Spectrometers Detect. Assoc. Equip.* **1996**, *375*, 6–9. [CrossRef]
49. Minehara, E.J.; Sugimoto, M.; Sawamura, M.; Nagai, R.; Kikuzawa, N.; Yamanouchi, T.; Nishimori, N. A 0.1 kW operation of the JAERI superconducting RF linac-based FEL. *Nucl. Instrum. Methods Phys. Res. Sect. A Accel. Spectrometers Detect. Assoc. Equip.* **1999**, *429*, 9–11. [CrossRef]
50. Neil, G.R.; Benson, S.; Biallas, G.; Bohn, C.L.; Douglas, D.; Dylla, H.F.; Evans, R.; Fugitt, J.; Gubeli, J.; Hill, R.; et al. First operation of an FEL in same-cell energy recovery mode. *Nucl. Instrum. Methods Phys. Res. Sect. A Accel. Spectrometers Detect. Assoc. Equip.* **2000**, *445*, 192–196. [CrossRef]
51. Lumpkin, A.H.; Tokar, R.L.; Dowell, D.H.; Lowrey, A.R.; Yeremian, A.D.; Justice, R.E. Improved performance of the Boeing/LANL FEL experiment. *Nucl. Instrum. Methods Phys. Res. Sect. A Accel. Spectrometers Detect. Assoc. Equip.* **1990**, *296*, 169–180. [CrossRef]
52. Jeong, Y.U.; Lee, B.C.; Kim, S.K.; Cho, S.O.; Cha, B.H.; Lee, J.; Kazakevitch, G.M.; Vobly, P.D.; Gavrilov, N.G.; Kubarev, V.V.; et al. First lasing of the KAERI compact far-infrared free-electron laser driven by a magnetron-based microtron. *Nucl. Instrum. Methods Phys. Res. Sect. A Accel. Spectrometers Detect. Assoc. Equip.* **2001**, *475*, 47–50. [CrossRef]
53. Wu, D.; Li, M.; Yang, X.; Wang, H.; Luo, X.; Shen, X.; Xiao, D.; Wang, J.; Li, P.; Li, X.; et al. First Lasing of the CAEP THz FEL facility driven by a superconducting accelerator. *J. Phys. Conf. Ser.* **2018**, *1067*, 032010. [CrossRef]
54. Oepts, D.; van der Meer, A.F.G.; Bakker, R.J.; van Amersfoort, P.W. Selection of single-mode radiation from a short-pulse free-electron laser. *Phys. Rev. Lett.* **1993**, *70*, 3255–3258. [CrossRef] [PubMed]
55. Billardon, M.; Elleaume, P.; Lapierre, Y.; Ortega, J.M.; Bazin, C.; Bergher, M.; Marilleau, J.; Petroff, Y. The Orsay storage ring free electron laser: New results. *Nucl. Instrum. Methods Phys. Res. Sect. A Accel. Spectrometers Detect. Assoc. Equip.* **1986**, *250*, 26–34. [CrossRef]
56. Kulipanov, G.; Litvinenko, V.N.; Pinaev, I.; Popik, V.; Skrinsky, A.N.; Sokolov, A.S.; Vinokurov, N.A. The VEPP-3 storage-ring optical klystron: Lasing in the visible and ultraviolet regions. *Nucl. Instrum. Methods Phys. Res. Sect. A Accel. Spectrometers Detect. Assoc. Equip.* **1990**, *296*, 1–3. [CrossRef]
57. Yamada, K.; Yamazaki, T.; Sugiyama, S.; Tomimasu, T.; Ohgaki, H.; Noguchi, T.; Mikado, T.; Chiwaki, M.; Suzuki, R. Visible oscillation of storage-ring free electron laser on TERAS. *Nucl. Instrum. Methods Phys. Res. Sect. A Accel. Spectrometers Detect. Assoc. Equip.* **1992**, *318*, 33–37. [CrossRef]
58. Yamazaki, T.; Yamada, K.; Sugiyama, S.; Ohgaki, H.; Sei, N.; Mikado, T.; Noguchi, T.; Chiwaki, M.; Suzuki, R.; Kawai, M.; et al. First lasing of the NIJI-IV storage-ring free-electron laser. *Nucl. Instrum. Methods Phys. Res. Sect. A Accel. Spectrometers Detect. Assoc. Equip.* **1993**, *331*, 27–33. [CrossRef]
59. Takano, S.; Hama, H.; Isoyama, G. Gain Measurement of a free electron laser with an optical klystron on the UVSOR storage ring. *Jpn. J. Appl. Phys.* **1993**, *32*, 1285–1289. [CrossRef]
60. Couprie, M.E.; Garzella, D.; Billardon, M. Operation of the Super-ACO free-electron laser in the UV range at 800 MeV. *Europhys. Lett. (EPL)* **1993**, *21*, 909–914. [CrossRef]
61. Trovò, M.; Clarke, J.A.; Couprie, M.E.; Dattoli, G.; Garzella, D.; Gatto, A.; Giannessi, L.; Günster, S.; Kaiser, N.; Marsi, M.; et al. Operation of the European storage ring FEL at ELETTRA down to 190 nm. *Nucl. Instrum. Methods Phys. Res. Sect. A Accel. Spectrometers Detect. Assoc. Equip.* **2002**, *483*, 157–161. [CrossRef]
62. Nölle, D.; Garzella, D.; Geisler, A.; Gianessi, L.; Hirsch, M.; Quick, H.; Ridder, M.; Schmidt, T.; Wille, K. First lasing of the FELICITA I FEL at DELTA. *Nucl. Instrum. Methods Phys. Res. Sect. A Accel. Spectrometers Detect. Assoc. Equip.* **2000**, *445*, 128–133. [CrossRef]
63. Sei, N.; Ogawa, H.; Yamada, K. Lasing of infrared free-election lasers using the storage ring NIJI-IV. *Opt. Lett.* **2009**, *34*, 1843–1845. [CrossRef]
64. Benson, S.; Biallas, G.; Bohn, C.; Douglas, D.; Dylla, H.F.; Evans, R.; Fugitt, J.; Hill, R.; Jordan, K.; Krafft, G.; et al. First lasing of the Jefferson Lab IR Demo FEL. *Nucl. Instrum. Methods Phys. Res. Sect. A Accel. Spectrometers Detect. Assoc. Equip.* **1999**, *429*, 27–32. [CrossRef]
65. Neil, G.R.; Bohn, C.L.; Benson, S.V.; Biallas, G.; Douglas, D.; Dylla, H.F.; Evans, R.; Fugitt, J.; Grippo, A.; Gubeli, J.; et al. Sustained kilowatt lasing in a free-electron laser with same-cell energy recovery. *Phys. Rev. Lett.* **2000**, *84*, 662–665. [CrossRef]

66. Nishimori, N.; Hajima, R.; Nagai, R.; Minehara, E.J. High extraction efficiency observed at the JAERI free-electron laser. *Nucl. Instrum. Methods Phys. Res. Sect. A Accel. Spectrometers Detect. Assoc. Equip.* **2001**, *475*, 266–269. [CrossRef]
67. Hajima, R.; Shizuma, T.; Sawamura, M.; Nagai, R.; Nishimori, N.; Kikuzawa, N.; Minehara, E.J. First demonstration of energy-recovery operation in the JAERI superconducting linac for a high-power free-electron laser. *Nucl. Instrum. Methods Phys. Res. Sect. A Accel. Spectrometers Detect. Assoc. Equip.* **2003**, *507*, 115–119. [CrossRef]
68. Antokhin, E.A.; Akberdin, R.R.; Arbuzov, V.S.; Bokov, M.A.; Bolotin, V.P.; Burenkov, D.; Bushuev, A.A.; Veremeenko, V.F.; Vinokurov, N.A.; Vobly, P.D.; et al. First lasing at the high-power free electron laser at Siberian center for photochemistry research. *Nucl. Instrum. Methods Phys. Res. Sect. A Accel. Spectrometers Detect. Assoc. Equip.* **2004**, *528*, 15–18. [CrossRef]
69. Benson, S.; Beard, K.; Biallas, G.; Boyce, J.; Bullard, D.; Coleman, J.; Douglas, D.; Dylla, F.; Evans, R.; Evtushenko, P.; et al. High power operation of the JLab IR FEL driver accelerator. In *Proceedings of the 2007 IEEE Particle Accelerator Conference (PAC)*; IEEE: Piscataway, NJ, USA, 2007; pp. 79–81. [CrossRef]
70. Shevchenko, O.A.; Vinokurov, N.A.; Arbuzov, V.S.; Chernov, K.N.; Deichuly, O.I.; Dementyev, E.N.; Dovzhenko, B.A.; Getmanov, Y.V.; Gorbachev, Y.I.; Knyazev, B.A.; et al. The Novosibirsk free electron laser facility. In *Proceedings of the AIP Conference Proceedings 2299-Synchrotron and Free Electron Laser Radiation*; AIP: Novosibirsk, Russia, 2020; p. 020001. [CrossRef]
71. Vinokurov, N.A.; Sknnsky, A.N. *Optical Range Klystron Oscillator Using Ultrarelativistic Electrons*; Preprint 77-59; Institute of Nuclear Physics: Novosibirsk, Russia, 1977.
72. Deacon, D.A.G.; Billardon, M.; Elleaume, P.; Ortega, J.M.; Robinson, K.E.; Bazin, C.; Bergher, M.; Velghe, M.; Madey, J.M.J.; Petroff, Y. Optical klystron experiments for the ACO storage ring free electron laser. *Appl. Phys. B Photophys. Laser Chem.* **1984**, *34*, 207–219. [CrossRef]
73. Yamazaki, T.; Yamada, K.; Sugiyama, S.; Ohgaki, H.; Tomimasu, T.; Noguchi, T.; Mikado, T.; Chiwaki, M.; Suzuki, R. Lasing in visible of a storage-ring free electron laser at ETL. *Nucl. Instrum. Methods Phys. Res. Sect. A Accel. Spectrometers Detect. Assoc. Equip.* **1991**, *309*, 343–347. [CrossRef]
74. Takano, S.; Hama, H.; Isoyama, G. Lasing of a free electron laser in the visible on the UVSOR storage ring. *Nucl. Instrum. Methods Phys. Res. Sect. A Accel. Spectrometers Detect. Assoc. Equip.* **1993**, *331*, 20–26. [CrossRef]
75. Yamazaki, T.; Yamada, K.; Sei, N.; Ohgaki, H.; Sugiyama, S.; Mikado, T.; Suzuki, R.; Noguchi, T.; Chiwaki, M.; Ohdaira, T.; et al. Lasing in the ultraviolet region with the NIJI-IV storage-ring free-electron laser. *Nucl. Instrum. Methods Phys. Res. Sect. A Accel. Spectrometers Detect. Assoc. Equip.* **1995**, *358*, 353–357. [CrossRef]
76. Wu, Y.K.; Mikhailov, S.; Li, J.; Popov, V.; Vinokurov, N.A.; Gavrilov, N.G.; Shevchenko, O.A.; Vobly, P.D.; Kulipanov, G.N. First lasing and initial operation of a circularly polarized optical klystron OK-5 fel and a variably polarized distributed optical klystron DOK-1 FEL at DUKE. In *Proceedings of the 27th International Free Electron Laser Conference*; Nuhn, H.D., Ed.; JACoW Publishing: Paolo Alto, CA, USA, 2005; pp. 407–410.
77. Cutolo, A.; Benson, S.V.; Schultz, J.F.; Madey, J.M. Cavity dumping for free electron lasers. *Appl. Opt.* **1989**, *28*, 3177–3182. [CrossRef]
78. Benson, S.V.; Madey, J.M.J.; Szarmes, E.B.; Bhowmik, A.; Metty, P.; Curtin, M. A demonstration of loss modulation and cavity dumping in a free-electron-laser oscillator. *Nucl. Instrum. Methods Phys. Res. Sect. A Accel. Spectrometers Detect. Assoc. Equip.* **1990**, *296*, 762–768. [CrossRef]
79. Bhowmik, A.; Curtin, M.S.; McMullin, W.A.; Benson, S.V.; Madey, J.M.J.; Richman, B.A.; Vintro, L. Initial results from the free-electron-laser master oscillator/power amplifier experiment. *Nucl. Instrum. Methods Phys. Res. Sect. A Accel. Spectrometers Detect. Assoc. Equip.* **1990**, *296*, 20–24. [CrossRef]
80. Takahashi, S.; Ramian, G.; Sherwin, M.S. Cavity dumping of an injection-locked free-electron laser. *Appl. Phys. Lett.* **2009**, *95*, 234102. [CrossRef]
81. Rana, R.; Klopf, J.M.; Ciano, C.; Singh, A.; Winnerl, S.; Schneider, H.; Helm, M.; Pashkin, A. Gold implanted germanium photoswitch for cavity dumping of a free-electron laser. *Appl. Phys. Lett.* **2021**, *118*, 011107. [CrossRef]
82. Burghoorn, J.; Kaminski, J.P.; Strijbos, R.C.; Klaassen, T.O.; Wenckebach, W.T. Generation of subnanosecond high power far infrared pulses using a FEL pumped passive resonator. *Nucl. Instrum. Methods Phys. Res. Sect. A Accel. Spectrometers Detect. Assoc. Equip.* **1992**, *318*, 85–86. [CrossRef]
83. Smith, T.I.; Haar, P.; Schwettman, H.A. Pulse stacking in the SCA/FEL external cavity. *Nucl. Instrum. Methods Phys. Res. Sect. A Accel. Spectrometers Detect. Assoc. Equip.* **1997**, *393*, 245–251. [CrossRef]
84. Faatz, B.; Haselhoff, E.H.; Zhulin, V.I.; van Amersfoort, P.W. Pulse stacking in FELIX. *Nucl. Instrum. Methods Phys. Res. Sect. A Accel. Spectrometers Detect. Assoc. Equip.* **1994**, *341*, ABS136. [CrossRef]
85. Marks, H.S.; Lurie, Y.; Dyunin, E.; Gover, A. Enhancing electron beam radiative energy extraction efficiency in free-electron laser oscillators through beam energy ramping. *IEEE Trans. Microw. Theory Tech.* **2017**, *65*, 4218–4224. [CrossRef]
86. Xu, Y.; Jia, Q.; Li, H. Efficiency enhancement of RF-linac based free electron laser oscillator with electron beam energy ramping. *Nucl. Instrum. Methods Phys. Res. Sect. A Accel. Spectrometers Detect. Assoc. Equip.* **2019**, *940*, 448–452. [CrossRef]
87. Jaroszynski, D.A.; Oepts, D.; van der Meer, A.F.G.; van Amersfoort, P.W.; Colson, W.B. Consequences of short electron-beam pulses in the FELIX project. *Nucl. Instrum. Methods Phys. Res. Sect. A Accel. Spectrometers Detect. Assoc. Equip.* **1990**, *296*, 480–484. [CrossRef]

88. Bakker, R.J.; van der Geer, C.A.J.; Jaroszynski, D.A.; van der Meer, A.F.G.; Oepts, D.; van Amersfoort, P.W.; Anderegg, V.; van Son, P.C. Agility of FELIX regarding wavelength and micropulse shape. *Nucl. Instrum. Methods Phys. Res. Sect. A Accel. Spectrometers Detect. Assoc. Equip.* **1993**, *331*, 79–83. [CrossRef]
89. Knippels, G.M.H.; Bakker, R.J.; van der Meer, A.F.G.; Jaroszynski, D.A.; Oepts, D.; van Amersfoort, P.W.; Hovenier, J.N. Dynamic cavity desynchronisation in FELIX. *Nucl. Instrum. Methods Phys. Res. Sect. A Accel. Spectrometers Detect. Assoc. Equip.* **1994**, *341*, ABS26–ABS27. [CrossRef]
90. Song, S.B.; Kim, S.K.; Choi, J.S.; Hahn, S.J. Dynamic cavity desynchronization in a shout pulse free-electron laser resonator. *J. Korean Phys. Soc.* **2000**, *37*, 209–214.
91. Sumitomo, Y.; Hajima, R.; Hayakawa, Y.; Sakai, T. Simulation of short-pulse generation from a dynamically detuned IR-FEL oscillator and pulse stacking at an external cavity. *J. Phys. Conf. Ser.* **2019**, *1350*, 012040. [CrossRef]
92. Zen, H.; Ohgaki, H.; Hajima, R. High-extraction-efficiency operation of a midinfrared free electron laser enabled by dynamic cavity desynchronization. *Phys. Rev. Accel. Beams* **2020**, *23*, 070701. [CrossRef]
93. Sprangle, P.; Tang, C.M.; Manheimer, W.M. Nonlinear formulation and efficiency enhancement of free-electron lasers. *Phys. Rev. Lett.* **1979**, *43*, 1932–1936. [CrossRef]
94. Kroll, N.; Morton, P.; Rosenbluth, M. Free-electron lasers with variable parameter wigglers. *IEEE J. Quantum Electron.* **1981**, *17*, 1436–1468. [CrossRef]
95. Bosco, P.; Colson, W.B. Spontaneous radiation from relativistic electrons in a tapered undulator. *Phys. Rev. A* **1983**, *28*, 319–327. [CrossRef]
96. Edighoffer, J.A.; Neil, G.R.; Hess, C.E.; Smith, T.I.; Fornaca, S.W.; Schwettman, H.A. Variable-wiggler free-electron-laser oscillation. *Phys. Rev. Lett.* **1984**, *52*, 344–347. [CrossRef]
97. Curtin, M.; Bhowmik, A.; Brown, J.; McMullin, W.; Metty, P.; Benson, S.V.; Madey, J.M.J. Initial results of operating the Rocketdyne undulator in a tapered configuration. *Nucl. Instrum. Methods Phys. Res. Sect. A Accel. Spectrometers Detect. Assoc. Equip.* **1990**, *296*, 69–74. [CrossRef]
98. Jaroszynski, D.A.; Prazeres, R.; Glotin, F.; Ortega, J.M.; Oepts, D.; van der Meer, A.F.G.; Knippels, G.M.H.; van Amersfoort, P.W. Free-electron laser efficiency enhancement, gain enhancement, and spectral control using a step-tapered undulator. *Phys. Rev. Lett.* **1995**, *74*, 2224–2227. [CrossRef]
99. Benson, S.; Gubeli, J.; Neil, G.R. An experimental study of an FEL oscillator with a linear taper. *Nucl. Instrum. Methods Phys. Res. Sect. A Accel. Spectrometers Detect. Assoc. Equip.* **2001**, *475*, 276–280. [CrossRef]
100. Asgekar, V.; Lehnert, U.; Michel, P. A tapered undulator experiment at the ELBE far infrared hybrid-resonator oscillator free electron laser. *Rev. Sci. Instrum.* **2012**, *83*, 015116. [CrossRef]
101. Saldin, E.L.; Schneidmiller, E.A.; Yurkov, M.V. The features of an FEL oscillator with a tapered undulator. *Opt. Commun.* **1993**, *103*, 297–306. [CrossRef]
102. Christodoulou, A.; Lampiris, D.; Polykandriotis, K.; Colson, W.B.; Crooker, P.P.; Benson, S.; Gubeli, J.; Neil, G.R. Free-electron-laser oscillator with a linear taper. *Phys. Rev. E* **2002**, *66*, 056502. [CrossRef]
103. Dattoli, G.; Pagnutti, S.; Ottaviani, P.L.; Asgekar, V. Free electron laser oscillators with tapered undulators: Inclusion of harmonic generation and pulse propagation. *Phys. Rev. Spec. Top. Accel. Beams* **2012**, *15*, 030708. [CrossRef]
104. Ottaviani, P.L.; Pagnutti, S.; Dattoli, G.; Sabia, E.; Petrillo, V.; van der Slot, P.J.M.; Biedron, S.G.; Milton, S.V. Deep saturated free electron laser oscillators and frozen spikes. *Nucl. Instrum. Methods Phys. Res. Sect. A Accel. Spectrometers Detect. Assoc. Equip.* **2016**, *834*, 108–117. [CrossRef]
105. Colson, W.B. Free-electron lasers operating in higher harmonics. *Phys. Rev. A* **1981**, *24*, 639–641. [CrossRef]
106. Colson, W.B. The nonlinear wave equation for higher harmonics in free-electron lasers. *IEEE J. Quantum Electron.* **1981**, *17*, 1417–1427. [CrossRef]
107. Becker, W. Increasing the frequency of a free electron laser by means of a linearly polarized magnetic field. *Z. Phys. B Condens. Matter* **1981**, *42*, 87–94. [CrossRef]
108. Benson, S.V.; Madey, J.M.J. Demonstration of harmonic lasing in a free-electron laser. *Phys. Rev. A* **1989**, *39*, 1579–1581. [CrossRef] [PubMed]
109. Bamford, D.J.; Deacon, D.A.G. Harmonic-generation experiments on the Mark III free electron laser. *Nucl. Instrum. Methods Phys. Res. Sect. A Accel. Spectrometers Detect. Assoc. Equip.* **1990**, *296*, 89–97. [CrossRef]
110. Prazeres, R.; Ortega, J.M. Enhancement of the free-electron coherent harmonic generation by use of the dispersive function on a storage ring. *Nucl. Instrum. Methods Phys. Res. Sect. A Accel. Spectrometers Detect. Assoc. Equip.* **1990**, *296*, 436–441. [CrossRef]
111. Prazeres, R.; Guyot-Sionnest, P.; Ortega, J.M.; Jaroszynski, D.; Billardon, M.; Couprie, M.E.; Velghe, M.; Petroff, Y. Production of VUV coherent light by harmonic generation with the optical klystron of super-ACO. *IEEE J. Quantum Electron.* **1991**, *27*, 1061–1068. [CrossRef]
112. Jaroszynski, D.A.; Prazeres, R.; Glotin, F.; Marcouillé, O.; Ortega, J.M. Coherent harmonic production using a two-section undulator FEL. *Nucl. Instrum. Methods Phys. Res. Sect. A Accel. Spectrometers Detect. Assoc. Equip.* **1996**, *375*, 456–459. [CrossRef]
113. Hayakawa, Y.; Sato, I.; Hayakawa, K.; Tanaka, T.; Yokoyama, K.; Sakai, T.; Kanno, K.; Ishiwata, K.i.; Hashimoto, E. Simultaneous measurement of the fundamental and third harmonic FEL at LEBRA. *Jpn. J. Appl. Phys.* **2002**, *41*, 54–57. [CrossRef]

114. Yamada, K.; Yamazaki, T.; Sei, N.; Ohgaki, H.; Mikado, T.; Sugiyama, S.; Kawai, M.; Yokoyama, M. Observation of higher harmonics in the NIJI-IV FEL. *Nucl. Instrum. Methods Phys. Res. Sect. A Accel. Spectrometers Detect. Assoc. Equip.* **1998**, *407*, 193–197. [CrossRef]
115. Neil, G.R.; Benson, S.V.; Biallas, G.; Gubeli, J.; Jordan, K.; Myers, S.; Shinn, M.D. Second harmonic FEL oscillation. *Phys. Rev. Lett.* **2001**, *87*, 084801. [CrossRef]
116. Hajima, R.; Nagai, R.; Nishimori, N.; Kikuzawa, N.; Minehara, E.J. Third-harmonic lasing at JAERI-FEL. *Nucl. Instrum. Methods Phys. Res. Sect. A Accel. Spectrometers Detect. Assoc. Equip.* **2001**, *475*, 43–46. [CrossRef]
117. Litvinenko, V.N. New results and prospects for harmonic generation in storage ring FELs. *Nucl. Instrum. Methods Phys. Res. Sect. A Accel. Spectrometers Detect. Assoc. Equip.* **2003**, *507*, 265–273. [CrossRef]
118. Hayakawa, Y.; Sato, I.; Hayakawa, K.; Tanaka, T.; Yokoyama, K.; Kanno, K.; Sakai, T.; Ishiwata, K.; Nakao, K.; Hashimoto, E. Characteristics of the fundamental FEL and the higher harmonic generation at LEBRA. *Nucl. Instrum. Methods Phys. Res. Sect. A Accel. Spectrometers Detect. Assoc. Equip.* **2003**, *507*, 404–408. [CrossRef]
119. De Ninno, G.; Danailov, M.B.; Diviacco, B.; Ferianis, M.; Trovo, M.; Giannessi, L. Coherent harmonic generation using the ELETTRA storage-ring optical klystron. In *Proceedings of the Proceedings of the 26th International Free Electron Laser Conference*; JACoW Publishing: Trieste, Italy, 2004; pp. 237–240.
120. Sei, N.; Ogawa, H.; Yamada, K. Third harmonic lasing in a storage ring free-electron laser. *J. Phys. Soc. Jpn.* **2010**, *79*, 093501. [CrossRef]
121. Kubarev, V.V.; Kulipanov, G.N.; Shevchenko, O.A.; Vinokurov, N.A. Third harmonic lasing on terahertz NovoFEL. *J. Infrared Millim. Terahertz Waves* **2011**, *32*, 1236–1242. [CrossRef]
122. Jaroszynski, D.A.; Prazeres, R.; Glotin, F.; Ortega, J.M. Two-color free-electron laser operation. *Phys. Rev. Lett.* **1994**, *72*, 2387–2390. [CrossRef]
123. Prazeres, R.; Glotin, F.; Insa, C.; Jaroszynski, D.A.; Ortega, J.M. Two-colour operation of a free-electron laser and applications in the mid-infrared. *Eur. Phys. J. At. Mol. Opt. Phys.* **1998**, *3*, 87–93. [CrossRef]
124. Wu, Y.K.; Yan, J.; Hao, H.; Li, J.Y.; Mikhailov, S.F.; Popov, V.G.; Vinokurov, N.A.; Huang, S.; Wu, J. Widely tunable two-color free-electron laser on a storage ring. *Phys. Rev. Lett.* **2015**, *115*, 184801. [CrossRef]
125. Yan, J.; Hao, H.; Li, J.Y.; Mikhailov, S.F.; Popov, V.G.; Vinokurov, N.A.; Huang, S.; Wu, J.; Günster, S.; Wu, Y.K. Storage ring two-color free-electron laser. *Phys. Rev. Accel. Beams* **2016**, *19*, 070701. [CrossRef]
126. Zako, A.; Kanazawa, Y.; Konishi, Y.; Yamaguchi, S.; Nagai, A.; Tomimasu, T. Simultaneous two-color lasing in the mid-IR and far-IR region with two undulators and one RF linac at the FELI. *Nucl. Instrum. Methods Phys. Res. Sect. A Accel. Spectrometers Detect. Assoc. Equip.* **1999**, *429*, 136–140. [CrossRef]
127. Swent, R.L.; Berryman, K.W.; Schwettman, H.A.; Smith, T.I. Applications of wavelength agility in an FEL facility. *Nucl. Instrum. Methods Phys. Res. Sect. A Accel. Spectrometers Detect. Assoc. Equip.* **1991**, *304*, 272–275. [CrossRef]
128. Smith, T.I.; Crosson, E.R.; James, G.E.; Schwettman, H.A.; Swent, R.L. Multi-color, multi-user operation at the Stanford free electron laser center. *Nucl. Instrum. Methods Phys. Res. Sect. A Accel. Spectrometers Detect. Assoc. Equip.* **1998**, *407*, 151–156. [CrossRef]
129. Knippels, G.M.H.; Mols, R.F.X.A.M.; van der Meer, A.F.G.; Oepts, D.; van Amersfoort, P.W. Intense far-infrared free-electron laser pulses with a length of six optical cycles. *Phys. Rev. Lett.* **1995**, *75*, 1755–1758. [CrossRef] [PubMed]
130. Knippels, G.M.H.; van der Meer, A.F.G.; Oepts, D.; van Amersfoort, P.W. Generation of frequency-chirped optical pulses in a large-slippage free-electron laser. *IEEE J. Quantum Electron.* **1997**, *33*, 10–17. [CrossRef]
131. Calderón, O.G.; Kimura, T.; Smith, T.I. Modulated desynchronism in short pulse free-electron laser oscillators. *Phys. Rev. Spec. Top. Accel. Beams* **2000**, *3*, 090701. [CrossRef]
132. Hajima, R.; Nagai, R. Generation of a self-chirped few-cycle optical pulse in a FEL oscillator. *Phys. Rev. Lett.* **2003**, *91*, 024801. [CrossRef]
133. McNeil, B.W.J.; Thompson, N.R. Cavity resonator free electron lasers as a source of stable attosecond pulses. *EPL (Europhys. Lett.)* **2011**, *96*, 54004. [CrossRef]
134. Hajima, R. Few-cycle infrared pulse evolving in FEL oscillators and its application to high-harmonic generation for attosecond ultraviolet and X-ray pulses. *Atoms* **2021**, *9*, 15. [CrossRef]
135. Bonifacio, R.; Pellegrini, C.; Narducci, L. Collective instabilities and high-gain regime in a free electron laser. *Opt. Commun.* **1984**, *50*, 373–378. [CrossRef]
136. Hahn, S.J.; Lee, J.K. Bifurcations in a short-pulse free-electron laser oscillator. *Phys. Lett. A* **1993**, *176*, 339–343. [CrossRef]
137. Bakker, R.J.; Jaroszynski, D.A.; van der Meer, A.F.G.; Oepts, D.; van Amersfoort, P.W. Short-pulse effects in a free-electron laser. *IEEE J. Quantum Electron.* **1994**, *30*, 1635–1644. [CrossRef]
138. Piovella, N.; Chaix, P.; Shvets, G.; Jaroszynski, D.A. Analytical theory of short-pulse free-electron laser oscillators. *Phys. Rev. E* **1995**, *52*, 5470–5486. [CrossRef]
139. Jaroszynski, D.A.; Chaix, P.; Piovella, N.; Oepts, D.; Knippels, G.M.H.; van der Meer, A.F.G.; Weits, H.H. Superradiance in a short-pulse free-electron-laser oscillator. *Phys. Rev. Lett.* **1997**, *78*, 1699–1702. [CrossRef]
140. Hajima, R.; Nishimori, N.; Nagai, R.; Minehara, E.J. Analyses of superradiance and spiking-mode lasing observed at JAERI-FEL. *Nucl. Instrum. Methods Phys. Res. Sect. A Accel. Spectrometers Detect. Assoc. Equip.* **2001**, *475*, 270–275. [CrossRef]

141. Nishimori, N.; Hajima, R.; Iijima, H.; Kikuzawa, N.; Minehara, E.; Nagai, R.; Nishitani, T.; Sawamura, M. FEL oscillation with a high extraction efficiency at JAEA ERL FEL. In *Proceedings of the 28th International Free Electron Laser Conference*; JACoW Publishing: Berlin, Germany, 2006; pp. 265–272.
142. Duris, J.; Musumeci, P.; Sudar, N.; Murokh, A.; Gover, A. Tapering enhanced stimulated superradiant oscillator. *Phys. Rev. Accel. Beams* **2018**, *21*, 080705. [CrossRef]
143. Jaroszynski, D.A.; Bakker, R.J.; van der Meer, A.F.G.; Oepts, D.; van Amersfoort, P.W. Experimental observation of limit-cycle oscillations in a short-pulse free-electron laser. *Phys. Rev. Lett.* **1993**, *70*, 3412–3415. [CrossRef]
144. Knippels, G.M.H.; van der Meer, A.F.G.; Mols, R.F.X.A.M.; Oepts, D.; van Amersfoort, P.W.; Jaroszynski, D.A. Influence of a step-tapered undulator field on the optical pulse shape of a far-infrared free-electron laser. *IEEE J. Quantum Electron.* **1996**, *32*, 896–904. [CrossRef]
145. De Ninno, G.; Fanelli, D.; Bruni, C.; Couprie, M.E. Chaotic dynamics in a storage-ring free electron laser. *Eur. Phys. J. D* **2003**, *22*, 269–277. [CrossRef]
146. Kiessling, R.; Colson, W.B.; Gewinner, S.; Schöllkopf, W.; Wolf, M.; Paarmann, A. Femtosecond single-shot timing and direct observation of subpulse formation in an infrared free-electron laser. *Phys. Rev. Accel. Beams* **2018**, *21*, 080702. [CrossRef]
147. Colson, W.B. Optical pulse evolution in the Stanford free-electron laser and in a tapered wiggler. In *Free-Electron Generators of Coherent Radiation (Physics of Quantum Electronics)*; Jacobs, S.F., Moore, G., Pilloff, H.S., Sargent, M., III, Scully, M.O., Spitzer, R., Eds.; Addison-Wesley Publishing Co: Reading, MA, USA, 1982; Volume 8, pp. 457–488.
148. Blau, J.; Wong, R.K.; Colson, W.B. Ultra-short pulse free electron laser oscillators. *Nucl. Instrum. Methods Phys. Res. Sect. A Accel. Spectrometers Detect. Assoc. Equip.* **1995**, *358*, 441–443. [CrossRef]
149. Blau, J.; Cohn, K.; Colson, W.B. Four-dimensional models of free-eletron laser amplifiers and oscillators. In *Proceedings of the 37th International Free Electron Laser Conference*; Kang, H., Kim, D.E., Schaa, V.W., Eds.; JACoW Publishing: Daejeon, Korea, 2015; pp. 607–614. [CrossRef]
150. Amir, A.; Knox-Seith, J.F.; Warden, M. Bandwidth narrowing of the UCSB FEL by injection seeding with a cw laser. *Nucl. Instrum. Methods Phys. Res. Sect. A Accel. Spectrometers Detect. Assoc. Equip.* **1991**, *304*, 12–16. [CrossRef]
151. Oepts, D.; Bakker, R.J.; Jaroszynski, D.A.; van der Meer, A.F.G.; van Amersfoort, P.W. Induced and spontaneous interpulse phase locking in a free-electron laser. *Phys. Rev. Lett.* **1992**, *68*, 3543–3546. [CrossRef]
152. Szarmes, E.B.; Madden, A.D.; Madey, J.M.J. Optical phase locking of a 286-GHz harmonically mode-locked free-electron laser. *J. Opt. Soc. Am. B* **1996**, *13*, 1588–1597. [CrossRef]
153. Takahashi, S.; Ramian, G.; Sherwin, M.S.; Brunel, L.C.; van Tol, J. Submegahertz linewidth at 240 GHz from an injection-locked free-electron laser. *Appl. Phys. Lett.* **2007**, *91*, 174102. [CrossRef]
154. Evain, C.; Szwaj, C.; Bielawski, S.; Couprie, M.E.; Hosaka, M.; Mochihashi, A.; Katoh, M. Suppression of self-pulsing instabilities in free-electron lasers using delayed optical feedback. *Phys. Rev. Spec. Top. Accel. Beams* **2012**, *15*, 040701. [CrossRef]
155. Hajima, R.; Nagai, R. Generating carrier-envelope-phase stabilized few-cycle pulses from a free-electron laser oscillator. *Phys. Rev. Lett.* **2017**, *119*, 204802. [CrossRef]
156. Shvets, G.; Wurtele, J.S. Generation of ultrashort radiation pulses by injection locking a regenerative free-electron-laser amplifier. *Phys. Rev. E* **1997**, *56*, 3606–3610. [CrossRef]
157. Boehmer, H.; Caponi, M.Z.; Munch, J. Fel operation with prebunched electron beam. In *Proceedings of the 4th International Topical Conference on High-Power Electron and Ion Beam Research & Technology*; Doucet, H., Buzzi, J.M., Eds.; EcolePolytechnique: Palaiseau, France, 1981; pp. 947–952.
158. Boscolo, I.; Stagno, V. A study of a transverse optical klystron experiment in Adone (TOKA). *Nucl. Instrum. Methods Phys. Res.* **1982**, *198*, 483–496. [CrossRef]
159. Schnitzer, I.; Gover, A. The prebunched free electron laser in various operating gain regimes. *Nucl. Instrum. Methods Phys. Res. Sect. A Accel. Spectrometers Detect. Assoc. Equip.* **1985**, *237*, 124–140. [CrossRef]
160. Yu, L.H. Generation of intense uv radiation by subharmonically seeded single-pass free-electron lasers. *Phys. Rev. A* **1991**, *44*, 5178–5193. [CrossRef]
161. Allaria, E.; Appio, R.; Badano, L.; Barletta, W.A.; Bassanese, S.; Biedron, S.G.; Borga, A.; Busetto, E.; Castronovo, D.; Cinquegrana, P.; et al. Highly coherent and stable pulses from the FERMI seeded free-electron laser in the extreme ultraviolet. *Nat. Photonics* **2012**, *6*, 699–704. [CrossRef]
162. Kim, K.J.; Shvyd'ko, Y.V.; Reiche, S. A proposal for an X-ray free-electron laser oscillator with an energy-recovery linac. *Phys. Rev. Lett.* **2008**, *100*, 244802. [CrossRef]
163. Sheffield, R.L.; Gray, E.R.; Fraser, J.S. The Los Alamos photoinjector program. *Nucl. Instrum. Methods Phys. Res. Sect. A Accel. Spectrometers Detect. Assoc. Equip.* **1988**, *272*, 222–226. [CrossRef]
164. Dowell, D.H.; Davis, K.J.; Friddell, K.D.; Tyson, E.L.; Lancaster, C.A.; Milliman, L.; Rodenburg, R.E.; Aas, T.; Bemes, M.; Bethel, S.Z.; et al. First operation of a photocathode radio frequency gun injector at high duty factor. *Appl. Phys. Lett.* **1993**, *63*, 2035–2037. [CrossRef]
165. Arnold, N.D.; Attig, J.; Banks, G.; Bechtold, R.; Beczek, K.; Benson, C.; Berg, S.; Berg, W.; Biedron, S.G.; Biggs, J.; et al. Observation and analysis of self-amplified spontaneous emission at the APS low-energy undulator test line. *Nucl. Instrum. Methods Phys. Res. Sect. A Accel. Spectrometers Detect. Assoc. Equip.* **2001**, *475*, 28–37. [CrossRef]

166. Rossbach, J.; Schneider, J.R.; Wurth, W. 10 years of pioneering X-ray science at the free-electron laser FLASH at DESY. *Phys. Rep.* **2019**, *808*, 1–74. [CrossRef]
167. Allaria, E.; Badano, L.; Bassanese, S.; Capotondi, F.; Castronovo, D.; Cinquegrana, P.; Danailov, M.B.; D'Auria, G.; Demidovich, A.; De Monte, R.; et al. The FERMI free-electron lasers. *J. Synchrotron Radiat.* **2015**, *22*, 485–491. [CrossRef] [PubMed]
168. Saldin, E.L.; Schneidmiller, E.A.; Yurkov, M.V. Similarity techniques in a one-dimensional theory of a FEL oscillator. *Opt. Commun.* **1993**, *102*, 360–378. [CrossRef]
169. Dattoli, G.; Giannessi, L.; Ottaviani, P.L.; Renieri, A. A model for the saturation of a storage ring free electron laser. *Nucl. Instrum. Methods Phys. Res. Sect. A Accel. Spectrometers Detect. Assoc. Equip.* **1995**, *365*, 559–563. [CrossRef]
170. Dattoli, G.; Ottaviani, P.L.; Pagnutti, S. Pulse propagation and nonlinear harmonic generation in free electron laser oscillators. *J. Appl. Phys.* **2007**, *101*, 024914. [CrossRef]
171. Curcio, A.; Dattoli, G.; Di Palma, E.; Petralia, A. Free electron laser oscillator efficiency. *Opt. Commun.* **2018**, *425*, 29–37. [CrossRef]
172. Madey, J.M.J. Stimulated emission of Bremsstrahlung in a periodic magnetic field. *J. Appl. Phys.* **1971**, *42*, 1906–1913. [CrossRef]
173. Madey, J.M.J.; Schwettman, H.A.; Fairbank, W.M. A free electron laser. *IEEE Trans. Nucl. Sci.* **1973**, *20*, 980–983. [CrossRef]
174. Hopf, F.A.; Meystre, P.; Scully, M.O.; Louisell, W.H. Classical theory of a free-electron laser. *Phys. Rev. Lett.* **1976**, *37*, 1215–1218. [CrossRef]
175. Colson, W.B.; Richardson, J.L. Multimode theory of free-electron laser oscillators. *Phys. Rev. Lett.* **1983**, *50*, 1050–1053. [CrossRef]
176. Colson, W.B.; Freedman, R.A. Synchrotron instability for long pulses in free electron laser oscillators. *Opt. Commun.* **1983**, *46*, 37–42. [CrossRef]
177. McVey, B.D.; Goldstein, J.C.; Tokar, R.L.; Elliott, C.J.; Gitomer, S.J.; Schmitt, M.J.; Thode, L.E. Numerical simulations of free electron laser oscillators. *Nucl. Instrum. Methods Phys. Res. Sect. A Accel. Spectrometers Detect. Assoc. Equip.* **1989**, *285*, 186–191. [CrossRef]
178. Parazzoli, C.G. FELEXN, Boeing simulation code, version B08. In *Proceedings of the X-ray FEL Theory and Simulation Codes Workshop (SLAC Report no. LCLS-TN-00-1)*; SLAC: Stanford, CA, USA, 1999; p. 161.
179. Dattoli, G.; Ottaviani, P.L. Design considerations for X-ray free electron lasers. *J. Appl. Phys.* **1999**, *86*, 5331–5336. [CrossRef]
180. Dattoli, G.; Ottaviani, P.L.; Renieri, A.; Biedron, S.G.; Freund, H.P.; Milton, S.V. A compact free electron laser device operating in the UV-soft X-ray region. *Opt. Commun.* **2004**, *232*, 319–326. [CrossRef]
181. Dattoli, G.; Ottaviani, P.L.; Pagnutti, S. High gain oscillators: Pulse propagation and saturation. *J. Appl. Phys.* **2007**, *101*, 103109. [CrossRef]
182. Dattoli, G.; Ottaviani, P.L.; Pagnutti, S. The PROMETEO code: A flexible tool for free electron laser study. *Nuovo C. Della Soc. Ital. Fis. C* **2009**, *32*, 283–287. [CrossRef]
183. van der Slot, P.J.M.; Freund, H.P.; Miner, W.H., Jr.; Benson, S.V.; Shinn, M.D.; Boller, K.J. Time-dependent, three-dimensional simulation of free-electron-laser oscillators. *Phys. Rev. Lett.* **2009**, *102*. [CrossRef]
184. Freund, H.P.; Biedron, S.G.; Milton, S.V. Nonlinear harmonic generation in free electron lasers. *IEEE J. Quantum Electron.* **2000**, *36*, 275–281. [CrossRef]
185. Karssenberg, J.G.; van der Slot, P.J.M.; Volokhine, I.V.; Verschuur, J.W.J.; Boller, K.J. Modeling paraxial wave propagation in free-electron laser oscillators. *J. Appl. Phys.* **2006**, *100*, 093106. [CrossRef]
186. Reiche, S. GENESIS 1.3: a fully 3D time-dependent FEL simulation code. *Nucl. Instrum. Methods Phys. Res. Sect. A Accel. Spectrometers Detect. Assoc. Equip.* **1999**, *429*, 243–248. [CrossRef]
187. Campbell, L.T.; McNeil, B.W.J. Puffin: A three dimensional, unaveraged free electron laser simulation code. *Phys. Plasmas* **2012**, *19*, 093119. [CrossRef]
188. McNeil, B.W.J.; Thompson, N.R.; Dunning, D.J.; Karssenberg, J.G.; van der Slot, P.J.M.; Boller, K.J. A design for the generation of temporally-coherent radiation pulses in the VUV and beyond by a self-seeding high-gain free electron laser amplifier. *New J. Phys.* **2007**, *9*, 239. [CrossRef]
189. Pongchalee, P.; McNeil, B.W. Unaveraged simulation of a regenerative amplifier free electron laser. In *Proceedings of the 39th International Free-Electron Laser Conference*; JACoW Publishing: Hamburg, Germany, 2019; pp. 106–109. [CrossRef]
190. Freund, H.P.; van der Slot, P.J.M.; Grimminck, D.L.A.G.; Setija, I.D.; Falgari, P. Three-dimensional, time-dependent simulation of free-electron lasers with planar, helical, and elliptical undulators. *New J. Phys.* **2017**, *19*, 023020. [CrossRef]
191. Freund, H.P.; van der Slot, P.J.M. Variable polarization states in free-electron lasers. *J. Phys. Commun.* **2021**, submitted.
192. FEL Simulation Code MINERVA. Available online: https://gitlab.utwente.nl/tnw/ap/lpno/public-projects/MINERVA (accessed on 25 May 2021).
193. Sprangle, P.; Ting, A.; Tang, C.M. Analysis of radiation focusing and steering in the free-electron laser by use of a source-dependent expansion technique. *Phys. Rev. A* **1987**, *36*, 2773–2781. [CrossRef]
194. Born, M.; Wolf, E. *Principles of Optics: Electromagnetic Theory of Propagation, Interference and Diffraction of Light*, 7th ed.; Cambridge University Press: Cambridge, UK, 1999.
195. Lee, J.S.; Gensch, M.; Hinrichs, K.; Seidel, W.; Schade, U. Determination of the polarization characteristics of the ELBE free electron laser. *Infrared Phys. Technol.* **2008**, *51*, 537–540. [CrossRef]
196. Allaria, E.; Diviacco, B.; Callegari, C.; Finetti, P.; Mahieu, B.; Viefhaus, J.; Zangrando, M.; De Ninno, G.; Lambert, G.; Ferrari, E.; et al. Control of the polarization of a vacuum-ultraviolet, high-gain, free-electron laser. *Phys. Rev. X* **2014**, *4*, 041040. [CrossRef]

197. Giannessi, L.; Alesini, D.; Antici, P.; Bacci, A.; Bellaveglia, M.; Boni, R.; Boscolo, M.; Briquez, F.; Castellano, M.; Catani, L.; et al. Self-amplified spontaneous emission for a single pass free-electron laser. *Phys. Rev. Spec. Top. Accel. Beams* **2011**, *14*, 060712. [CrossRef]
198. Emma, P.; Akre, R.; Arthur, J.; Bionta, R.; Bostedt, C.; Bozek, J.; Brachmann, A.; Bucksbaum, P.; Coffee, R.; Decker, F.J.; et al. First lasing and operation of an ångstrom-wavelength free-electron laser. *Nat. Photonics* **2010**, *4*, 641–647. [CrossRef]
199. Optical Propagation Code (OPC). Available online: https://gitlab.utwente.nl/tnw/ap/lpno/public-projects/Physics-OPC (accessed on 25 May 2021).
200. Siegman, A.E. *Lasers*; University Science Books: Mill Valley, CA, USA, 1986.
201. Haus, H. *Waves and Fields in Optoelectronics*; Prentice-Hall: Englewood Cliffs, NJ, USA, 1984.
202. Goodman, J.W. *Introduction to Fourier Optics*; McGraw-Hill: New York, NY, USA, 1996.
203. van der Slot, P.J.M.; Karssenberg, J.G.; Boller Mesa, K.J. Modelling mirror aberrations in FEL oscillators using OPC. In *Proceedings of the 29th International Free Electron Laser Conference*; JACoW Publishing: Novosibirsk, Russia, 2007; pp. 207–210.
204. van der Slot, P.J.M.; Freund, H.P.; van der Meer, R.; Boller, K.J. Mirror aberrations in a low gain FEL oscillator. In *Proceedings of the 30th International Free Electron Laser Conference*; JACoW Publishing: Gyeongju, Korea, 2008; pp. 63–66.
205. Shvyd'ko, Y.V. *X-ray Optics: High-Energy Resolution Applications*; Optical Sciences; Springer: Berlin, Germany, 2004; Volume 98,
206. Fox, A.G.; Li, T. Resonant modes in a maser interferometer. *Bell Syst. Tech. J.* **1961**, *40*, 453–488. [CrossRef]
207. van der Slot, P.J.M.; Biedron, S.G.; Milton, S.V. Design of a resonator for the CSU THz FEL. In *Proceedings of the 35th International Free-Electron Laser Conference*; JACoW Publishing: New York, NY, USA, 2013; pp. 719–722.
208. Benson, S.V.; Davidson, P.S.; Jain, R.; Kloeppel, P.K.; Neil, G.R.; Shinn, M.D. Optical modeling of the Jefferson laboratory IR demo FEL. *Nucl. Instrum. Methods Phys. Res. Sect. A Accel. Spectrometers Detect. Assoc. Equip.* **1998**, *407*, 401–406. [CrossRef]
209. Shinn, M.D.; Baker, G.R.; Behre, C.P.; Benson, S.V.; Bevins, M.E.; Dillon-Townes, L.; Dylla, H.F.; Feldl, E.J.; Gubeli, J.F.; Lassiter, R.D.; et al. Design of the Jefferson Lab IR Upgrade FEL optical cavity. *Nucl. Instrum. Methods Phys. Res. Sect. A Accel. Spectrometers Detect. Assoc. Equip.* **2003**, *507*, 196–199. [CrossRef]
210. Nguyen, D.C.; Sheffield, R.L.; Fortgang, C.M.; Goldstein, J.C.; Kinross-Wright, J.M.; Ebrahim, N.A. First lasing of the regenerative amplifier FEL. *Nucl. Instrum. Methods Phys. Res. Sect. A Accel. Spectrometers Detect. Assoc. Equip.* **1999**, *429*, 125–130. [CrossRef]
211. Madey, J.M.J. Relationship between mean radiated energy, mean squared radiated energy and spontaneous power spectrum in a power series expansion of the equations of motion in a free-electron laser. *Il Nuovo C. B Ser. 11* **1979**, *50*, 64–88. [CrossRef]
212. Freund, H.P.; Nguyen, D.C.; Sprangle, P.A.; van der Slot, P.J.M. Three-dimensional, time-dependent simulation of a regenerative amplifier free-electron laser. *Phys. Rev. Spec. Top. Accel. Beams* **2013**, *16*, 010707. [CrossRef]
213. Freund, H.P.; van der Slot, P.J.M.; Shvyd'ko, Y.V. An X-ray regenerative amplifier free-electron laser using diamond pinhole mirrors. *New J. Phys.* **2019**, *21*, 093028. [CrossRef]
214. Xie, M. Design optimization for an X-ray free electron laser driven by SLAC linac. In *Proceedings of the Particle Accelerator Conference*; IEEE: Dallas, TX, USA, 1995; Volume 1, pp. 183–185. [CrossRef]
215. Huang, Z.; Kim, K.J. Review of x-ray free-electron laser theory. *Phys. Rev. Spec. Top. Accel. Beams* **2007**, *10*, 034801. [CrossRef]
216. Saldin, E.L.; Schneidmiller, E.A.; Yurkov, M.V. *The Physics of Free Electron Lasers*; Advanced Texts in Physics; Springer: Berlin/Heidelberg, Germany, 2000; [CrossRef]
217. Ishikawa, T.; Aoyagi, H.; Asaka, T.; Asano, Y.; Azumi, N.; Bizen, T.; Ego, H.; Fukami, K.; Fukui, T.; Furukawa, Y.; et al. A compact X-ray free-electron laser emitting in the sub-ångström region. *Nat. Photonics* **2012**, *6*, 540–544. [CrossRef]
218. Milne, C.; Schietinger, T.; Aiba, M.; Alarcon, A.; Alex, J.; Anghel, A.; Arsov, V.; Beard, C.; Beaud, P.; Bettoni, S.; et al. SwissFEL: The Swiss X-ray free electron laser. *Appl. Sci.* **2017**, *7*, 720. [CrossRef]
219. Kang, H.S.; Min, C.K.; Heo, H.; Kim, C.; Yang, H.; Kim, G.; Nam, I.; Baek, S.Y.; Choi, H.J.; Mun, G.; et al. Hard X-ray free-electron laser with femtosecond-scale timing jitter. *Nat. Photonics* **2017**, *11*, 708–713. [CrossRef]
220. Ko, I.; Kang, H.S.; Heo, H.; Kim, C.; Kim, G.; Min, C.K.; Yang, H.; Baek, S.; Choi, H.J.; Mun, G.; et al. Construction and commissioning of PAL-XFEL facility. *Appl. Sci.* **2017**, *7*, 479. [CrossRef]
221. Weise, H.; Decking, W. Commissioning and first lasing of the European XFEL. In *Proceedings of the 38th International Free-Electron Laser Conference*; JACoW Publishing: Santa Fe, NM, USA, 2017; pp. 9–13. [CrossRef]
222. Tanaka, T. Proposal for a pulse-compression scheme in X-ray free-electron lasers to generate a multiterawatt, attosecond X-ray pulse. *Phys. Rev. Lett.* **2013**, *110*, 084801. [CrossRef]
223. Prat, E.; Reiche, S. Simple method to generate terawatt-attosecond X-ray free-electron-laser pulses. *Phys. Rev. Lett.* **2015**, *114*, 244801. [CrossRef]
224. Prat, E.; Löhl, F.; Reiche, S. Efficient generation of short and high-power X-ray free-electron-laser pulses based on superradiance with a transversely tilted beam. *Phys. Rev. Spec. Top. Accel. Beams* **2015**, *18*, 100701. [CrossRef]
225. Emma, C.; Fang, K.; Wu, J.; Pellegrini, C. High efficiency, multiterawatt X-ray free electron lasers. *Phys. Rev. Accel. Beams* **2016**, *19*, 020705. [CrossRef]
226. Freund, H.P.; van der Slot, P.J.M. Studies of a terawatt X-ray free-electron laser. *New J. Phys.* **2018**, *20*. [CrossRef]
227. Shim, C.H.; Parc, Y.W.; Kumar, S.; Ko, I.S.; Kim, D.E. Isolated terawatt attosecond hard X-ray pulse generated from single current spike. *Sci. Rep.* **2018**, *8*, 7463. [CrossRef]
228. Lindberg, R.R.; Kim, K.J. Mode growth and competition in the X-ray free-electron laser oscillator start-up from noise. *Phys. Rev. Spec. Top. Accel. Beams* **2009**, *12*, 070702. [CrossRef]

229. Kim, K.J.; Shvyd'ko, Y.V. Tunable optical cavity for an X-ray free-electron-laser oscillator. *Phys. Rev. Spec. Top. Accel. Beams* **2009**, *12*, 030703. [CrossRef]
230. Lindberg, R.R.; Kim, K.J.; Shvyd'ko, Y.V.; Fawley, W.M. Performance of the X-ray free-electron laser oscillator with crystal cavity. *Phys. Rev. Spec. Top. Accel. Beams* **2011**, *14*, 010701. [CrossRef]
231. Kim, K.J.; Shvyd'ko, Y.V.; Lindberg, R.R. An X-ray free-electron laser oscillator for record high spectral purity, brightness, and stability. *Synchrotron Radiat. News* **2012**, *25*, 25–31. [CrossRef]
232. Kim, K.J. A harmonic X-ray FEL oscillator. In *High-Brightness Sources and Light-Driven Interactions*; OSA: Washington, DC, USA, 2016; ES2A.2. [CrossRef]
233. Qin, W.; Huang, S.; Liu, K.X.; Kim, K.J.; Lindberg, R.R.; Ding, Y.; Huang, Z.; Maxwell, T.; Bane, K.; Marcus, G. Start-to-end simulations for an X-ray FEL oscillator at the LCLS-II and LCLS-II-HE. In *Proceedings of the 38th International Free-Electron Laser Conference*; JACoW Publishing: Santa Fe, NM, USA, 2017; pp. 247–250. [CrossRef]
234. Shvyd'ko, Y.V.; Stoupin, S.; Cunsolo, A.; Said, A.H.; Huang, X. High-reflectivity high-resolution X-ray crystal optics with diamonds. *Nat. Phys.* **2010**, *6*, 196–199. [CrossRef]
235. Shvyd'ko, Y.V.; Stoupin, S.; Blank, V.; Terentyev, S. Near-100 *Nat. Photonics* **2011**, *5*, 539–542. [CrossRef]
236. Shvyd'ko, Y.V. Feasibility of X-ray cavities for free electron laser oscillators. *Beam Dyn. News Lett.* **2013**, *60*, 68–83.
237. Kolodziej, T.; Vodnala, P.; Terentyev, S.; Blank, V.; Shvyd'ko, Y.V. Diamond drumhead crystals for X-ray optics applications. *J. Appl. Crystallogr.* **2016**, *49*, 1240–1244. [CrossRef]
238. Kolodziej, T.; Shvyd'ko, Y.V.; Shu, D.; Kearney, S.; Stoupin, S.; Liu, W.; Gog, T.; Walko, D.A.; Wang, J.; Said, A.; et al. High Bragg reflectivity of diamond crystals exposed to multi-kW/mm^2 X-ray beams. *J. Synchrotron Radiat.* **2018**, *25*, 1022–1029. [CrossRef]
239. LCLS-II Final Design Report; SLAC Pub LCLSII-1.1-DR-0251-R0. 2014. Available online: https://portal.slac.stanford.edu/sites/ad_public/people/galayda/Shared_Documents/FDR.png (accessed on 27 May 2021).
240. Huang, Z.; Ruth, R.D. Fully coherent X-ray pulses from a regenerative-amplifier free-electron laser. *Phys. Rev. Lett.* **2006**, *96*, 144801. [CrossRef]
241. Marcus, G.; Halavanau, A.; Huang, Z.; Krzywinski, J.; MacArthur, J.; Margraf, R.; Raubenheimer, T.; Zhu, D. Refractive guide switching a regenerative amplifier free-electron laser for high peak and average power hard X-rays. *Phys. Rev. Lett.* **2020**, *125*, 254801. [CrossRef]
242. Snigirev, A.; Kohn, V.; Snigireva, I.; Lengeler, B. A compound refractive lens for focusing high-energy X-rays. *Nature* **1996**, *384*, 49–51. [CrossRef]
243. Lengeler, B.; Schroer, C.; Tümmler, J.; Benner, B.; Richwin, M.; Snigirev, A.; Snigireva, I.; Drakopoulos, M. Imaging by parabolic refractive lenses in the hard X-ray range. *J. Synchrotron Radiat.* **1999**, *6*, 1153–1167. [CrossRef]
244. Li, H.; Jia, Q. Commissioning and first lasing of the FELiChEM: A new IR and THz FEL oscillator in China. In *Proceedings of the 39th International Free-Electron Laser Conferenc*; JACoW Publishing: Hamburg, Germany, 2019; pp. 15–19. [CrossRef]
245. Lee, T.Y. Storage ring based X-ray FEL oscillator. In *Proceedings of the AIP Conference Proceedings 2054*; AIP: Taipei, Taiwan, 2019; p. 030021. [CrossRef]
246. Petrillo, V.; Opromolla, M.; Bacci, A.; Broggi, F.; Drebot, I.; Ghiringhelli, G.; Puppin, E.; Rossetti Conti, M.; Rossi, A.R.; Ruijter, M.; et al. Coherent, high repetition rate tender X-ray free-electron laser seeded by an extreme ultra-violet free-electron laser oscillator. *New J. Phys.* **2020**, *22*, 073058. [CrossRef]
247. Yan, J.; Hao, H.; Huang, S.; Li, J.; Litvinenko, V.N.; Liu, P.; Mikhailov, S.F.; Popov, V.G.; Swift, G.; Vinokurov, N.A.; et al. Polarization control of a free-electron laser oscillator using helical undulators of opposite helicities. *Phys. Rev. Accel. Beams* **2020**, *23*, 060702. [CrossRef]
248. Paraskaki, G.; Grattoni, V.; Lang, T.; Zemella, J.; Faatz, B.; Hillert, W. Optimization and stability of a high-gain harmonic generation seeded oscillator amplifier. *Phys. Rev. Accel. Beams* **2021**, *24*, 034801. [CrossRef]
249. Campbell, L.T.; Freund, H.P.; Henderson, J.R.; McNeil, B.W.J.; Traczykowski, P.; van der Slot, P.J.M. Analysis of ultra-short bunches in free-electron lasers. *New J. Phys.* **2020**, *22*, 073031. [CrossRef]

Article

Two-Color TeraHertz Radiation by a Multi-Pass FEL Oscillator

Michele Opromolla [1,2],* and Vittoria Petrillo [1,2]

1. Dipartimento di Fisica, Universitá degli Studi di Milano, Via Celoria 16, 20133 Milano, Italy; vittoria.petrillo@mi.infn.it
2. INFN-Sezione di Milano, Via Celoria 16, 20133 Milano, Italy
* Correspondence: michele.opromolla@mi.infn.it

Abstract: In this paper, we show that an electron beam produced by a super-conducting linac, driven in a sequence of two undulator modules of different periods, can generate two-color Terahertz radiation with wavelengths ranging from 100 µm to 2 µm. The generated pulses are synchronized, both MW-class, and highly coherent. Their specific properties and generation will be discussed in detail. Besides the single-spike pulse structure, usually observed in oscillators, we show that both the THz pump and probe can be modulated in a coherent comb of pulses, enabling periodic excitation and stroboscopic measurements.

Keywords: two-color; TeraHertz radiation; Free-Electron Laser Oscillators

1. Introduction

TeraHertz (THz) radiation is a frontier research area in physics, chemistry, medicine, and biological and material sciences. The increasing number of advanced and exciting applications of THz waves in all these fields demands versatile and tunable sources combining high-power and excellent output performances. Traditional microwave sources in the THz region, like backward wave oscillators, orotrons, vircators, and klinotrons suffer from simple physical scaling problems, metallic wall losses, the need for higher static magnetic, electric fields, and electron current densities with increasing frequency, and have already achieved saturation in their developments. A summary of these sources and their main properties can be found in [1]. Other sources, like IMPATT-diodes, are low-cost, reliable, and compact, but characterized by moderately efficient mW power levels.

THz sources of high quality are scarce, this lack being often referred to in the literature as the 'THz gap'. Considerable efforts have been put towards the development of novel sources of THz radiation and the aforementioned gap has recently begun to be filled by a wide choice of new technologies capable of generating high-power and tunable radiation. In particular, the THz range of the electromagnetic spectrum can be covered by Free-Electron Lasers (FELs), whose widely tunable radiation shows optimal performances in terms of pulse energy stability, polarization, and spectrum and spatial distribution in this domain. The key parameters of several operating FELs with an exhaustive comparative analysis can be found in [2]. The THz FELs in operation produce coherent radiation characterized by very short pulse lengths and up to MW-level peak intra-cavity powers with continuously tunable wavelengths from 10 µm to 0.2 mm. The THz wave is now available in both the continuous wave (CW) and the pulsed form, down to single cycles or less.

Mainly, infrared (IR) and far-IR FELs are designed to operate as oscillators, that is, they are equipped with resonators confined by metal-coated mirrors [3], one of which is translucent or contains outcoupling apertures for radiation extraction. Some of the advantages of the FEL oscillator mode with respect to other FEL configurations, like single-pass FELs operating in Self-Amplified Spontaneous Emission (SASE), seeded, or superradiant modes, are its compactness, the relaxed requirements for the electron bunch quality, and the fact that oscillators are suitable for super-conducting linacs enabling the generation of powerful quasi-CW light. Few devices exploiting this scheme operate worldwide [4–6] or have been proposed [7,8]. Similar to the multi-pass FEL oscillator configuration is the storage-ring FEL oscillator [9], where the electron beam circulating in the storage ring participates in the FEL interaction during each pass through a FEL undulator.

The envisioned applications of such a source include high-repetition-rate pump-probe experiments and investigation of reactions with very small quantum yield [10]. Two-color operation could widely increase the number and the interest of the applications. A pioneering experiment for the production of two-color far Infrared-THz radiation has been shown in the Ref. [11]. In particular, IR pump-THz probe configuration can elucidate phenomena such as the response of low-frequency collective solvent modes in liquids, and transient photoconductivity in a variety of semiconductor systems, such as bulk GaAs, low-temperature grown GaAs, nanocrystalline colloidal TiO_2, and CdSe quantum dots. Other specific measurements instead need a Terahertz pump–Terahertz probe scheme.

In this paper, we show that the electron beam produced by a super-conducting linac (as, for instance, the one described in [12]), driven in a sequence of two undulator modules of different periods, can generate two-color Terahertz radiation with wavelengths ranging from 100 µm to 2 µm. The two pulses of different wavelengths are synchronized, both MW-class and highly coherent.

The paper is organized as follows: in Section 2 we describe the source and discuss the basic requirements for its operation; in Section 3 we summarize the working points and report the simulation results for a specific wavelength range of interest, while Section 4 draws some conclusions and outlooks on future implementations.

2. Materials and Methods

We describe here the behaviour and the potentiality of an FEL oscillator conceived as two undulator modules separated by a drift, where optical elements and diagnostics can be possibly allocated, and embedded into an optical cavity equipped with mirrors suitable to the frequency range. The two modules can have different periods for permitting a more versatile two-color operation. The wavelength of the produced radiation pulses is given by the FEL resonance condition $\lambda_{1,2} = \lambda_{w_{1,2}}(1 + a_{w_{1,2}}^2)/(2\gamma^2)$, where $\lambda_{w_{1,2}}$ and $a_{w_{1,2}} = 0.657 \lambda_{w_{1,2}}(cm) B_{1,2}(T)$ are the periods and adimensional parameters of the two undulator modules, with $B_{1,2}(T)$ being their peak on-axis magnetic field. Therefore, for a certain period of the two undulators, the wavelengths can be tuned either simultaneously by varying the electron Lorentz factor, or independently by changing the undulator magnetic fields. With $\lambda_{w_1} = 2.8$ cm being constant, the achievable ratio λ_2/λ_1 as a function of the period λ_{w_2} of the second module is shown in Figure 1 for different magnetic field values $B_{1,2}$ between 0.75 and 1.2 T. As shown in this plot, a period larger than 4 cm for the second module allows to efficiently generate with the same electron beam two colours with a wavelength ratio larger than 5. The darkest region in the plot corresponds to a large undulator magnetic field for both undulators, thus leading to higher FEL emission.

Figure 2 shows the scheme of the source. It is composed of two undulator modules (a) and (b), separated by a quadrupole (c) for electron-beam matching and embedded in a cavity. Given the repetition rate of 92.86 MHz of the electron beam, the cavity length $L_c = 12.9$ m corresponds to 4 times the bunch separation. The two undulator modules, each 3 m long, have variable gaps for flexible tuning of the radiation. A further degree of versatility may be guaranteed by the use of modules constituted by subsections which can be tuned independently.

The radiation beam is amplified and propagates within the undulator and the resonator optical line. Considering a Gaussian beam, its radius evolves along the propagation axis z according to $\sigma_r(z) = \sigma_{r,0}\sqrt{1 + (z/z_R)^2}$, where $\sigma_{r,0}$ is the beam waist and $z_R = \pi \sigma_{r,0}^2 / \lambda$ is its Rayleigh length. Therefore, strong diffraction affects long wavelength radiation pulses, and the operation at THz wavelengths requires gaps of about 1 cm or larger, for permitting the transport of a transversely large electron beam and containing the propagation of the highly diffracted radiation. This can limit the minimum value of periods and gaps that can be used; if necessary, propagation in waveguides could be foreseen, as, for instance, conceived in other devices [4]. In our scheme, the electron beam is driven in a beam pipe, whose vertical size should be of the order of 1 cm within the undulator gaps. The horizontal dimension of the pipe (orthogonal to the undulator magnetic field) could be larger and allow the free expansion of the radiation pulse along this direction.

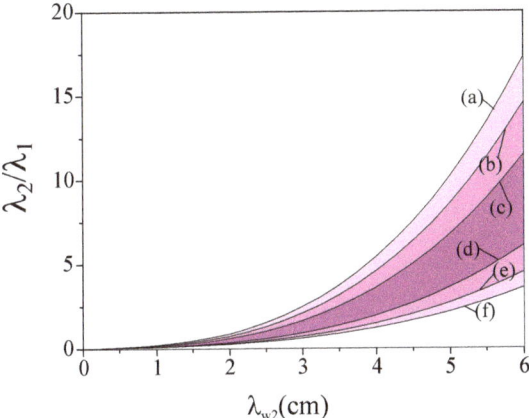

Figure 1. Ratio λ_2/λ_1 as a function of the period of the second undulator module, fixing the first one to $\lambda_{w_1} = 2.8$ cm. The sequence of lines is obtained by scanning over the magnetic field values $(B_1(T), B_2(T))$: a (0.75, 1.2), b (0.85, 1.2), c (1, 1.2), d (1.2, 1), e (1.2, 0.85), f (1.2, 0.75). The most efficient condition in terms of output power is represented by the darkest region, corresponding to large magnetic field values for both modules.

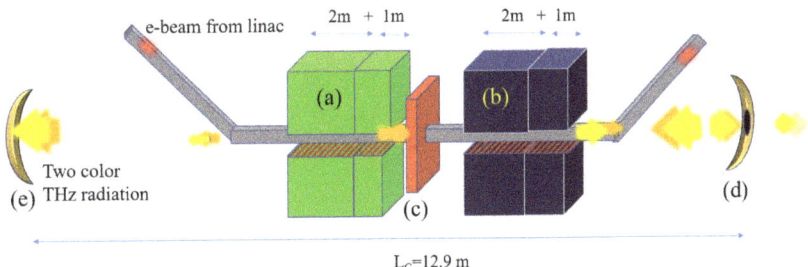

Figure 2. Scheme of the two-color radiation source. (**a**,**b**) Undulator modules (2 + 1 m long), (**c**) quadrupole for electron-beam matching, (**d**) front mirror, (**e**) rear mirror. Cavity length $L_c = 12.9$ m. Metal-coated mirrors: curvature radius about 15–25 m, reflectivity about 95%.

Moreover, the different velocity of light and electrons causes their detachment as they propagate within the undulator. The slippage length of the radiation with respect to the electron beam is estimated to be $L_s = N\lambda$, N being the number of undulator periods. Long wavelength radiation pulses lead to larger slippage lengths. In order to compensate this effect and synchronize the radiation and the electron beam at the undulator entrance, the radiation needs to be delayed with respect to the electron bunches at each round trip. Furthermore, for maintaining this synchronization along the whole undulator, the electron bunch length σ_e should be at least two times the slippage length, leading to the condition: $\sigma_e \geq 2L_s$. Furthermore, in two-color operation, the two produced pulses slip with different rates, and the previous condition should hold for the longest slippage length. Following the road map proposed in [13] and the references therein, another condition on the electron beam related to the threshold of operation is $4\sqrt{3}\pi\rho N >$ Loss, where ρ is the FEL Pierce parameter [14–16]. In our case, the radiation Rayleigh length Z_R is of the order of the undulator length, so that the dimension of the radiation beam σ_r turns out to be of the order of $\sqrt{\frac{Z_R \lambda}{2\pi}} \gg \sigma_e$. Even if the radiation losses along the trajectory outside the undulator and on the mirrors are small, the portion of the radiation coupling to the electron beam at the undulator entrance is scarce, and we can estimate loss to be close to 100%. A conservative choice of undulator length should then satisfy the constraint $N\lambda_w > \frac{\lambda_w}{4\sqrt{3}\pi\rho}$.

The plot in Figure 3 reports the required number N of undulator periods as a function of the beam current for two typical cases, where three-dimensional and inhomogeneity effects have been taken into account in the calculation of the Pierce parameter [17]. Sustainable undulator lengths (<3 m) and reasonable peak currents (<30 A) are needed.

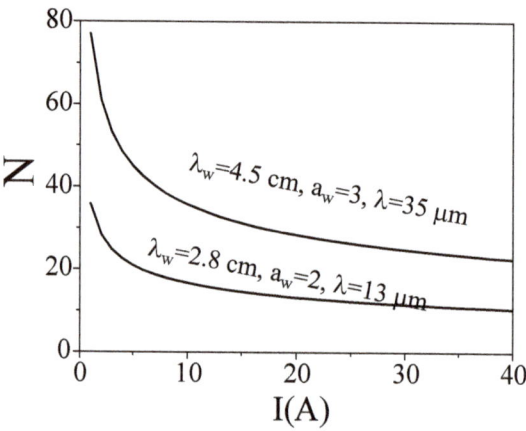

Figure 3. Required undulator period number N for successful FEL oscillator operation as a function of electron beam current I(A) for two typical cases.

3. Working Points and Simulation Results

This section contains the working points of the source and reports the simulation results in a wavelength range where the FEL efficiency is robust. The parameters of the electron beam used in the simulations are summarized in Table 1, being the typical output of a super-conducting accelerator suitable for this kind of application.

Table 1. Electron beam parameters.

Energy	MeV	15–50
Bunch charge	pC	100–250
Repetition rate	MHz	100
Peak Current	A	15–30
Slice normalized emittance	mm mrad	1.5–2
Slice energy Spread	%	0.1
Bunch length	mm	1–2

Considering $\lambda_{w,2} = 4.5$ cm for the second module, a possible choice of undulator parameters deduced by the resonance graph of Figure 4 is reported in Table 2. By using such undulator periods and parameters, this source has the best performance in correspondence of a range of relatively short wavelengths between 10 μm and 40 μm. Longer wavelengths up to 300 μm would require longer undulator periods, being at the limit of our device.

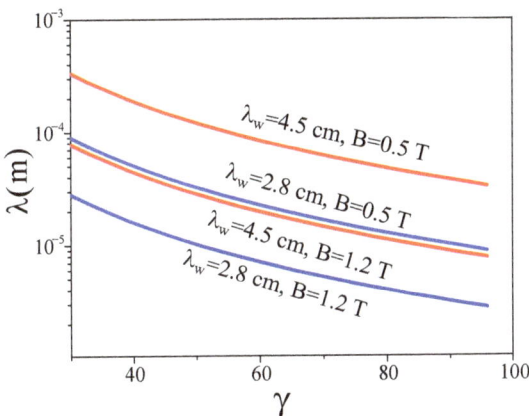

Figure 4. Radiation wavelength λ vs electron Lorentz factor γ for $\lambda_w = 2.8$ cm in blue, and 4.5 cm in red. B = 1.2 T and 0.5 T.

Table 2. Two color set-up: undulator parameters.

Color 1			Color 2		
λ_{w_1}	cm	2.8	λ_{w_2}	cm	4.5
B	T	0.5–1.2	B	T	0.5–1.2
λ_1	µm	3–90	λ_2	µm	7–300
gap	cm	1.0	gap	cm	1.7
Length	m	3	Length	m	3

The numerical modeling of the two-color source has been performed by using the three-dimensional, time-dependent FEL code GENESIS 1.3 [18]. Starting from the electron beam parameters listed in Table 1 and in order to simulate the fluctuations of the bunch train, we have injected into the undulators a sequence of randomly prepared electron beams, which are different from each other both microscopically and macroscopically. This was done by randomly changing the seeds of the Hammersley sequences loading the particle phase space from shot to shot. Furthermore, the values of the macroscopic electron beam parameters, such as energy, current, emittance, and energy spread, have been varied to reproduce the shot-to-shot jitters. Each radiation output result is obtained by maximizing the output power as a function of the delay time compensating the slippage, and cycling the radiation within the cavity, taking into account the details of the optical line that returns the radiation to the undulator entrance [19,20]. Mirror reflectivities of the order of 95–97% have been assumed. A 40 MeV electron beam, propagating inside the long period undulator, emits radiation at $\lambda = 35$ µm. At the end of this first module, the radiation has slipped with respect to the electron beam by a length $N\lambda$ of a few mm. The radiation is synchronized to a fresh electron bunch at the beginning of the first undulator module after each round trip. The fraction of energy extracted from the electron beam is moderate, so its phase space is substantially not deteriorated, permitting considerable emission in the second short period undulator tuned at $\lambda = 13$ µm. The delay between the two pulses is equal to the slippage after the first module, corresponding to about 10 ps. This temporal separation could be compensated or increased by suitable radiation transfer lines. Apart from this time delay, the two pulses generated by the same electron beam are naturally synchronized, while the shot-to-shot jitters of the accelerator affect the radiation.

Figure 5 shows the generation of radiation at 35 µm, with an undulator of a 4.5 cm period. Radiation energy growth along the undulator axis as a function of the number of successive shots generated by the superconducting accelerator is shown in Plot (a) for an undulator length $L_w = 2$ m, with the corresponding power and spectral distributions in Plots (b) and (c). The case with $L_w = 3$ m is shown in the right column. In Figure 6, the same quantities are shown for the short period module tuned at 13 µm.

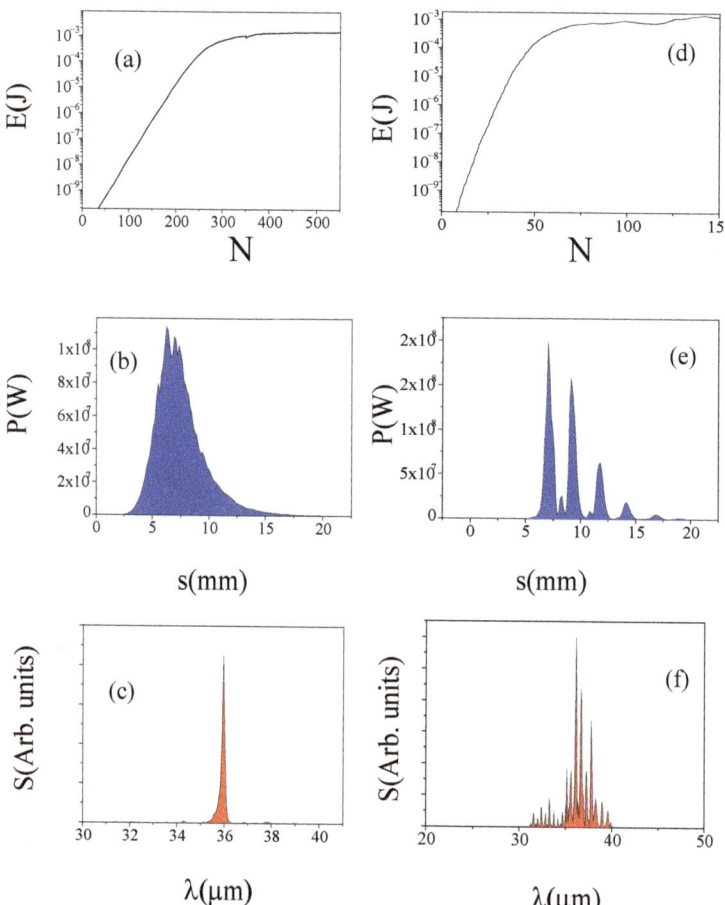

Figure 5. Radiation at $\lambda = 35$ µm from an electron beam of 40 MeV with an undulator of period $\lambda_w = 4.5$ cm. Left column: undulator length $L_w = 2$ m. Right column: undulator length $L_w = 3$ m. (**a**,**d**) Energy growth (J) as a function of the number N of shots; (**b**,**e**) power profile (W) vs. s (mm). (**c**,**f**) Spectral profile in arbitrary units vs. λ (µm).

These cases can be run with the same device by closing the undulator gaps according to the magnetic length needed. The operation with a short portion of the undulator (left columns of Figures 5 and 6) gives rise to single-spiked pulses both in the temporal and spectral domains, while deep-saturation frozen fringes, stable in time from shot to shot, appear when operating with the whole undulator length (right columns of the same figures). This second interesting regime, constituted by a statistically stable sequence of spikes, has been widely discussed in [21]. Since each spike of the pulse train is considerably narrower than the corresponding one in the single-spike situation and spectral and power distributions are connected by the Fourier Transform operator, the spectrum is conversely larger.

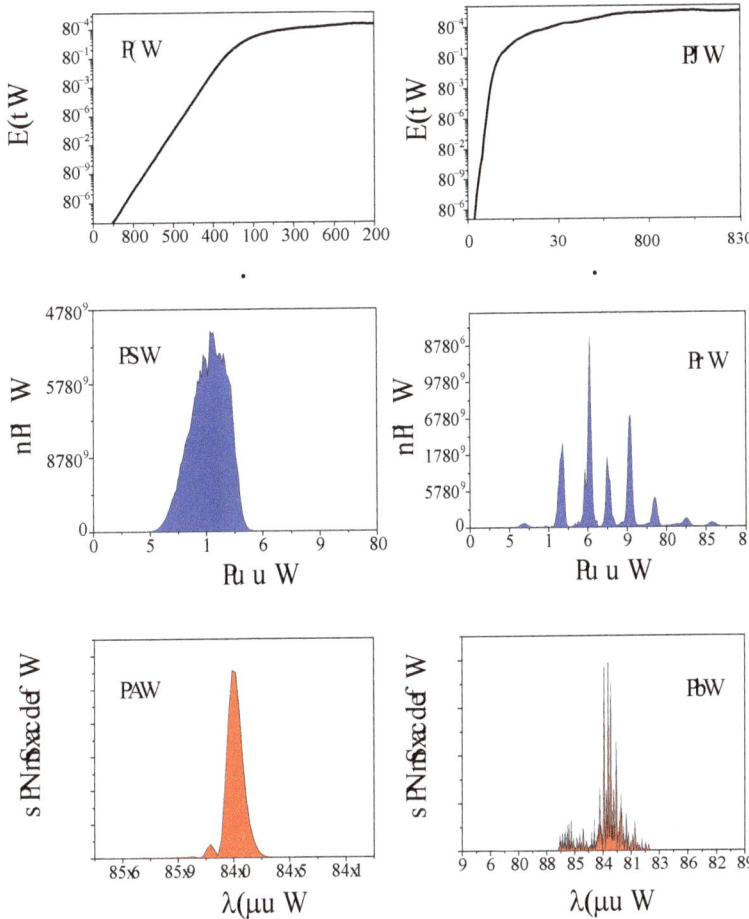

Figure 6. Radiation at $\lambda = 13\ \mu m$ from an electron beam of 40 MeV with an undulator of period $\lambda_w = 2.8$ cm. Left column: undulator length $L_w = 2$ m. Right column: undulator length $L_w = 3$ m. (**a,d**) Energy growth (J) as a function of the number N of shots; (**b,e**) power profile (W) vs. s (mm). (**c,f**) Spectral profile in arbitrary units vs. λ (μm).

A two-color source of this kind, whose radiation properties are summarized in Table 3, would enable the generation of both pump and probe radiation that is either single- or multi-spiked. In the latter case, the excitation and stroboscopic measurements of processes lasting a few picoseconds could be performed with a statistically coherent sequence of spikes. The distance between two successive peaks is 8 ps for the longer wavelength and 4 ps for the shorter one.

Table 3. Radiation properties of the two-color source. IC = intracavity, EC = extra-cavity.

Color 1				Color 2			
Undulator length	m	2	3	Undulator length	m	2	3
λ_1	μm	13	13	λ_2	μm	35	35
IC energy	mJ	1.4	2.6	IC energy	mJ	1.4	1.1
EC energy	μJ	42	79	EC energy	μJ	44	34
Bandwidth	%	0.9	4.9	Bandwidth	%	3	2.9
Size	mm	2	2	Size	mm	2.2	3.5
Divergence	mrad	2.4	2.2	Divergence	mrad	3.7	4
Spike duration	ps	3	0.4	Spike duration	ps	7	0.97
Spike number		1	6	Spike number		1	8
Spike separation	ps		4	Spike separation	ps		8
Coherence degree		0.93	0.5			0.92	0.5

The stability and coherence degree of the oscillator pulses of the same color has been estimated through the cross-correlation between two generic consecutive pulses after saturation:

$$\Gamma_{12}(\tau) = \left| \frac{\int dt E_1(t) E_2^*(t-\tau)}{\sqrt{\int dt |E_1|^2} \sqrt{\int dt |E_2|^2}} \right|,$$

where $E_{1,2}$ is the complex field of the radiation of the pulses. In Table 3, the equal time coherence degree $\Gamma_{12}(\tau = 0)$ has been reported, showing a large coherence for the single-spike case, and a considerable value also in the case of multiple peaks.

4. Discussion

We showed that the electron beam produced by a state-of-the-art CW super-conducting linac, driven in a sequence of two undulator modules of different periods, can generate two-color Terahertz radiation. The generated THz pulses are synchronized and highly stable. Depending on the undulator length, both the THz pump and probe can be modulated in a coherent comb of pulses, permitting periodic excitation of the sample under investigation and stroboscopic measurements, as already done in the optical/IR regime [22]. The data presented in this work are based on realistic and state-of-the-art parameters, and could be experimentally implemented in operating THz FEL oscillators. A dedicated project is going to be designed and will be realized in the near future [23,24], covering the so-called Short THz radiation range, corresponding to wavelengths between 10 and 50 μm, whereas different wavelength regimes would require longer undulator periods.

Author Contributions: The authors equally contributed to the manuscript. All authors have read and agreed to the published version of the manuscript.

Funding: This research received no external funding.

Institutional Review Board Statement: Not applicable.

Informed Consent Statement: Informed consent was obtained from all subjects involved in the study.

Conflicts of Interest: The authors declare no conflict of interest.

References

1. Xu, W.; Xu, H. Review of the High-Power Vacuum Tube Microwave Sources Based on Cherenkov Radiation. Available online: https://arxiv.org/ftp/arxiv/papers/2003/2003.04288.pdf (accessed on 20 June 2021).
2. Table of Parameters and Information about IR/THz FELs around the World from 'Electron Linear Accelerator with High Brilliance and Low Emittance' (ELBE). Available online: https://www.hzdr.de/db/Cms?pOid=56940 (accessed on 1 May 2021).

3. Naftaly, M.; Dudley, R. Terahertz reflectivities of metal-coated mirrors. *Appl. Opt.* **2011**. [CrossRef] [PubMed]
4. Free-Electron Laser (FEL) at the Electron Linear Accelerator with High Brilliance and Low Emittance. Available online: https://www.hzdr.de/FELBE (accessed on 1 April 2021).
5. Free-Electron Laser at Jefferson Laboratory. Available online: https://www.jlab.org/FEL/ (accessed on 1 April 2021).
6. Bolotin, V.P.; Vinokurov, N.A.; Kayran, D.A.; Knyazev, A.; Kolobanov, E.I.; Kotenkov, V.V.; Kubarev, V.V.; Kulipanov, G.N.; Matveenko, A.N.; Medvedev, L.E.; et al. Status of the Novosibirsk Terahertz FEL. In Proceedings of the 26th International Free Electron Laser Conference and 11th FEL User Workshop (FEL 04), Trieste, Italy, 29 August–3 September 2004; pp. 226–228.
7. Dou, Y.; Shu, X.; Yang, X.; Li, M.; Deng, D.; Wang, H.; Lu, X.; Xu, Z. Present status of CAEP THz FEL facility. In Proceedings of the 40th International Conference on Infrared, Millimeter, and Terahertz Waves (IRMMW-THz), Hong Kong, China, 23–28 August 2015; pp. 1–2. [CrossRef]
8. Serafini, L.; Bacci, A.; Bellandi A.; Bertucci, M.; Bolognesi, M.; Bosotti, A.; Rossi, G. MariX, an advanced MHz-class repetition rate X-ray source for linear regime time-resolved spectroscopy and photon scattering. *Nucl. Instr. Meth. Phys. Res. Sect. A* **2019**, *930*, 167. [CrossRef]
9. Wu, Y.K.; Yan, J.; Hao, H.; Li, J.Y.; Mikhailov, S.F.; Popov, V.G.; Vinokurov, N.A.; Huang, S.; Wu, J. 'Widely tunable two-color free-electron laser on a storage ring. *Phys. Rev. Lett.* **2015**, *115*, 184801. [CrossRef]
10. Kawasaki, T.; Tsukiyama, K.; Irizawa, A. Dissolution of a fibrous peptide by terahertz free electron laser. *Sci. Rep.* **2019**, *9*, 10636. [CrossRef] [PubMed]
11. Prazeres, R.; Glotin, F.; Insa, C.; Jaroszynski, D.A.; Ortega, J.M. Two-colour operation and applications of the CLIO FEL in the mid-infrared range. *Nucl. Instr. Meth. Phys. Res. Sect. A* **1998**, *407*, 464–469. [CrossRef]
12. Bacci, A.; Rossetti Conti, M.; Bosotti, A.; Cialdi, S.; Dimitri, S.; Drebot, I.; Faillace, L. et al. Two-pass two-way acceleration in a super-conducting CW linac to drive low jitters X-ray FELs. *Phys. Rev. Accel. Beams* **2019**, *22*, 111304 . [CrossRef]
13. Curcio, A.; Dattoli, G.; Di Palma, E.; Petralia, A. Free electron laser oscillator efficiency. *Opt. Comm.* **2018**, *425*, 29–37. [CrossRef]
14. Bonifacio, R.; Pellegrini, C.; Narducci, L. Collective instabilities and high-gain regime in a free-electron Laser. *Opt. Comm.* **1984**, *50*, 373–378. [CrossRef]
15. Dattoli, G.; Ottaviani, P.L.; Pagnutti, S. Booklet for FEL Design: A Collection of Practical Formulae, ENEA RT/2007/40/FIM. Available online: www.fel.enea.it/booklet/pdf/Booklet_for_FEL_design.pdf (accessed on 1 March 2020).
16. Dattoli, G.; Ottaviani, P.L.; Pagnutti, S. High gain amplifiers: Power oscillations and harmonic generation. *J. Appl. Phys.* **2007**, *102*, 033103. [CrossRef]
17. Xie, M. Design Optimization for an X-ray Free Electron Laser Driven by SLAC Linac. Available online: https://accelconf.web.cern.ch/p95/ARTICLES/TPG/TPG10.PDF (accessed on 1 January 2020).
18. Reiche, S. GENESIS 1.3: A fully 3D time-dependent FEL simulation code. *Nucl. Instr. Meth. Phys. Res. Sect. A* **1999**, *429*, 243. [CrossRef]
19. Petrillo, V.; Opromolla, M.; Bacci, A.; Broggi, F.; Drebot, I.; Ghiringhelli, G.; Puppin, E.; Rossetti Conti, M.; Rossi, A.R.; Ruijter, M.; et al. Coherent, high repetition rate tender X-ray Free-Electron Laser seeded by an Extreme Ultra-Violet Free-Electron Laser Oscillator. *New J. Phys.* **2020**, *22*, 073058. [CrossRef]
20. Opromolla, M.; Bacci, A.; Rossetti Conti, M.; Rossi, A.R.; Rossi, G.; Serafini, L.; Tagliaferri, A.; Petrillo, V. High Repetition Rate and Coherent Free-Electron Laser Oscillator in the Tender X-ray Range Tailored for Linear Spectroscopy. *Appl. Sci.* **2021**, *11*, 5892. [CrossRef]
21. Ottaviani, P.L.; Pagnutti, S.; Dattoli, G.; Sabia, E.; Petrillo, V.; van der Slot, P.J.M.; Biedron, S.; Milton, S. Deep saturated Free Electron Laser oscillators and frozen spikes. *Nucl. Instr. Meth. Phys. Res. Sect. A* **2016**, *834*, 108–117. [CrossRef]
22. Petrillo, V.; Anania, M.P.; Artioli, M.; Bacci, A.; Bellaveglia, M.; Chiadroni, E.; Cianchi, A.; Ciocci, F.; Dattoli, G.; Di Giovenale, D.; et al. Observation of time-domain modulation of free-electron-laser pulses by multipeaked electron-energy spectrum. *Phys. Rev. Lett.* **2013**, *111*, 114802. [CrossRef] [PubMed]
23. Piccirillo, B.; Paparo, D.; Rubano, A.; Andreone, A.; Giove, D.; Hernez, V.-V.; Koral, C.; Masullo, M.R.; Mettivier, G.; et al. Geometric Phase-Enhanced Platform for Polarization and Wavefront analysis techniques with the short-TeraHertz FEL Oscillator TerRa@BriXSinO. *Front. Phys.* **2021**, submitted.
24. Koral, C.; Mazaheri, Z.; Papari, G.P.; Andreone, A.; Drebot, I.; Giove, D.; Masullo, M.R.; Mettivier, G.; Opromolla, M.; Paparo, D.; et al. Multi-pass Free-Electron Laser-assisted spectral and imaging applications in the THz/FIR range using the future superconducting electron source BriXSinO. *Front. Phys.* **2021**, submitted.

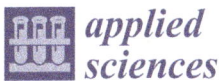

Article

Recirculated Wave Undulators for Compact FELs

Alessandro Curcio

Centro de Laseres Pulsados (CLPU), Edificio M5, Parque Científico, C/Adaja, 8, 37185 Villamayor, Spain; acurcio@clpu.es

Abstract: Particular schemes of Free Electron Lasers (FELs) are designed to exploit wave undulators. We consider a system employing a recirculated electromagnetic undulator provided by a high-power laser in a resonator cavity. The aim is to establish from calculations a set of realizable parameters for such a device. Indeed, novel generation electron accelerators push forward the limits on the accelerating fields, reducing to the sub-meter scale the length over which the electrons can gain enough energy for lasing in the VUV/X-ray region of the electromagnetic spectrum. On the other hand, these innovative technologies do not solve yet the problem associated with the saturation length and therefore of the undulator length, which can be as long as several tens of meters. The option of a FEL based on a wave undulator might provide a valid solution in this respect.

Keywords: recirculated undulator; free electron lasers

1. Introduction

Free Electron Lasers (FELs) are indeed one of the most interesting devices belonging to the realm of the radiation sources [1–14]. Lasers are presently the most diffuse and best-working radiation sources in terms of brilliance, monochromaticity, coherence, directionality and polarization. A future perspective would be that of realizing FEL facilities in the VUV-X region exploiting compact accelerators and short undulator sections. Novel electron acceleration schemes [15–17] can provide high gradient (GV/m) acceleration. Even though the latter might solve the problem of the accelerator length, it still does not solve the issue associated with the saturation length and therefore to the undulator length. Wave undulator-based FELs might provide a valid solution [18–27]. In the wave undulator scheme the undulator is replaced by a laser, thus the associated period is much shorter than that of conventional undulator magnet in existing FELs, paving the way to the reduction of the saturation length. Another advantage is that the electron beam energy necessary to reach the short wavelength region scales as the square root of the undulator period: a wave undulator would permit the operational beam energy to be reduced by several orders of magnitude, as well as it would lead to a reduction in the accelerator size. The conditions for FEL operation of a wave undulator have been studied [26] without too much attention to the laser and electron beams transport. More focus on the laser beam transport has been given in Ref. [27], where a compact VUV-X FEL device has been proposed consisting of an electron LINAC and a resonator cavity to recirculate the wave undulator, used for multiple interactions with the electron beam. Conversely, in this paper we focus on the electron beam transport in the recirculated undulator, both through the interaction points and in the magnetic chicane, while considering the same design for the optical cavity used in [27]. In particular we study the evolution of the longitudinal phase-space during the beam transport and during the interaction with the wave undulator, leading to the electron microbunching responsible for coherent FEL power emission. The paper first consists of a short introduction to the ring cavity design considered for the recirculated wave undulator. Then, the exact solution of the Liouville equation for the longitudinal dynamics of particle beams is derived concerning the phase-space evolution in magnetic chicanes [28], adding corrections due to the emission of synchrotron radiation. The dynamics of relativistic

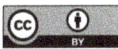

electrons undergoing oscillations in the wave undulator is developed by means of the Hamilton-Jacobi formalism. The electron trajectories are obtained, from which the 1D FEL equations are derived. Simulation results based on the numerical solution of the 1D FEL equations via an in-house Python script combined with the Liouville analytic theory for the electron beam transport in the chicane are shown, in order to demonstrate the electron microbunching with the subsequent FEL emission, as well as for quantitatively characterizing the output power from the recirculated undulator under analysis. Finally, an analytic approach is presented for the wave undulator scaling laws and the FEL power evolution, showing the pros and cons of exploiting a fully analytic model for the FEL emission while comparing numerical and analytic results relative to the same scientific case.

2. The Optical Cavity

We consider an optical cavity [29] which is the same as in Ref. [27], composed by two Flat Mirrors (FM1, FM2), two Parabolic Mirrors (PM1, PM2) and one focusing lens. The design of such ring cavity is shown in Figure 1.

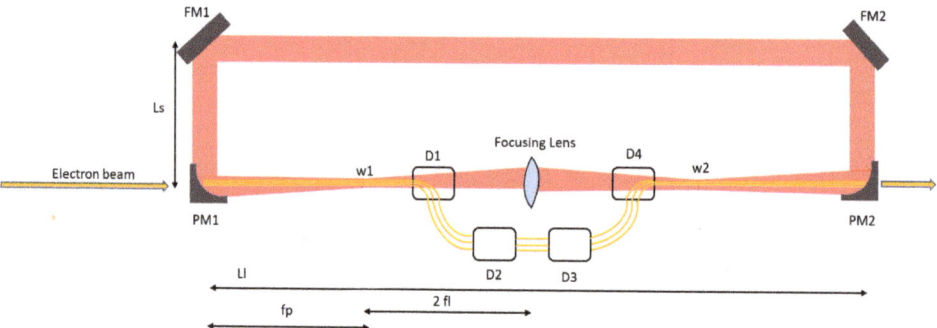

Figure 1. Design of the ring cavity for the wave undulator. The laser circulates clockwise.

This design allows obtaining two waists of the laser beam along a straight line, which is as well the direction where an electron beam is injected while counter-propagating with respect to the laser. The electron beam interacts at the first laser waist w_1 and then at the second waist w_2, with the emission of FEL radiation. The length of the cavity is $L_c = 2L_l + 2L_s$, the long side being L_l and the short one L_s. A focusing lens is placed between two parabolic mirrors at a distance $L_l/2$ from both. Denoting with f_p the focal length of the parabolic mirrors and with f_l the focal length of the central focusing lens, the relative distance between one laser waist and the central focusing lens is $d = 2f_l$. Furthermore, the following equation must hold $L_l = 2f_p + 4f_l$. After the first interaction the electron beam passes through the magnetic chicane (composed by the four dipoles D1, D2, D3, D4) during the time T_{mc}, finally reaching the second interaction point. This time must be synchronized to the laser pulse in such a way that the two beams can "meet" at the waist w_2, in formulas we obtain $cT_{mc} = 2f_p + 2L_s + L_l$, with c the speed of light in vacuum. The strength parameter of the wave undulator is defined as:

$$a_0 = \frac{\lambda_0 e E_p}{2\pi mc^2} \quad (1)$$

where e is the elementary charge, m is the electron's mass and λ_0 is the period of the wave undulator. The peak electric field E_p associated with the laser can be expressed in terms of the laser intensity at the waist:

$$E_p = \sqrt{2Z_0 I_p} \quad (2)$$

where the vacuum impedance has been denoted as Z_0 and I_p is the laser peak intensity calculated as $I_p = P_L/\pi w_0^2$ where P_L is the peak power of the laser.

3. Solution of the Liouville Equation for Longitudinal Beam Dynamics in Magnetic Chicanes

In this section, we develop the theory that will be used to calculate the phase-space evolution of the electron beam passing from the first to the second interaction point through the magnetic chicane, as shown in Figure 2 at the end of this section. We study the longitudinal dynamics of relativistic electron beams in magnetic chicanes [28,30]. The traveling direction is denoted by z. The 1D Liouville equation describing the evolution of the longitudinal phase-space of an electron beam is:

$$\frac{\partial \rho}{\partial t}(z, p_z; t) = \hat{L}\rho(z, p_z; t) \tag{3}$$

where ρ is the longitudinal phase-space density, p_z is the electron longitudinal momentum and the expression of the Liouville operator is:

$$\hat{L} = \left[\frac{\partial H}{\partial z} \frac{\partial}{\partial p_z} - \frac{\partial H}{\partial p_z} \frac{\partial}{\partial z} \right] \tag{4}$$

The Hamiltonian function has been denoted as H and the respective Hamilton equations are:

$$\begin{aligned} \frac{dp_z}{dt} &= -\frac{\partial H}{\partial z} = F_z \\ \frac{dz}{dt} &= \frac{\partial H}{\partial p_z} = v_z \end{aligned} \tag{5}$$

where F_z is the longitudinal force acting on the electrons and $v_z = p_z/\gamma mc$ the longitudinal velocity, with γ the Lorentz factor of the particle. Equation (3) admits the integral solution:

$$\rho(z, p_z; t) = e^{\int_0^t dt \hat{L}} \rho(z, p_z; 0) \tag{6}$$

Equation (6) states that the action of the exponential operator $\exp\left(\int_0^t dt\hat{L}\right)$ on the phase-space density ρ at the initial time $t = 0$ yields the phase-space density at time t. Moreover, using Equation (5), Equation (6) can be further reduced to a more explicit form:

$$\rho(z, p_z; t) = e^{-\int_0^t dt F_z \frac{\partial}{\partial p_z} - \int_0^t dt v_z \frac{\partial}{\partial z}} \rho(z, p_z; 0) = \rho\left(z - \int_0^t dt v_z, p_z - \int_0^t dt F_z; 0\right) \tag{7}$$

Indeed, in Equation (7) we have used the definition of unitary displacement-operator for both the coordinate and the momentum subspaces [30]. The power of this solution lays in the fact that the knowing the single-particle dynamics allows for a complete description of the whole beam in the phase-space at any time. A magnetic chicane consists of dipole magnets usually with the same field-strengths and magnetic lengths. For the study of the recirculated wave undulator under consideration it is preferable to exploit the ponderomotive phase-energy deviation ($\psi - \delta$) space instead than the coordinate-momentum space ($z - p_z$), where $\delta = (\gamma - \gamma_r)/\gamma_r$ with γ_r the Lorentz factor of the reference particle (the one with energy equal to the beam average energy). The meaning of the ponderomotive phase ψ will be clearer in Section 5, where the 1D FEL theory is presented. The transformation matrix associated with a magnetic chicane composed by four dipoles, up to the second-order in the energy deviation, reads:

$$\begin{pmatrix} \psi \\ \delta \end{pmatrix} = \begin{pmatrix} 1 & \frac{2\pi}{\lambda_0} R_{56} \\ 0 & 1 \end{pmatrix} \begin{pmatrix} \psi_0 \\ \delta_0 \end{pmatrix} \tag{8}$$

where

$$R_{56} = \frac{4L}{\sin\theta}(\tan\theta - \theta) + 2d\frac{\tan\theta^2}{\cos\theta} \tag{9}$$

is the linear longitudinal dispersion, θ is bending angle, d is distance between the dipoles and L is the dipole length [31]. These transformations are useful to express the dynamical shifts of the phase-space density:

$$\Delta \psi = \frac{2\pi}{\lambda_0} R_{56} \delta_0,$$
$$\Delta \delta = 0, \tag{10}$$

The longitudinal phase-space density at the exit of the magnetic chicane, say at the time t, is calculated by means of Equations (7) and (10):

$$\rho(\psi, \delta; t) = \rho(\psi - \Delta\psi, \delta - \Delta\delta; 0) = \rho\left(\psi - \frac{2\pi}{\lambda_0} R_{56} \delta_0, \delta; 0\right) \tag{11}$$

where $t = 0$ is the time of entrance into the chicane.

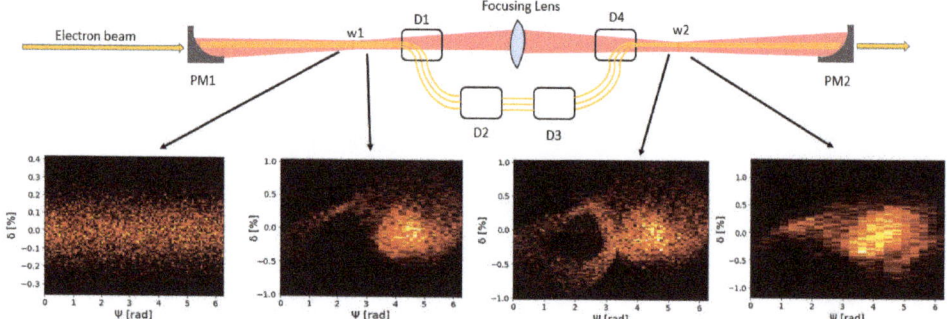

Figure 2. Evolution of the longitudinal phase-space of the electron beam passing from one interaction point to the other. The evolution through the magnetic chicane is calculated via the analytic solution of the Liouville equation. The longitudinal phase spaces shown above will be commented in Section 8.

4. Dynamics of Relativistic Electrons Inside an Electromagnetic Undulator

In this section, we calculate the electron trajectories from first principles of relativistic mechanics when they interact with an electromagnetic plane wave. The formalism of Hamilton-Jacobi will be adopted here, as in [32]. The four-dimensional form of Hamilton-Jacobi equation for the interaction of our interest is:

$$g^{ik}\left(\frac{\partial S}{\partial x^i} - \frac{e}{c} A_i\right)\left(\frac{\partial S}{\partial x^k} - \frac{e}{c} A_k\right) = m^2 c^2 \tag{12}$$

where g^{ik} is the Minkowski tensor with $(1,3)$ signature, S the Hamilton function, x^i the radius four-vector. We make explicit the planar symmetry in the argument of the four-vector potential by setting $A_i \equiv A_i(\zeta)$, with $\zeta = k_i x^i = \omega_0(t + z/c)$, where the sign + in the phase expression stands for the head-on interaction on the z-direction; then we impose the Lorentz gauge condition:

$$\frac{\partial A^i}{\partial x^i} = \frac{\partial A^i}{\partial \zeta} k_i = 0 \tag{13}$$

that is equivalent to $A^i k_i = 0$. To find the Hamilton principal function, we look for a solution of the kind:

$$S = -p_i x^i + F(\zeta) \tag{14}$$

where p_i is the four-vector who satisfies the condition $p_i p^i = m^2 c^2$, and $F(\xi)$ is an unknown function to determine. Substituting (14) into (12) yields:

$$2\eta \frac{\partial F}{\partial \xi} + 2\frac{e}{c} p_i A^i - \frac{e^2}{c^2} A_i A^i = 0 \tag{15}$$

where $\eta = p_i k^i$. From the above we can infer the expression for F and therefore for S:

$$S = -p_i x^i - \frac{ep_i}{\eta} \int A^i d\xi + \frac{e^2}{2\eta} \int A^i A_i d\xi \tag{16}$$

Being $k^i = (\omega_0/c, 0, 0, -\omega_0/c)$ with $\omega_0 = 2\pi c/\lambda_0$, we obtain $\eta = (\omega_0/c)(p_0 + p_3)$. Expanding the square of p_i, we obtain $p_0^2 - p_3^2 - p_{\perp 0}^2 = m^2 c^2$, where we have denoted by $p_{\perp 0}$ the modulus of the generalized transverse four-momentum: $\vec{p}_{\perp 0}$ is a constant of motion, and it will be naturally interpreted as the electron initial transverse moment just before impacting on the photons. It is straightforward to deduce at this point the following equation:

$$p_0 - p_3 = \left(\frac{\omega_0}{c}\right) \frac{p_{\perp 0}^2 + m^2 c^2}{\eta} \tag{17}$$

Now, by means of the algebra below:

$$p^3 x^3 - p^0 x^0 = \frac{(p^3 + p^0)(x^3 - x^0)}{2} + \frac{(p^3 - p^0)(x^3 + x^0)}{2} \tag{18}$$

and using Equations (16) and (17), one obtains the following expression for S:

$$S = \vec{p}_{\perp 0} \cdot \vec{r}_\perp - \frac{c\eta}{2\omega_0}(ct - z) - \frac{p_{\perp 0}^2 + m^2 c^2}{2\eta}\xi - \frac{ep_i}{\eta}\int A^i d\xi + \frac{e^2}{2\eta}\int A_i A^i d\xi \tag{19}$$

By equating the S derivatives with respect to the $\vec{p}_{\perp 0}$ components and to the η parameter to zero, valid for a suitable choice of reference frame, we achieve the useful results for the electron trajectories:

$$\vec{r}_\perp = \frac{\vec{p}_{\perp 0}}{\eta}\xi + \frac{e}{\eta}\int \vec{A} d\xi$$

$$z = \left[\frac{c}{2\omega_0} - \frac{p_{\perp 0}^2 + m^2 c^2}{2\eta^2}\left(\frac{\omega_0}{c}\right)\right]\xi - \frac{\omega_0 e}{c\eta^2}\vec{p}_{\perp 0} \cdot \int \vec{A} d\xi + \frac{\omega_0 e^2}{2c\eta^2}\int A_i A^i d\xi \tag{20}$$

Carrying out the time derivative $\partial S/\partial t = -\gamma(t)mc^2$, yields an expression for the invariant η, evaluated at the origin of times: $\eta = (\omega_0/c)(\gamma_0 mc + p_{z0})$, with γ_0 the initial Lorentz factor. Equations (20) describe the motion of a free electron under the influence of the wave undulator. In the case of a circularly polarized wave undulator the electron trajectory is of the kind shown in Figure 3, obtained plotting Equation (20) for arbitrary parameters to provide a visual example.

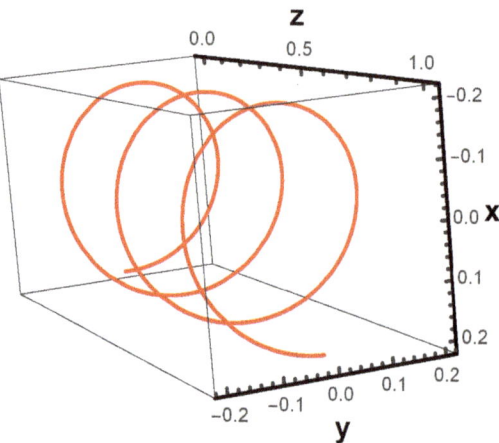

Figure 3. Electron trajectory in a circularly polarized wave undulator (arbitrary units).

5. 1D FEL Equations

In the most of relevant cases $p_{z0} \sim \gamma_0 mc$, we obtain $\eta = 2\gamma_0 \omega_0 m$. Thus, the electron laws of motion can be recast into:

$$\vec{r}_\perp = \frac{\lambda_0}{4\pi}\vec{\theta}_0 \xi + \frac{\lambda_0}{4\pi}\frac{1}{\gamma_0}\int \vec{a}_0 d\xi$$

$$z = \frac{\lambda_0}{4\pi}\left[1 - \frac{(1+\gamma_0^2\theta_0^2)}{2\gamma_0^2}\right]\xi - \frac{\lambda_0}{8\pi}\frac{\vec{\theta}_0}{\gamma_0}\cdot\int \vec{a}_0 d\xi + \frac{\lambda_0}{16\pi}\frac{1}{\gamma_0^2}\int a_0^2 d\xi \quad (21)$$

where $\vec{\theta}_0$ is the vector representing the initial divergence of the electron. For sake of simplicity in this paper we focus on the 1D FEL model, justified by the condition $\theta_0 \ll 1$ for any electron, i.e., low-divergence beams at the interaction region. Moreover, we consider $a_0 \ll 1$ and $\gamma_0 \gg 1$. The laws of motion can be further simplified into:

$$\vec{r}_\perp \simeq \frac{\lambda_0}{4\pi}\frac{1}{\gamma_0}\int \vec{a}_0 d\xi$$

$$z \simeq \frac{\lambda_0}{4\pi}\xi \quad (22)$$

Given the above equations of motion, and choosing a circularly polarized vector potential, the one-dimensional FEL equations are finally (see Appendix A for the derivation):

$$\frac{dE}{dz} = \left(\frac{ea_0}{4\pi\varepsilon_0\gamma_r}\right)n_e\langle e^{-i\psi_j}\rangle$$

$$\frac{d\psi_j}{dz} = \left(\frac{4\pi}{\lambda_0}\right)\delta_j$$

$$\frac{d\delta_j}{dz} = \left(\frac{ea_0}{4\gamma_r^2 mc^2}\right)\left[E(z)e^{i\psi_j} + E^*(z)e^{-i\psi_j}\right] \quad (23)$$

where we have introduced the ponderomotive phase $\psi_j = \omega z/c + \xi_j - (\omega_0 + \omega)t + \phi_j$, i.e., the coordinate identifying the longitudinal position of a particle inside a bucket of physical size determined by the radiation wavelength $\lambda_r \sim \lambda_0/2\gamma_r^2$. ϕ_j is an arbitrary initial phase, and we have defined the relative energy deviation δ_j of an arbitrary j-particle with Lorentz factor γ_j:

$$\delta_j = \frac{\gamma_j - \gamma_r}{\gamma_r} = \frac{\Delta\gamma_j}{\gamma_r} \quad (24)$$

The particles' density of the electron bunch has been denoted as n_e. An important quantity has been introduced as well, which is the bunching factor:

$$b = \langle e^{-i\psi_j} \rangle \qquad (25)$$

where the angular brackets indicate the average over the electron ensemble composing one FEL bucket (more details in Appendix A). The strength parameter K associated with a circularly polarized wave undulator of intensity I_p and wavelength λ_0, in practical units reads:

$$K = a_0 = 0.85 \times 10^{-5} \lambda_0[m] \sqrt{I_p(W/m^2)} \qquad (26)$$

The choice made in this paper of using a circularly polarized wave undulator is based on the fact that doing so, the strength parameter (a_0) is increased with respect to the case of a linearly polarized wave undulator ($a_0/\sqrt{2}$).

6. Discussions on the Recirculated Wave Undulator FEL Scheme

As already discussed and demonstrated in Ref. [27], a CO_2 laser ($\lambda_0 = 10.6$ μm), with an intensity $I_p = 4.2 \times 10^{18}$ W/m^2, corresponding to an energy per pulse of 40 J delivered in 300 ps ($P_L = 130$ GW) over an effective area $\Sigma_0 = \pi w_0^2 \sim \pi \times 10^{-8}$ m^2 would be enough to provide a wave undulator with sufficiently large K to support the FEL SASE operation [33–35]. The value for the strength parameter under these operational conditions is $K \sim 0.186$. This K value is too low for standard FEL, but sufficiently high for the emission of coherent radiation in the wave undulator scheme. The energy for the electron beam we consider is around 35 MeV corresponding to a $\gamma_r \sim 70$. We choose an electron current value $I_e = j_e \Sigma_e = 3$ kA, where $\Sigma_e = 0.075 \Sigma_0$, which means that the electron beam is focused more tightly than the laser beam: this can allow a greater output flux of X-ray photons and eases the spatial overlap of the two beams practically speaking. Moreover, the initial relative energy spread is 10^{-4}. Even if the considered energy of the electron beam is quite low and the beam focusing rather tight, space charge effects can be neglected. The extension of the interaction region Z_i is evaluated as the minimum between two times the Rayleigh length $Z_R = \pi w_0^2/\lambda_0$ and the laser pulse length $c\tau$ where τ is the FWHM pulse duration. In formulas:

$$Z_i = \min\{c\tau, 2Z_R\} \qquad (27)$$

In our case $2Z_R/c\tau \ll 1$, so the interaction region is determined by the Rayleigh length. The number of periods per wave undulator both in the waist w_1 and w_2 are $2Z_R/\lambda_0$, which is many hundreds. As anticipated in the previous section, the working principle of the compact FEL based on the wave undulator is the following: the electron beam is injected into the ring cavity interacting at the laser waists w_1 and w_2. The electron bunches are microbunched at the radiation wavelength's period which is in our case $\lambda_r \sim 1$ nm, falling in the soft X-ray region. When this occurs, coherent radiation power is emitted. A further and important aspect to discuss is the interaction between the electron beams and the wakefields in the machine. The laser can circulate in the ring cavity and interact with the electrons thanks to hollow parabolic mirrors, while the beam passing through the holes generates wakefields (only the first mirror encountered by the electron beam is significant). Given the shortness of the electron bunches considered here, a single bunch of electrons might be not able to efficiently interact with the wakefields. On the other hand, the wakefields might interact with trailing bunches for a certain time structure of the electron bunches in the machine. For facing this issue, the use of dielectric mirrors to suppress the effect of wakefields might be more favorable than metallic-coated optics. Furthermore, for the parameters considered here, the laser diameter at the hollow parabolic mirror is expected to be about 10 cm, therefore the hole would not need to be extremely small.

7. Coherent Synchrotron Radiation

To take into account for the Coherent Synchrotron Radiation (CSR) emitted in the magnetic chicane and to which extent this affects the longitudinal electron beam dynamics, the longitudinal phase-space density at the exit of the magnetic chicane must be expressed with a correction term:

$$\rho(\psi, \delta; t) = \rho(\psi - \Delta\psi, \delta - \Delta\delta; 0) = \rho\left(\psi - \frac{2\pi}{\lambda_0} R_{56}\delta_0, \delta - \kappa\delta_0; 0\right) \quad (28)$$

which is different than Equation (11) because of the factor κ which explains the relative energy losses due to the emission of CSR. The synchrotron radiation spectrum at low frequencies is proportional to the $\omega^{1/3}$ where ω is the angular frequency of the photons. The total CSR energy E_{CSR} emitted by a bunch with gaussian envelope over one full circle is calculated as:

$$E_{CSR} = \frac{N_e^2 e^2}{4\pi\varepsilon_0 c} \int e^{-\omega^2 \tau_e^2} \left(\frac{\omega R}{c}\right)^{1/3} d\omega = \Gamma\left(\frac{2}{3}\right) \frac{N_e^2 e^2}{8\pi\varepsilon_0 c \tau_e} \left(\frac{R}{c\tau_e}\right)^{1/3} \quad (29)$$

where $\Gamma(x)$ is the Gamma function, τ_e is the rms electron bunch length, N_e is the number of electrons in the bunch and R is the bending radius. The total beam energy is calculated as $E_{beam} = N_e \gamma_r m c^2$. The CSR correction is therefore found to be:

$$\kappa = \frac{E_{CSR}}{E_{beam}} = \frac{4\theta}{2\pi} \Gamma\left(\frac{2}{3}\right) \frac{N_e e^2}{8\pi\varepsilon_0 \tau_e \gamma_r m c^3} \left(\frac{R}{c\tau_e}\right)^{1/3} \quad (30)$$

where the factor $4\theta/2\pi$ takes into account for the fact that the CSR emitted in the four bending magnets composing the chicane corresponds to a total bending angle which is smaller than the full circle. For a better evaluation of the κ parameter the microbunching should be taken into account beyond the bunch envelope (in this case gaussian), nevertheless this is not relevant for the design considered here since the critical energy of the synchrotron radiation spectrum falls in a range of frequencies much lower than the microbunching frequency.

8. FEL Radiation: Numerical Simulations

We have developed a numerical code in Python for solving the 1D FEL Equation (23) and to propagate the electron beam from one interaction point to the other self-consistently via Equation (28). This choice has been made (instead of using other available codes) to have more control on the approximations done in the model and in such a way to easily extend it for the forthcoming works where the design will be reconsidered including further effects towards an even more realistic description of the machine. In this section we report on simulation results, in particular showing the longitudinal phase-space evolution of the electron beam while interacting with the electromagnetic undulator and with the magnetic chicane. The parameters used for the chicane considered in this paper are $L_c = 2.1$ m, $f_p = 150$ mm, $f_l = 300$ mm, $L_s = 150$ mm, $B = 1.16$ T and $\theta = 72°$. The chosen length of the dipoles has been $d = 200$ mm and the reciprocal distance $L = 100$ mm. Considering an electron bunch of duration 300 fs and charge 1 nC the correction due to CSR is $\kappa = 1.6\%$, which is not fully negligible, and it has been implemented in the Python code. The effect of the energy losses due to CSR in the magnetic chicane onto the bandwidth of the wave undulator FEL spectrum is not the main goal of the present paper, but it shall be addressed in a future work. The first result is given in Figure 4, showing the randomly distributed initial longitudinal phase-space relative to one bucket of ponderomotive phase (top-left), the bunched longitudinal phase-space after the interaction with the laser at the waist w_1 of Figure 1 (top-right), the emitted FEL power during the interaction with the CO_2 laser over one Rayleigh length (bottom-left), and finally the evolution of the bunching factor over the same length (bottom-right). The pixel level in the top-left and top-right figure is in arbitrary units but the two plots are normalized on the same scale.

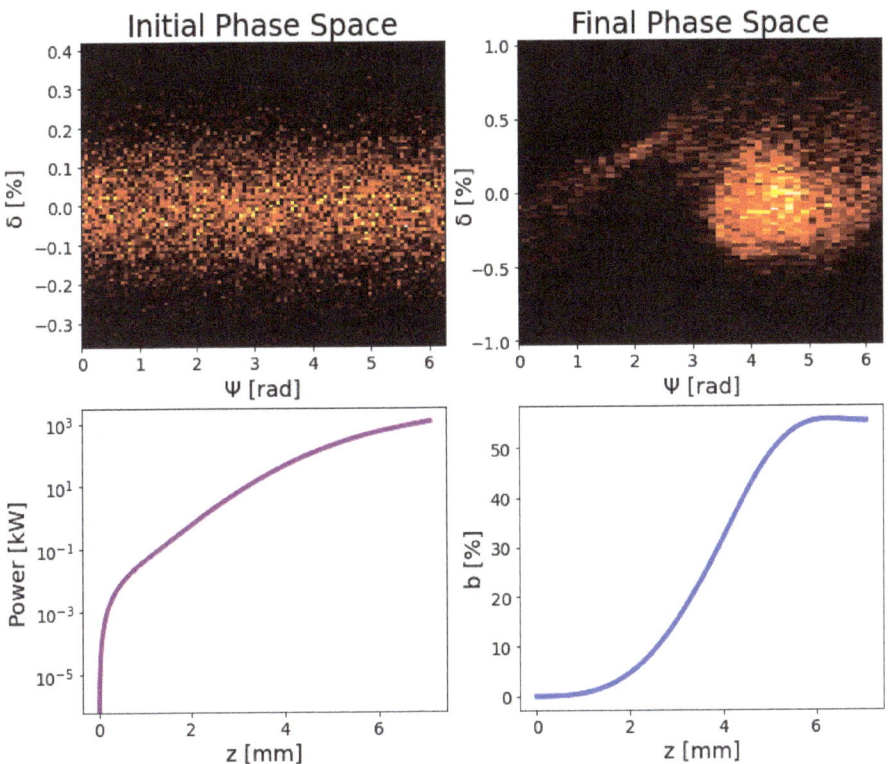

Figure 4. Simulation results with FEL1D code in Python, concerning the first interaction point of Figure 2.

Figure 5 shows the longitudinal phase-space of the electron beam after passing through the magnetic chicane. In order to calculate it, the top-right phase-space of Figure 4 has been propagated according to Equation (28), i.e., for every particle individuated by the pair (ψ, δ) the relative energy deviation has been shifted due to CSR and the ponderomotive phase has been shifted by a quantity depending on the element R_{56}. The result is shown in Figure 5, where it is possible to observe that the electron microbunching is preserved to some extent. The last simulation result is reported in Figure 6, showing the same distribution in Figure 5 (top-left), the bunched longitudinal phase-space after the interaction with the laser at the waist w_2 of Figure 2 (top-right), the emitted FEL power during the interaction with the CO_2 laser over one Rayleigh length (bottom-left), and finally the evolution of the bunching factor over the same length (bottom-right). The second interaction is evidently more efficient in terms of the FEL power emitted. This is essentially due to the preservation of some order in the longitudinal phase-space after the magnetic chicane which favors the FEL mechanism at the interaction point w_2 even more than at w_1. The laser is considered essentially not affected by the roundtrip, since the cavity losses are reasonably supposed negligible. Nevertheless, the presence of two interaction points is overall of great advantage since it increases the average output power. Indeed, the time structure of the FEL radiation is a two-pulse structure, and it is worth noting that the fact of having two interaction points does not affect the peak power, but only the average one.

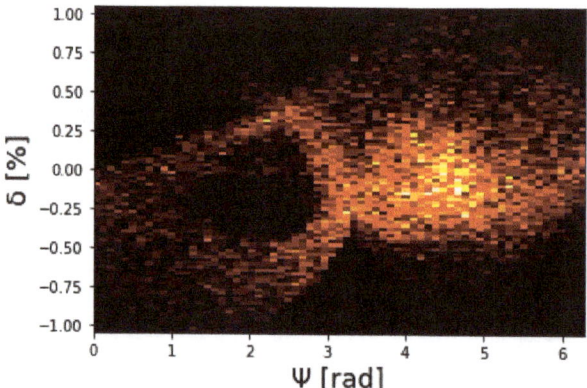

Figure 5. Simulation results with FEL1D code in Python, at the entrance of the second interaction point.

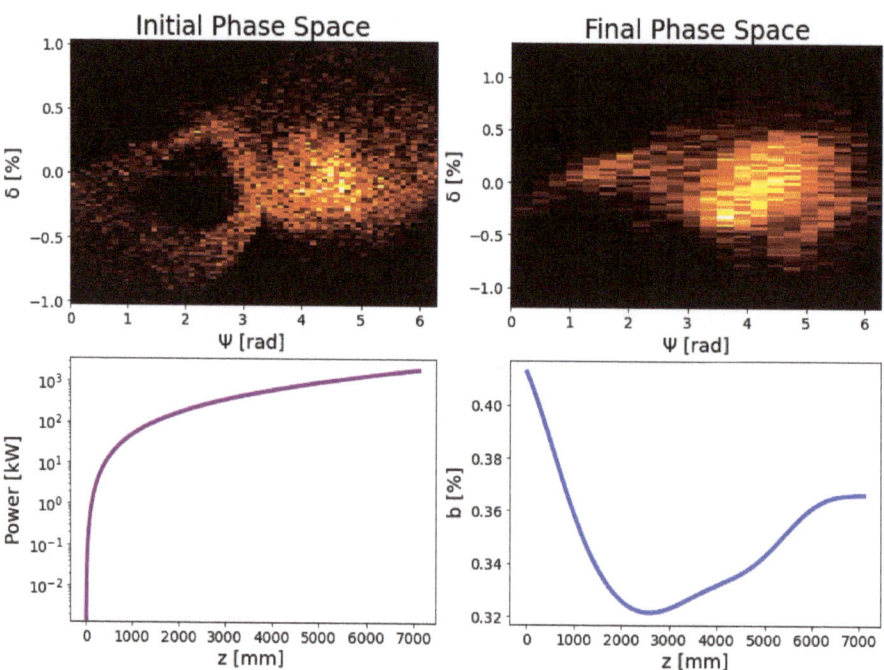

Figure 6. Simulation results with FEL1D code in Python, after the second interaction point.

9. FEL Radiation: Comparison with the Analytic Model

In this section, we finally review a fully analytical approach to the FEL power evolution [27], in order to make a comparison with the numerical approach used above while highlighting the main differences. The FEL intensity evolution is ruled by the so-called Pierce parameter, which, for the purposes of this paper, can be cast in the following form:

$$\varrho = \frac{8.36 \times 10^{-3}}{\gamma_e} \left(j_e[A/m^2] \lambda_0^2[m] K^2 \right)^{1/3} \tag{31}$$

where j_e is the electron beam density current. The saturation length can be roughly expressed in terms of a few gain lengths. The "full saturation" condition on the emitted power is usually achieved after several times the gain length, the latter given by:

$$L_g = \frac{\lambda_0}{4\pi\sqrt{3}\varrho} \tag{32}$$

The saturation power is:

$$P_F = \sqrt{2\varrho}P_e \tag{33}$$

where $P_e = \gamma_r mc^2 j_e \Sigma_e / e$. As a consequence of the previous equations, the FEL saturated power reads:

$$P_F(MW) = 1.7 \times 10^{16} \frac{(\gamma_r \varrho)^4}{I_p[W/m^2]\lambda_0[m]^4} \Sigma_e[m^2] \tag{34}$$

Beside the scaling formulas above, a more complete and analytic description of the SASE intensity growth can be specified by the following logistic-like function:

$$P(z) = \frac{P_0}{9} \frac{B(z)}{1 + \frac{P_0}{9P_F}B(z)} \tag{35}$$

$$B(z) = 2\left[\cosh\left(\frac{z}{L_g}\right) - e^{z/2L_g}\cos\left(\frac{\pi}{3} + \frac{\sqrt{3}z}{L_g}\right) - e^{-z/2L_g}\cos\left(\frac{\pi}{3} - \frac{\sqrt{3}z}{L_g}\right)\right] \tag{36}$$

The radiated FEL power analytically calculated by Formulas (35) and (36) under the same operational conditions used for the numerical simulations in Section 8 is shown in Figure 7. For the sake of rigor, Figure 7 should be compared to the bottom-left plot of Figure 4, since it is related to the assumption of no initial correlation (or bunching) in the phase-space. Therefore, the power level and the power trend after the first interaction point analytically calculated is in good agreement with the one numerically simulated. The same cannot be said at the second interaction point, since the pre-bunching preserved after the magnetic chicane makes the analytic model not longer comparable to the bottom-left plot of Figure 6. In conclusion, the above presented analytic model can be used for evaluating the power emitted at the first interaction point, but to be reliable as well at the second interaction point should be generalized to a situation of pre-bunching, which is not in the focus of this paper. In Ref. [27] the FEL emission was studied only analytically and the free parameter P_0 was set to an arbitrarily small value to obtain reasonable output power. On the other hand, in the current paper we have managed to fix this free parameter to a value ($P_0 = 21$ kW) such that the analytic model coincides in terms of final output power with the more rigorous numerical approach. Therefore, here we demonstrate that actually the performance of the proposed design can be higher than the one already shown in [27]. At the same time we show the limitation of the analytic approach, which cannot be used for more than one interaction point (unless for the case that the pre-bunching is completely destroyed by the chicane), since it does not consider the effects related to the pre-bunching.

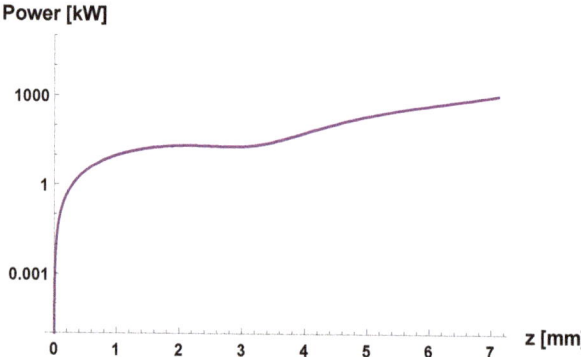

Figure 7. The FEL radiated power versus the propagation distance inside of the wave undulator.

10. Conclusions

In this paper, we have considered an unconventional scheme of wave undulator FEL. The system we have proposed employs a radiation pulse serving as undulator provided by a high-power laser. A feasibility study has been reported with particular focus on the electron beam dynamics. The device is compact, and the relevant technology will be available in the next future. We have faced the aspects related to the electron beam transport in the wave undulator design previously proposed in Ref. [27]. It has been found that the interaction in the first interaction point is efficient, but the interaction in the second point can be even more efficient provided that the electron beam dynamics in the magnetic chicane is properly controlled to preserve the microbunching to some extent. Conceptual tools for the electron transport have been here provided, also considering losses due to coherent synchrotron radiation. A more realistic design of the whole machine will be topic for a future work, including effects related to the electron beam optics, to the transport of the transverse and longitudinal phase spaces together, to the beam interactions with the wakefields and to the evaluation and optimization of the FEL radiation spectral features.

Funding: This research received no external funding.

Institutional Review Board Statement: Not applicable.

Informed Consent Statement: Not applicable.

Conflicts of Interest: The author declares no conflict of interest.

Appendix A. Derivation of the 1D FEL Equations for the Wave Undulator

The wave equation for the electric field E generated by a current density j is:

$$\frac{1}{c^2}\frac{\partial^2 E}{\partial t^2} - \frac{\partial^2 E}{\partial z^2} = -\mu_0 \frac{\partial j}{\partial t} \tag{A1}$$

where the electric field is assumed complex and scalar (this can still cover the case of circular polarization) and the current density is considered along the field polarization direction. With a standard procedure, assuming slowly varying envelope, a forward propagation of the electromagnetic wave and a single-mode oscillation such that $\partial_t \ll c\partial_z$, Equation (A1) can be reduced to:

$$\frac{\partial E}{\partial z} \sim \frac{i\mu_0 c}{2\omega} e^{-i\psi(t)} \frac{\partial j}{\partial t} \tag{A2}$$

In the same framework of assumptions above, we average the current density over a period of rapid oscillation of the radiation field, i.e., within one FEL bucket, while considering $\gamma_r \gg 1$:

$$e^{-i\psi(t)}\frac{\partial j}{\partial t} \sim \frac{i\omega^2}{2\pi}\int_{-\frac{\pi}{\omega}}^{\frac{\pi}{\omega}} j e^{-i\psi(t)} dt = -\frac{ie\omega^2 a_0}{4\pi\gamma_r \Sigma_e}\sum_{j=1}^{N_e}\int_{-\frac{\pi}{\omega}}^{\frac{\pi}{\omega}} e^{-i\psi(t)}\delta[z-z_j(t)]dt \sim -\frac{ie\omega^2 a_0}{2\pi\gamma_r \Sigma_e}\sum_{j=1}^{N_e} e^{-i\psi(t_j)} \quad (A3)$$

where for the last passage we have used the second of Equation (21). We recognize $n_e = N_e \omega / \Sigma_e c$, therefore:

$$e^{-i\psi(t)}\frac{\partial j}{\partial t} \sim -\frac{i\omega a_0 n_e e c}{2\pi\gamma_r}\langle e^{-i\psi(t_j)}\rangle \equiv -\frac{i\omega a_0 n_e e c}{2\pi\gamma_r}\langle e^{-i\psi_j}\rangle \quad (A4)$$

where N_e is the number of electrons in the FEL bucket and the angular brackets denote an average over the particles composing the temporal slice of width $2\pi/\omega$. Thus, the first of Equation (23) is obtained combining Equations (A2) and (A4). The second and third of Equation (23) are the so-called pendulum equations, which are derived as shown below. First, we set the equation for the ponderomotive phase evolution recalling that $\omega \sim 2\gamma_r^2 \omega_0$:

$$\frac{d\psi_j}{dz} = \frac{\omega}{c^2}\frac{dz_j}{dt} + \frac{\omega_0}{c} + \frac{\omega_0}{c^2}\frac{dz_j}{dt} - \frac{\omega_0 + \omega}{c} + \frac{d\phi_j}{dz} = (\omega+\omega_0)\frac{\beta_j}{c} - \frac{\omega}{c} \sim \frac{\omega_0}{c}\left(1 - \frac{\gamma_r^2}{\gamma_j^2}\right) \quad (A5)$$

Since $\gamma_r^2/\gamma_j^2 = (\delta_j + 1)^{-2} \sim 1 - 2\delta_j$ for $\delta_j \ll 1$, the ponderomotive phase obeys to:

$$\frac{d\psi_j}{dz} = \frac{\omega_0}{c}\left(1 - \frac{\gamma_r^2}{\gamma_j^2}\right) \sim 2\frac{\omega_0}{c}\delta_j \quad (A6)$$

which coincides with the second of Equation (23). Concerning the energy deviation:

$$\frac{d\delta_j}{dz} = \frac{1}{\gamma_r}\frac{d\gamma_j}{dz} = \frac{1}{\gamma_r m c^2}\frac{dW_j}{dz} \quad (A7)$$

Where, by means of the first of Equation (21), the energy exchange rate dW_j/dz is given by:

$$\frac{dW_j}{dz} = -\frac{e}{c}\frac{d\vec{r}_\perp}{dt}\cdot Re\left[\vec{E}(z)e^{i\psi_j}\right] \sim -\frac{ea_0}{2\gamma_r}Re\left[E(z)e^{i\psi_j}\right] = -\frac{ea_0}{4\gamma_r}\left[E(z)e^{i\psi_j} + E^*(z)e^{-i\psi_j}\right] \quad (A8)$$

Finally, by combining Equation (A8) with Equation (A7) it is possible to obtain the last of Equation (23).

References

1. O'Shea, P.G.; Freund, H.P. Free-electron lasers: Status and applications. *Science* **2001**, *292*, 1853–1858. [CrossRef] [PubMed]
2. McNeil, B.W.; Thompson, N.R. X-ray free-electron lasers. *Nat. Photonics* **2010**, *4*, 814–821. [CrossRef]
3. Brau, C.A. Free-electron lasers. *Science* **1988**, *239*, 1115–1121. [CrossRef] [PubMed]
4. Barletta, W.A.; Bisognano, J.; Corlett, J.N.; Emma, P.; Huang, Z.; Kim, K.J.; Lindberg, R.; Murphy, J.B.; Neil, G.R.; Nguyen, D.C.; et al. Free electron lasers: Present status and future challenges. *Nucl. Instrum. Methods Phys. Res. Sect. A Accel. Spectrometers Detect. Assoc. Equip.* **2010**, *618*, 69–96. [CrossRef]
5. Colson, W.B.; Sessler, A.M. Free electron lasers. *Annu. Rev. Nucl. Part. Sci.* **1985**, *35*, 25–54. [CrossRef]
6. Allaria, E.; Badano, L.; Bassanese, S.; Capotondi, F.; Castronovo, D.; Cinquegrana, P.; Danailov, M.B.; D'Auria, G.; Demidovich, A.; Monte, R.D.; et al. The FERMI free-electron lasers. *J. Synchrotron Radiat.* **2015**, *22*, 485–491. [CrossRef]
7. Schmüser, P.; Dohlus, M.; Rossbach, J.; Behrens, C. *Free-Electron Lasers in the Ultraviolet and X-ray Regime*; Springer Tracts in Modern Physics; Springer: Berlin/Heidelberg, Germany, 2014; Volume 258.
8. Pellegrini, C.; Marinelli, A.; Reiche, S. The physics of X-ray free-electron lasers. *Rev. Mod. Phys.* **2016**, *88*, 015006. [CrossRef]
9. Feng, C.; Deng, H.X. Review of fully coherent free-electron lasers. *Nucl. Sci. Tech.* **2018**, *29*, 1–15. [CrossRef]
10. Pellegrini, C. The history of X-ray free-electron lasers. *Eur. Phys. J. H* **2012**, *37*, 659–708. [CrossRef]
11. Margaritondo, G.; Rebernik Ribic, P. A simplified description of X-ray free-electron lasers. *J. Synchrotron Radiat.* **2011**, *18*, 101–108. [CrossRef]
12. Curcio, A.; Dattoli, G.; Di Palma, E.; Petralia, A. Free electron laser oscillator efficiency. *Opt. Commun.* **2018**, *425*, 29–37. [CrossRef]
13. Honkavaara, K. Status of the FLASH FEL User Facility at DESY. In Proceedings of the 38th International Free Electron Laser Conference, Santa Fe, NM, USA, 20–25 August 2017.

14. Rönsch-Schulenburg, J.; Honkavaara, K.; Schreiber, S.; Treusch, R.; Vogt, M. FLASH-Status and Upgrades. In Proceedings of the 39th International Free Electron Laser Conference (FEL'19), Hamburg, Germany, 26–30 August 2019.
15. Corde, S.; Phuoc, K.T.; Lambert, G.; Fitour, R.; Malka, V.; Rousse, A.; Beck, A.; Lefebvre, E. Femtosecond X rays from laser-plasma accelerators. *Rev. Mod. Phys.* **2013**, *85*, 1–58. [CrossRef]
16. Esarey, E.; Shadwick, B.A.; Catravas, P.; Leemans, W.P. Synchrotron radiation from electron beams in plasma-focusing channels. *Phys. Rev. E* **2002** *65*, 056505. [CrossRef]
17. Aschikhin, A.; Behrens, C.; Bohlen, S.; Dale, J.; Delbos, N.; Di Lucchio, L.; Elsen, E.; Erbe, J.-H.; Felber, M.; Foster, B.; et al. The FLASHForward facility at DESY. *Nucl. Instrum. Methods Phys. Res. Sect. A Accel. Spectrometers Detect. Assoc. Equip.* **2016**, *806*, 175–183. [CrossRef]
18. Dobsiach, P.; Meystre, P.; Scully, M.O. Optical wiggler free-electron X-ray laser in the 5 Å region. *IEEE J. Quantum Electron.* **1983**, *19*, 1812–1820. [CrossRef]
19. Ciocci, F.; Dattoli, G.; Walsh, J. A short note on the wave-undulator FEL operation. *Nucl. Instrum. Methods A* **1985**, *237*, 401–403. [CrossRef]
20. Banacloche, J.G.; Moore, G.T.; Schlicher, R.R.; Scully, M.O.; Walther, H. Soft X-Ray freeelectron laser with a laser undulator. *IEEE J. Quantum Electron.* **1987**, *23*, 1558–1570. [CrossRef]
21. Tang, C.M.; Hafizi, B.; Ride, S.K. Thomson backscattered X-rays from an intense laser beam. *Nucl. Instrum. Methods A* **1993**, *331*, 371–378. [CrossRef]
22. Dattoli, G.; Letardi, T.; Vazquez, L.R. FEL SASE WAVE undulators. *Opt. Commun.* **2012**, *285*, 5341–5346. [CrossRef]
23. Bacci, A.; Ferrario, M.; Maroli, C.; Petrillo, V.; Serafini, L. Transverse effects in the production of x rays with a free-electron laser based on an optical undulator. *Phys. Rev. Spec. Top.-Accel. Beams* **2006**, *9*, 060704. [CrossRef]
24. Polyanskiy, M.N.; Pogorelsky, I.V.; Yakimenko, V. Picosecond pulse amplification in isotopic CO_2 active medium. *Opt. Express* **2011**, *19*, 7717–7725. [CrossRef] [PubMed]
25. Bazarov, I.V.; Dunham, B.M.; Sinclair, C.K. Maximum achievable beam brightness from photoinjectors. *Phys. Rev. Lett.* **2009**, *102*, 104801. [CrossRef] [PubMed]
26. Dattoli, G.; Petrillo, V.; Rau, J.V. FEL SASE and wave-undulators. *Opt. Commun.* **2012**, *285*, 5341–5346. [CrossRef]
27. Curcio, A.; Dattoli, G.; Ferrario, M.; Giulietti, D.; Nguyen, F. An optical cavity design for a compact wave-undulator based-FEL. *Opt. Commun.* **2017**, *405*, 197–200. [CrossRef]
28. Curcio, A.; Panas, R.; Knafel, M.; Wawrzyniak, A.I. Liouville theory for fully analytic studies of longitudinal beam dynamics and bunch profile reconstruction in dispersive lines. *Nucl. Instrum. Methods Phys. Res. Sect. A Accel. Spectrometers Detect. Assoc. Equip.* **2021**, *986*, 164755. [CrossRef]
29. Svelto, O. *Principles of Lasers*; Plenum Press, New York, NY, USA, 1976; p. 386.
30. Babusci, D.; Dattoli, G.; Quattromini, M. Relativistic equations with fractional and pseudodifferential operators. *Phys. Rev. A* **2011**, *83*, 062109. [CrossRef]
31. Di Mitri, S. Bunch length compressors. *CERN Yellow Rep. Sch. Proc.* **2018**, *1*, 363. [CrossRef]
32. Landau, L.D. (Ed.) *The Classical Theory of Fields*; Elsevier: Amsterdam, The Netherlands, 2013; Volume 2.
33. Dattoli, G.; Ottaviani, P.L.; Pagnutti, S. Nonlinear harmonic generation in high-gain free-electron lasers. *J. Appl. Phys.* **2005**, *97*, 113102. [CrossRef]
34. Dattoli, G.; Ottaviani, P.L.; Pagnutti, S. *Booklet for FEL Design*; ENEA-Edizioni Scientifiche: Frascati, Italy, 2007.
35. Lau, Y.Y.; He, F.; Umstadter, D.P.; Kowalczyk, R. Nonlinear Thomson scattering: A tutorial. *Phys. Plasmas* **2003**, *10*, 2155–2162. [CrossRef]

Article

Advanced Scheme to Generate MHz, Fully Coherent FEL Pulses at nm Wavelength

Georgia Paraskaki [1], Sven Ackermann [1], Bart Faatz [2], Gianluca Geloni [3,*], Tino Lang [1], Fabian Pannek [4], Lucas Schaper [1] and Johann Zemella [1]

[1] Deutsches Elektronen-Synchrotron DESY, Notkestraße 85, 22607 Hamburg, Germany; georgia.paraskaki@desy.de (G.P.); sven.ackermann@desy.de (S.A.); tino.lang@desy.de (T.L.); lucas.schaper@desy.de (L.S.); johann.zemella@desy.de (J.Z.)
[2] Shanghai Advanced Research Institute, Chinese Academy of Sciences, Haike Road 99, Shanghai 201210, China; faatzbart@sari.ac.cn
[3] European XFEL, Holzkoppel 4, 22869 Schenefeld, Germany
[4] Institute for Experimental Physics, University of Hamburg, Luruper Chaussee 149, 22761 Hamburg, Germany; fabian.pannek@desy.de
* Correspondence: gianluca.geloni@xfel.eu

Citation: Paraskaki, G.; Ackermann, S.; Faatz, B.; Geloni, G.; Lang, T.; Pannek, F.; Schaper, L.; Zemella, J. Advanced Scheme to Generate MHz, Fully Coherent FEL Pulses at nm Wavelength. *Appl. Sci.* **2021**, *11*, 6058. https://doi.org/10.3390/app11136058

Academic Editors: Giuseppe Dattoli, Alessandro Curcio and Danilo Giulietti

Received: 25 May 2021
Accepted: 19 June 2021
Published: 29 June 2021

Publisher's Note: MDPI stays neutral with regard to jurisdictional claims in published maps and institutional affiliations.

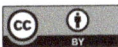

Copyright: © 2021 by the authors. Licensee MDPI, Basel, Switzerland. This article is an open access article distributed under the terms and conditions of the Creative Commons Attribution (CC BY) license (https://creativecommons.org/licenses/by/4.0/).

Abstract: Current FEL development efforts aim at improving the control of coherence at high repetition rate while keeping the wavelength tunability. Seeding schemes, like HGHG and EEHG, allow for the generation of fully coherent FEL pulses, but the powerful external seed laser required limits the repetition rate that can be achieved. In turn, this impacts the average brightness and the amount of statistics that experiments can do. In order to solve this issue, here we take a unique approach and discuss the use of one or more optical cavities to seed the electron bunches accelerated in a superconducting linac to modulate their energy. Like standard seeding schemes, the cavity is followed by a dispersive section, which manipulates the longitudinal phase space of the electron bunches, inducing longitudinal density modulations with high harmonic content that undergo the FEL process in an amplifier placed downstream. We will discuss technical requirements for implementing these setups and their operation range based on numerical simulations.

Keywords: seeded FEL; oscillator; amplifier; high repetition rate

1. Introduction

Free-electron lasers (FELs) have been making enormous improvements during the past decades, delivering high-brightness radiation to users all over the world at wavelengths from mm to hard x-rays, covering a wide range of experiments. At the same time, many experiments, for instance, those that depend on spectroscopic techniques to resolve electronic structure, require full coherence and high statistics, which can only be fulfilled with fully coherent radiation at high repetition rate. These two requirements are becoming important for scientific applications and are driving new FEL developments. Currently, superconducting accelerators are capable of providing thousands of bunches per second at MHz repetition rate. This potential is currently exploited in self-amplified spontaneous emission (SASE) mode [1]. However, in this case, the FEL process starts from random fluctuations of the electron beam charge density distribution [2] leading to a limited temporal coherence, which impacts the peak brightness. The longitudinal coherence can be improved by self-seeding [3,4] and single-mode [5,6] lasing schemes which are based on the SASE process. As a consequence, the stochastic nature of SASE is imprinted on the final FEL pulse as intensity fluctuations even though improved longitudinal coherence is achieved.

At wavelengths in the nanometer range and longer, alternatives to generate fully coherent radiation are based on external seeding. In this case, a seed laser of typically several tens MW of power is used to prepare an initial signal for a final FEL amplifier, usually tuned at a harmonic of its wavelength, thus imprinting its coherence properties upon the output FEL pulse. Many interesting experiments and methods are allowed due to the unique properties of seed radiation [7–10]. Two chief examples of external seeding schemes are the high-gain harmonic generation (HGHG) [11,12] and the echo-enabled harmonic generation (EEHG) [13–15]. As the harmonic conversion of seeding schemes is limited, it is advantageous to use short wavelength seed lasers. Currently, ultraviolet (UV) seed lasers are the most suitable candidates for such setups [14–16]. However, the requirements put on these laser systems in terms of peak power limit their repetition rate, which is usually in the kHz regime. As seeded radiation pulses can be generated at a maximum repetition rate defined by the seed laser repetition rate, not all electron bunches generated in superconducting accelerators can be seeded. This leads to high peak brightness FEL pulses, but limited average flux, in contrast to the number of electron bunches available. In order to address this limitation, alternatives have been recently studied to increase the repetition rate of seeding schemes by reducing the seed laser power requirements [17,18], and in this paper, we propose an oscillator–amplifier setup.

Here, we review and further discuss a scheme which can generate FEL pulses of both high peak brightness, compared to SASE, and of high average flux compared to standard seeding schemes, by generating high repetition rate seeded radiation pulses [19–22]. In this scheme, an FEL oscillator is employed and acts as a feedback system which recirculates a seed pulse, and seeds the electron bunches at high repetition rate. In this case, one may either use a low repetition rate seed laser, or start from shot noise. Starting from shot noise lets us be independent of seed laser systems both in terms of repetition rate and wavelength. Oscillator FELs are a well-studied topic, and their technology has been established for a long time. There is a wide range of oscillator FELs that were operated during the past decades, and detailed simulation studies were performed almost two decades ago [23–25]. These studies led, more recently, to the development of other ideas such as XFELOs [26] and Regenerative Amplifier Free-Electron Lasers (RAFELs) [27–30] (high-gain oscillators). Both these schemes aim at Angstrom radiation with Bragg crystals instead of conventional mirrors, and no harmonic conversion is used. However, at wavelengths in the nanometer range, where crystal optics cannot be used, mirror technology strongly limits the generation of wavelengths below the 190 nm demonstrated at ELETTRA [31]. In order to reach shorter wavelengths, one can exploit a resonator at a longer wavelength, together with harmonic conversion. Such cascades have been proposed in [32–35]. Earlier work on resonators in the EUV regime can be found in [36].

An overview of the seeding schemes that can employ an oscillator to increase the repetition rate of the FEL radiation is given in Section 2, together with comments on its implementation in continuous wave and burst-mode accelerators. Considerations on the implementation of a resonator and a simple model which can be used for its design are provided in Section 3. In Section 4, we introduce the methods used in simulations for power gain control in the cavity, when the start-up of the FEL process is based on random fluctuations of the initial electron beam distribution. In Section 5, we compare these results to the case of an oscillator where the start-up of the FEL process is based on a low repetition rate external seed laser, to the case of standard single-pass seeding, and to SASE simulations.

2. Overview of Methods

2.1. Employing an Oscillator in Standard Seeding Schemes

In this section, we review different schemes that can be implemented with an oscillator in order to provide high repetition rate seed pulses. In standard seeding techniques, an external seed laser is used to modulate the energy of the electron beam as a result of their interaction along an undulator (modulator). In this case, one seed laser pulse needs to be injected for each electron bunch. The purpose of adding an optical cavity to a seeding scheme is to replace the need for an external seed laser, because the cavity can recirculate a radiation pulse and maintain its peak power and pulse properties. In this case, in addition to the energy modulation process which happens along the modulator, an amplification process must also occur. This is important because the power gain is used to compensate for unavoidable cavity losses. Here, we define as net gain the difference between the peak power at the beginning of a pass n + 1 and the peak power at the beginning of pass n, divided by the peak power at pass n. If the power gain compensates exactly for the losses and the net gain is zero, the peak power per pass remains constant as long as the pulse properties remain stable. In this way, the seed pulse is reproducible and can support seeding schemes at high repetition rates.

In this paper we consider two approaches to generate and store a seed laser pulse in cavity.

1. An oscillator-FEL starting with an external seed laser pulse. An external seed laser initiates the modulation of the first electron bunch and the bunch amplifies the seed pulse to compensate for the power losses in the cavity. The optical cavity feeds back the seed pulse which is used to modulate the following bunches. The shortest wavelength of the modulator is determined by the low repetition rate seed laser source and by the mirror availability.

2. An oscillator-FEL starting from shot-noise. An electron bunch generates radiation along the modulator, which is amplified with the number of passes. This process can be divided into two phases. The "build-up regime", where the net gain per pass needs to be positive to build up the peak power required for seeding, and the "steady-state regime" where the net gain needs to go back to zero so that the resonator losses are equal to the power gain. In order to transition between these two phases, an active control on the gain per pass is required. In addition, starting from noise means that a SASE spectrum is generated. This needs to be monochromatized. In this case, the shortest wavelength of the modulator is determined by the mirror availability.

In the following, we consider the implementation of an oscillator-based FEL in support to HGHG and EEHG seeding schemes in order to further extend the tuning range to shorter wavelength and higher repetition rate.

2.1.1. High-Gain Harmonic Generation (HGHG)

HGHG is a method to achieve fully coherent and stable seeded radiation in high-gain FELs and was introduced in [11]. The components needed are a modulator, a seed laser resonant to the wavelength of the modulator, a dispersive section, and an FEL amplifier tuned at a harmonic of the seed laser wavelength. The seed laser is overlapped with the electron bunch in the modulator, and their interaction results in a longitudinal sinusoidal energy modulation along the electron bunch with the periodicity of the resonant wavelength. In the dispersive section placed downstream, the energy modulation is converted into density modulation that includes relevant harmonic content. The dispersive section is characterized by the R_{56} matrix element of the transfer matrix, which describes the evolution of the 6-D phase space (x, x', y, y', δ_γ, z) of the electrons. The R_{56} is closely related with the presence of longitudinal dispersion. When a correlation between the longitudinal position (z) and a relative energy offset (δ_γ) is established in the modulator, it is possible to choose an R_{56} to rotate the longitudinal phase space, and convert the energy modulation into longitudinal density modulation. The same matrix element is responsible for the so called bunch compression in accelerators, where we exploit an electron beam with an energy-longitudinal position correlation (electron beam energy chirp) to compress it longitudinally and increase its peak current. After the dispersive section, the bunched electron beam then enters the amplifier and emits coherent radiation. In the case of an HGHG oscillator-amplifier, an optical cavity which encloses the modulator is added as shown in Figure 1. Instead of injecting a seed laser pulse for each consecutive electron bunch, the optical cavity stores a radiation pulse which acts as a seed laser source. Because, as discussed above, a certain amount of power gain is required at each pass, the modulator is longer than in a conventional HGHG scheme.

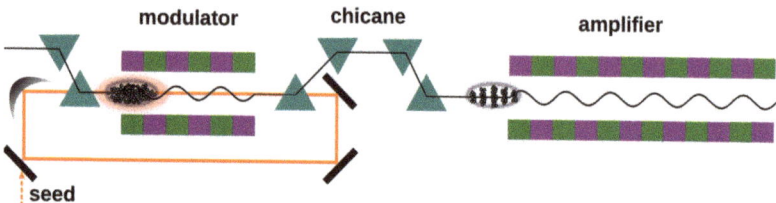

Figure 1. In an oscillator-based HGHG scheme, an optical cavity is added and encloses the modulator. The optical cavity acts as a feedback system which maintains the peak power of the stored radiation field and, under perfect synchronism, this field is used to seed consecutive electron bunches arriving from the linac upstream the cavity. Note that in reality, the optical cavity design will be more complex than this simplified sketch.

2.1.2. Echo-Enabled Harmonic Generation (EEHG)

HGHG schemes are characterized by a limited up-frequency conversion efficiency due to the fact that the nth harmonic requires the energy modulation to be n times larger than the slice energy spread to maximize the bunching. This is typically limiting the conversion to $n = 15$ and critically depends on the energy spread [37]. The EEHG scheme [13–15] was proposed to overcome this limitation, achieve higher harmonics and, thus, shorter wavelengths. In this scheme, there are two seed lasers with two modulators, two dispersive sections, and one radiator. The first modulator and seed laser are used to induce an energy modulation, and then the first dispersive section, which has a large longitudinal dispersion, shreds the longitudinal phase space of the electron beam creating thin energy bands. Each of these bands has a lower energy spread than the initial one, and this way a lower energy modulation is required in the second modulator compared to HGHG. The second dispersive section is weaker and compresses the energy bands. Similarly to what happens in HGHG, it converts the energy modulation from the second modulator into a density modulation, which in this case can have higher harmonic content.

In a regular single-pass EEHG, two modulators and two seed lasers are needed. In order to convert the classic scheme to a high repetition rate cavity-FEL, one possibility is to include two cavities, one for each modulator. In the case of two cavities, the wavelength can be chosen independently and the high repetition rate is secured. Another solution is to feed one modulator with an external seed laser and place the other modulator in a cavity. In this case, the repetition rate of the external seed laser source determines the overall repetition rate. This seed laser should have a longer wavelength which is at present already available at high repetition rate. Then, the other modulator which is enclosed in the optical cavity is resonant to a shorter wavelength.

It is important to investigate if it is more advantageous to have the shortest wavelength at the first or the second modulator. We study the specific case of a combination of two seed laser wavelengths of 300 nm and 50 nm by using an electron beam with a nominal energy of 1.35 GeV, energy spread of 120 keV, and energy modulation amplitudes of $A_1 = 3$ and $A_2 = 5$ times the energy spread in the first and second modulator, respectively. These parameters fit the choices of the FLASH2020+ project [38]. The resulting maximum bunching factor b [13] for final wavelengths between 2 nm and 6 nm is shown in Figure 2a. Using a seed with a wavelength of 50 nm in the first modulator and 300 nm in the second modulator is not beneficial in terms of bunching compared to the classic scheme with two seed lasers with a wavelength of 300 nm, whereas much higher bunching can be achieved by utilizing the shorter seed in the second modulator. Both 50 nm configurations drastically reduce the required longitudinal dispersion of the first chicane, as can be seen in Figure 2b. As the second chicane converts the energy modulation from the second modulator, a seed wavelength of 50 nm in this modulator results in an approximately six times smaller optimum dispersive strength than the one needed for a 300 nm seed.

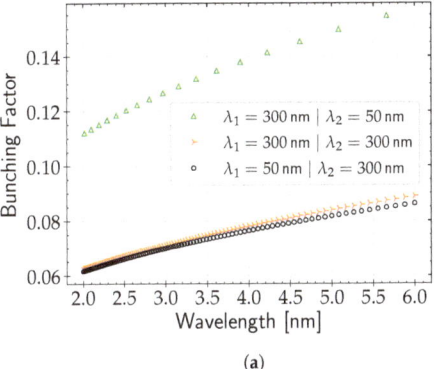 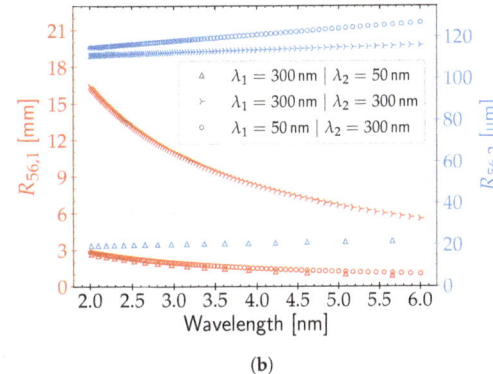

Figure 2. (**a**) Maximum bunching factor for different combinations of seed laser wavelengths. (**b**) Optimum setup of the chicanes to maximize the bunching factor. The working point resulting in a lower $R_{56,1}$ is shown for each configuration.

A tunable seed around 50 nm in the second modulator would allow to overcome the limitations of the wavelength separation of the harmonics and provide access to a continuous wavelength range and high bunching. For example, a final target wavelength of 4 nm with more than 13% bunching could be achieved either by a 47.4 nm or a 51.3 nm seed. The preferred setup with the second modulator enclosed in a cavity and thus being resonant to a shorter seed is shown in Figure 3. As a final remark, we note that one cavity could be employed for both modulators, which would be preferred in terms of cavity length requirements. However, in this case, the peak power of the radiation cannot be tuned independently at the two modulators which is an important aspect of the optimization of EEHG.

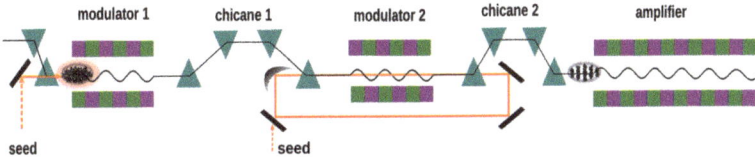

Figure 3. In an oscillator-based EEHG scheme, one or two optical cavities can be attached. In this figure, the first modulation occurs with a conventional external seed laser, while the second energy modulation is achieved by employing an optical cavity around the second modulator. The optical cavity is fed by a seed laser and maintains its properties in order to seed consecutive electron bunches.

To demonstrate the feasibility of the proposed EEHG configuration, a single-pass full simulation with the FEL code Genesis 1.3 [39] is carried out. The wavelengths of the first and the second seed laser are 300 nm and 50 nm, respectively. The electron beam parameters are the same as those used in the already presented analytical calculations above, and in addition, the normalized emittance is 0.6 mm mrad, the electron bunch length is 314 fs full width at half max (FWHM), and the current profile is Gaussian with a peak of 500 A. The duration of the Gaussian seed laser pulses is set to 150 fs and 50 fs FWHM for the first and second seed laser, respectively. The simulation is optimized for an output wavelength of 2.013 nm with longitudinal dispersions of $R_{56,1} = 2.649$ mm and $R_{56,2} = 17.50\,\mu$m. The radiator has a period length of $\lambda_u = 19$ mm and is tuned to the output wavelength. The bunching along the electron bunch upstream from the radiator, the evolution of the FEL peak power along the radiator, as well as the spectrum and power profile at the same position in the radiator are presented in Figure 4. The bunching amplitude is approximately 9.5% and thus slightly smaller than the 11.2% predicted by the simple analytical model (see Figure 2a), but still more than sufficient for an efficient amplification in the radiator.

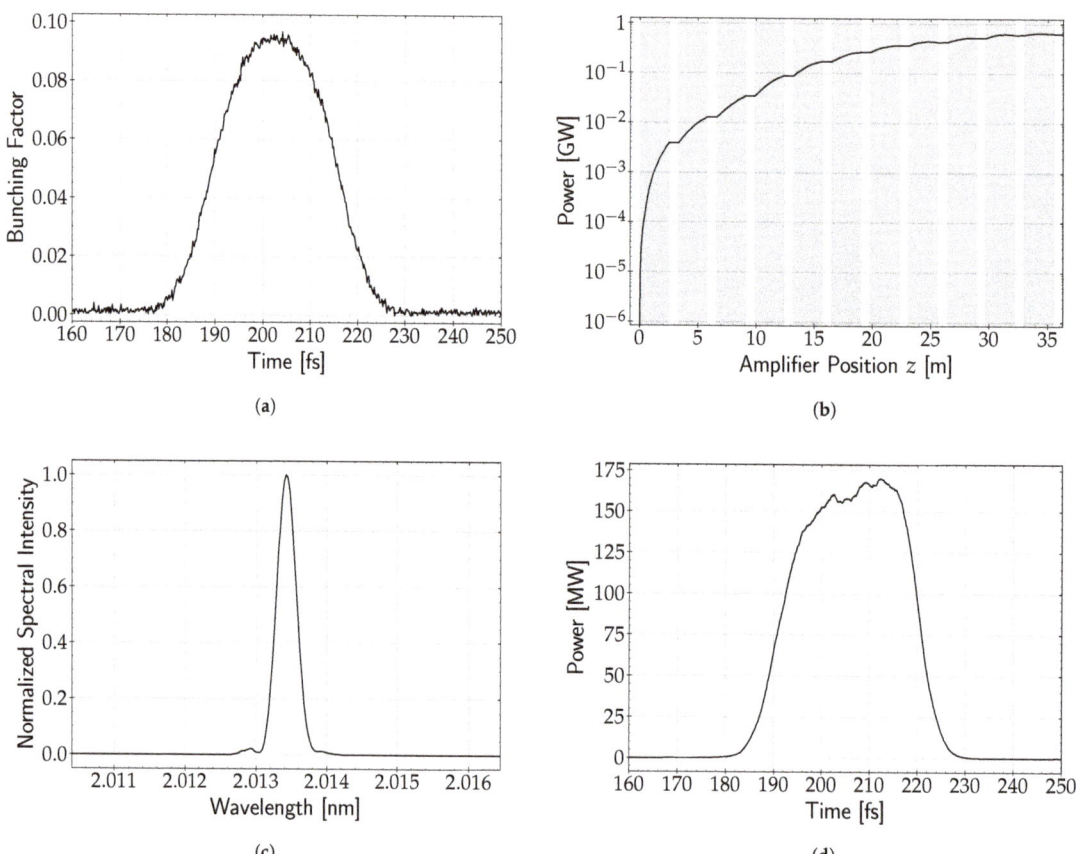

Figure 4. (**a**) Bunching along the electron bunch. (**b**) FEL peak power along the amplifier modules (gray). (**c**) Spectrum after the 5 modules of the amplifier. (**d**) Power profile after 5 modules of the amplifier.

2.2. Employing an Oscillator-Based Seeding Scheme in an Accelerator in Continuous-Wave or Burst-Mode Operation

A seeded oscillator-amplifier scheme is suitable for accelerators that can generate electron bunches at high repetition rates, as it requires a cavity length which matches the electron bunch repetition rate. The cavity roundtrip length should be $L_{cav} = c/(m \cdot f_{rep})$, where f_{rep} refers to the electron bunch separation and m is an integer which represents the number of roundtrips of the radiation before it meets again an electron bunch. For instance, when the electron bunches arrive with a frequency of 1 MHz, the total roundtrip cavity length should be $L_{cav} \approx 300$ m for $m = 1$. Alternatively, the radiation pulse can perform more than one roundtrip in between two consecutive bunches. However, in this case the total resonator reflectivity decreases with the number of passes m as R^m.

A superconducting accelerator can run in continuous wave (CW) or burst-mode operation. At FLASH [40,41], which operates in burst-mode, the bunch trains arrive with a repetition rate of 10 Hz with a flattop of 800 µs and a bunch spacing of 1 µs (1 MHz repetition rate). With a pulsed operation at 10 Hz as well, the flattop of the European XFEL is 600 µs with a 0.22 µs bunch separation (4.5 MHz) [42]. The exact number of bunches available depends on the operation mode and the sharing of those bunches among different undulator beamlines. In the case of burst-mode operation, there is a specific number of bunches available to build-up the peak power and stability needed to deliver seeded FEL pulses. This is not an issue when the process starts with a low repetition rate seed laser source because the steady-state regime is reached within a few passes [22] as shown in Figure 5a, but it is critical when starting from shot noise, as we show in Figure 5b. The build-up regime is marked with a green background color. During this process, there must be positive net gain, and the peak power in each pass increases. The steady-state regime is marked with blue color in the same figure, and refers to the passes in the oscillator where the net gain is zero and the peak power per pass is constant. Comparing Figure 5a,b, there are more power fluctuations in the case where we start with a seed laser. This might be due to the fact that in this case we do not use a monochromator.

In burst-mode operation, the more bunches are used during the build-up process, the less bunches will be part of the steady-state regime when seeded radiation is generated. The steady-state can be maintained for a maximum number of passes defined by the difference between the available bunches in one bunch train and the number of bunches used during the build-up process. Taking as an example FLASH and the build-up regime shown in Figure 5b, we would need 18 bunches to take part in the build-up of the power, and the remaining 782 bunches would be part of the steady-state regime where the seeded radiation is generated.

A machine operated in CW mode offers a continuous number of bunches with a constant separation between them. For instance, SHINE in Shanghai will be operated in a CW mode and is expected to provide bunches with a continuous 1 MHz repetition rate [43]. The same repetition rate is planned for LCLS-II [44] as well. In this case, the build-up time needed becomes less important. It is possible to increase the number of passes in the build-up regime and ensure a smooth transition to the steady state. However, it becomes more important to verify how long the steady-state regime can be maintained before the process needs to be initiated again.

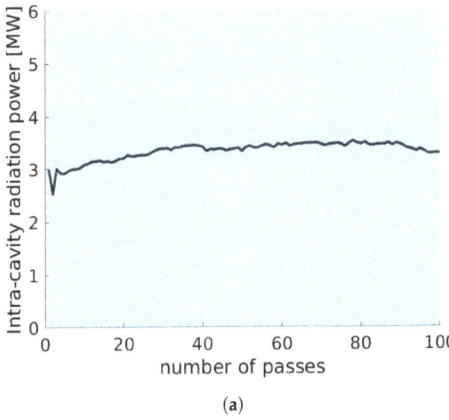
(a)

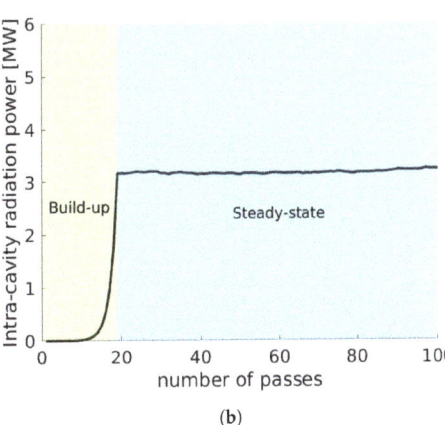
(b)

Figure 5. (a) Example of the peak power per pass in an oscillator starting with a low repetition rate seed laser. From the first pass already the net gain should be zero. In practice, it takes a few passes for the system to self-stabilize. (b) Example of the peak power per pass in an oscillator starting from shot-noise. For 19 passes the build-up regime where the net gain is positive is highlighted with a green color. At pass 19, the desired peak power level is reached and the steady state regime is entered, marked with a blue color. From this pass and onward, the net gain is reduced to zero and the peak power level is maintained in each pass.

3. Resonator Considerations

3.1. A Simple Model for the Reflectivity Requirements and Estimated Power Level in the Cavity

The transition between the build-up and the steady-state regime in the case of start-up from shot noise is discussed in more detail in Section 4, while here we focus on the steady-state operation of the modulator-amplifier. We maintain the generality of the discussion by using approximations to build a simple model that can be used to investigate the parameter space for the design requirements. In the steady-state regime, there is a number of conditions that need to be fulfilled:

- The input seed power needs to exceed the shot noise power of the electron beam by several orders of magnitude; otherwise, the SASE is not suppressed and the seeding process is not successful. Only a part of the seed power contributes to the exponential growth. Using for estimation the 1D cold FEL model this fraction amounts to 1/9. Assuming an excess of 3 orders of magnitude, the minimum input seed laser pulse peak power needs to be at least several 10 kW to 100 kW, depending on the exact electron beam parameters [45]. In addition, for seeding techniques it is required to induce an energy modulation of several times the initial energy spread which depends on the target harmonic to be amplified, the exact seeding scheme and the modulator length for given electron beam parameters. Typically, this requires a peak power that is larger than 100 kW.
- The saturation power downstream of the modulator needs to be well below the "natural" saturation to avoid large induced energy spread, which would suppress the amplification process at the amplifier. As a general rule, the energy spread downstream of the modulator σ_E relative to the electron beam energy E, should be considerably less than the FEL parameter of the amplifier ρ_{amp} [46], thus $\sigma_E/E \ll \rho_{amp}$ [45]. The maximum acceptable seed peak power after amplification in the modulator strongly depends on the length of the modulator with respect to the gain length, and thus on the power amplification and on the energy spread increase. For the sake of avoiding a specific parameter set, here we assume that saturation at the seed laser wavelength yields between 1 GW to several 10 GW. Assuming a margin of 3 orders of magnitude to avoid "heating" of the beam, the seed peak power after amplification needs to be limited to not more than several tens of MW.

The gain from shot noise to saturation of an FEL is around 9 orders of magnitude, which corresponds to about 20 power gain lengths (L_g). This means that there are 3 orders of magnitude between the minimum input peak power (P_{in}) and the maximum output peak power which are allowed to be lost in the cavity. Otherwise, either the minimum power is too close to shot noise or the maximum power too close to saturation. It is clear that these boundaries are not very strict and should only be seen as an approximation. It is known that the power along z develops as [46]:

$$P(z) = \frac{P_{in}}{9} \cdot e^{z/L_g}. \tag{1}$$

With a roundtrip reflectivity R, the power after a modulator length of L_{mod} should be $P(L_{mod}) = P_{in}/R$. This leads to

$$\frac{P_{in}}{R} = \frac{P_{in}}{9} \cdot e^{L_{mod}/L_g} \rightarrow L_{mod} = L_g \cdot \ln(\frac{9}{R}) \tag{2}$$

For the first approximately three power gain lengths we expect no FEL power amplification, and this is referred to as the lethargy regime. Assuming three orders of magnitude for the maximum allowed power amplification, the maximum modulator length is $9 \cdot L_g$ to compensate losses. The same equation can be used for design considerations; for instance, for a total reflectivity of 6%, the modulator should be roughly $5 \cdot L_g$. This result is independent of the input seed laser power, however, in practice, the energy modulation process depends on both the input seed peak power and the length of the modulator as [47]:

$$\Delta E = \sqrt{\frac{P_{in}}{P_0}} \frac{m_e 2 K L_{mod} JJ}{\gamma w_0}, \quad (3)$$

where w_0 is the seed waist size, K is the dimensionless undulator parameter, m_e is the electron mass in keV, $P_0 \approx 8.7\,GW$ [47], $JJ = J_0(\xi) - J_1(\xi)$, where $\xi = K^2/(4+2K^2)$ and $J_{0,1}$ the Bessel function of the zeroth and first order. As the modulator is used both for energy modulation and amplification, both these aspects need to be taken into account for the exact design. Let us consider an example of these analytical estimations by means of a reasonable set of parameters: $\lambda_{seed} = 50\,nm$, $K = 3.25$, $w_0 = 286\,\mu m$, $\gamma = 2641.9$, $L_g = 1.12\,m$. In Figure 6, we show the expected energy modulation for a combination of seed laser peak power and modulator length, calculated with Equation (3). In the same figure, we show the reflectivity required as expected by the 1D cold theory and Equation (1) with the dashed black vertical lines, as it is independent of the input seed laser power. It is clear that while the modulator length is fixed and is used to determine the amplification, for a given modulator length, it is still possible to use the seed laser peak power as a knob to adjust the energy modulation. In turn, the energy modulation is related to the energy spread which affects the FEL process in the amplifier, as already discussed. Note that while Equations (1) and (3) are well established approximations valid in the 1D case, diffraction effects should be also taken into account and the exact dependencies may deviate from this result.

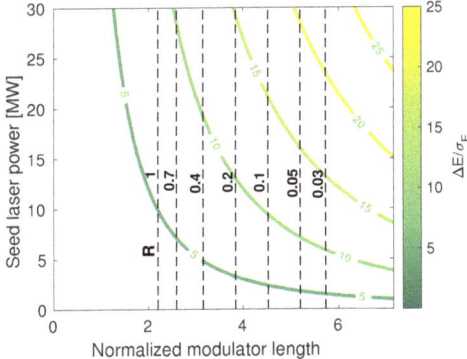

Figure 6. The color bar indicates the energy modulation achieved for combinations of seed laser peak powers (P_{in}) and modulator lengths (L_{mod}) and is calculated with Equation (3). The horizontal axis shows the normalized modulator length to the gain length (L_{mod}/L_g). The vertical dashed lines show the reflectivity R required for equilibrium between amplification and losses for different normalized modulator lengths, and is calculated with Equation (2).

3.2. Cavity Design Considerations

The numbers quoted so far are needed for the system to work, and should be complementary with a discussion on the technical feasibility of the resonator. The important questions here are if the downstream mirror, which will have the maximum power density, will be able to withstand it, and if mirrors with the required properties actually exist. We consider two operation regimes for the resonator: one at a wavelength between 200 nm and 300 nm, and one between 50 nm and 100 nm.

Regarding the reflectivity requirements, we expect that for wavelengths around 300 nm, the mirror choice will not pose an issue as there are options to choose from. Optics in this wavelength regime are used for current laser systems, such as dielectric mirrors, with reflectivity and damage threshold that guarantee sustainable operation and have been studied for other storage ring FELs in the past as well [48]. The main challenge is faced for the working point in the XUV range between 100 nm and 50 nm, where no commonly used options are available. Here, we consider the upper limit in gain, where the roundtrip loss should not exceed a factor 1000 to avoid electron beam heating. Under normal incidence, this means that each mirror should reflect at least $1/\sqrt{1000} \approx 1/33$ or 3%. In case of a ring resonator with mirrors at 45 degree incidence angle, each should reflect more than $1/\sqrt{\sqrt{1000}} \approx 1/5.6$ or 18%. For example, we consider Molybdenum mirrors. At normal incidence, the reflectivity at 40 nm is ~6%, at 45 degree around 40% [49]. Both values exceed the requirements. Note that a gain of 1000 is an upper limit that would require a relatively long modulator. However, it is preferred to operate at a lower gain if the reflectivity of mirrors allows it.

Here, we consider simple estimations in order to calculate the power density for a Gaussian beam. Assuming a Gaussian beam with a waist at the end of the undulator, the size of the spot at the mirror is [47]:

$$w^2(L) = w_0^2 \left(1 + \left(\frac{L}{\ell}\right)^2\right), \quad (4)$$

where L is the distance from the undulator to the mirror, w_0 is the spotsize at the waist and ℓ is the Rayleigh length. With the distance to the mirror much larger than the Rayleigh length and remembering that for a Gaussian beam $\pi w_0^2 = \lambda \ell$ with λ the radiation wavelength, the dependence of the beam radius on the distance becomes nearly linear and we can rewrite Equation (4) as

$$w^2(L) \approx \left(\frac{L\lambda}{\pi w_0}\right)^2 \approx \left(\frac{L\lambda}{\pi \sigma_b}\right)^2, \quad (5)$$

where we have approximated the spotsize of the radiation with the electron beam size σ_b. Since the mirror has an angle with respect to the radiation in one plane only, the area of the radiation on the mirror for a transversely symmetric beam can be approximated as:

$$S \approx \left(\frac{L\lambda}{\pi \sigma_b}\right)^2 \frac{1}{\sin \alpha}, \quad (6)$$

with α the glancing angle.

Assuming that the fraction of the pulse energy that is not reflected by the mirror is in fact absorbed, the power density P_d absorbed is

$$P_d = \frac{E_p}{S} \cdot (1 - R) = E_p(1 - R) \sin \alpha \left(\frac{\pi \sigma_b}{L\lambda}\right)^2, \quad (7)$$

with E_p the pulse energy.

Here, we take the example of FLASH2 and the existing mirrors commonly used in FLASH operation to demonstrate a feasible working point. For a wavelength of 15 nm with a mirror 15 m downstream of the undulator under a glancing angle of 1 degree, from Equation (6) the spot size is approximately 0.3 cm², assuming a 100 µm beam size. With a reflectivity of 99% ($R = 0.99$) and 1 mJ of pulse energy per second for a single pulse, the power density is around 1 mW/0.3 cm², or up to 17 W/cm² for a pulse train of 5000 pulses per second. Under these assumptions and taking into account the reflectivity, the absorbed power of FLASH2 on the mirror is up to 170 mW/cm² for 15 nm.

For a modulator with the mirror at normal incidence at the same distance of 15 m, the same electron beam size and a wavelength of 50 nm, the spot is from Equation (5) approximately 2.4 by 2.4 mm. Assuming again Molybdenum mirrors with 95% absorption, the pulse energy should not exceed 2 µJ in order to avoid an absorbed power density higher than 170 mW/cm². At 45 degrees with 60% absorption, the pulse energy would be approximately 5 µJ. Assuming a typical pulse duration of 100 fs, the peak power is therefore 20 MW (or 50 MW for the 45 degree mirror case), which is consistent with the values mentioned earlier for FLASH. For a CW-FEL, the numbers are more critical because of the larger number of bunches per second.

Finally, we would like to comment on the geometry of the optical feedback system. There is a number of components needed in order to maintain a stable operation and diagnose the radiation field properties. The intensity of the seed laser, which in this case is the intensity inside the resonator, needs to be regulated and therefore measured for a large wavelength range without significant distortion of the radiation field. Furthermore, with the system starting from noise, the noise needs to be suppressed, which is best done with a grating. Finally, the radiation needs to be refocused in the middle of the modulator. Therefore, the actual resonator will have a more complicated geometry than depicted earlier. A ring resonator could include all needed elements, but other geometries should be considered and compared depending on the wavelength requirements and space constraints of a specific facility. The technical design and specifications are, however, beyond the scope of this paper.

4. Simulation Results and Implementation Considerations for Oscillator-Based Seeding Starting from Shot Noise

In this section, we focus on an HGHG-based oscillator scheme as shown in Figure 1 and more specifically, in the case of an oscillator-FEL starting from shot noise. As shown in Figure 5b, when the process in the cavity starts from shot noise, there are two separate operation regimes to be considered. For a transition from positive net gain ("build-up") to zero net gain ("steady-state"), the gain has to be reduced. Here, we discuss different methods that could be applied in order to achieve control over the power gain in the resonator. In all cases we use the same set of simulation parameters, which is summarized in Table 1, and the modulator is resonant with 50 nm wavelength. For the sake of simplicity, here we restrict ourselves to the case of a relative energy modulation $A = \Delta E / \sigma_E = 7$, meaning that the amplitude of the energy modulation ΔE after the modulator is seven times larger than the initial energy spread σ_E in the steady-state regime. As seen in Equation (3), for given lattice, electron beam parameters and constant waist size, the energy modulation is stabilized if the input peak power in the modulator P_{in} is stable too. All simulations here are done with Genesis 1.3 for the FEL process [39], while the radiation field in the cavity is treated with ocelot [50], which accounts for the slippage, reflectivity, focusing, and monochromatization.

Table 1. Electron beam parameters used in simulations.

Electron Beam Parameters	
Energy	1350 MeV
Energy spread	120 keV
Peak current	1 kA (flat-top)
Pulse duration	300 fs
Normalized Emittance	1 mm · mrad

4.1. Reflectivity Adjustment

The most direct way to control the net gain is to adjust the resonator reflectivity. In this case, initially the reflectivity ($R_{build-up}$) is as high as possible to enable a fast build-up of the power and then, when the desired peak power level is reached, the reflectivity has to drop to the value R_{equil}, which ensures equilibrium between losses and power gain. The reflectivity applied during the build-up process, $R_{build-up}$, is determined by the maximum total reflectivity allowed by the mirrors, and the maximum change in reflectivity that can be supported by a filter within the time separation of two consecutive bunches. The larger the difference in reflectivity $\Delta R = R_{build-up} - R_{equil}$ is, the higher the net gain and the faster the steady-state regime will start, as shown in Figure 7a. For the present setup of resonator and beam parameters shown in at Table 1, the reflectivity at equilibrium is $R_{equil} = 10.6\%$, including the losses in the monochromator. With $R_{build-up} = 14\%$, 46 passes are required in the build-up regime in order to reach a relative energy modulation of $A = 7$, while a reflectivity of $R_{build-up} = 12\%$ requires 99 passes. It is also possible to apply the reflectivity change in steps if a fast change is not possible. For instance, for the reflectivity change required as shown in Figure 7b, it is possible to apply the $\Delta R = 3.4\%$ (from $R_{build-up} = 14\%$ to $R_{equil} = 10.6\%$) in steps of $\Delta R = 0.34\%$ in 10 passes. In the case of a burst-mode of operation, the number of steps must be reasonably small compared to the number of bunches at the steady-state. In the case of a continuous wave operation, these steps can be as small as required by the hardware limitations.

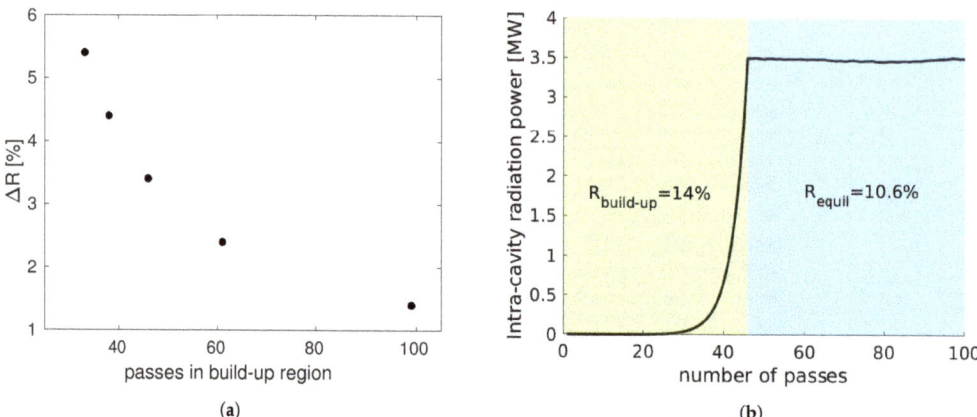

Figure 7. (a) In this plot, the number of passes needed to reach steady-state as function of reflectivity change, $\Delta R = R_{build-up} - R_{equil}$, is shown. We assume that the build-up process is over when the energy modulation is at least A = 7. (b) Example of $\Delta R = 3.4\%$. For the first 46 passes the reflectivity is set to $R_{build-up} = 14\%$ and from the 47th pass onward the reflectivity drops to $R_{equil} = 10.6\%$ and the net gain is zero. As a result, the peak power is stabilized.

In practice, the reflectivity change can be implemented by adding a filter in the return path of the radiation field. A total reflectivity change of several percent is currently not possible to be applied within 1 μs, but would be possible in several steps during a transition time. For this reason, this method would be an option in CW machines, as it is currently unlikely to function in burst-mode in view of time constraints.

4.2. Longitudinal Overlap between Electron Bunch and the Recirculating Light Pulses

Another method to obtain gain control is by affecting the longitudinal overlap between the electron bunch and the stored radiation field. A change in cavity length would change the arrival time of the radiation pulse, a procedure known as cavity detuning. The exact amount of the detuning or delay needed to transition between positive net gain and zero net gain depends on the electron bunch length. Here, we have assumed a 300 fs flat-top current distribution for the electron bunch as an example study.

For all passes, the reflectivity is set to a value R_{set} which is larger than R_{equil}, namely, the reflectivity, which leads to zero net gain when the longitudinal synchronism between the electron bunches and the recirculated seed pulse is optimum. Here, we define the cavity length L_{cav} for which the detuning is zero ($\Delta L_{cav} = 0$), as the cavity length for perfect synchronism between the radiation pulses and consecutive electron bunches for no slippage, thus it is the cold cavity length. Due to slippage effects, perfect synchronism is achieved for longer cavity lengths ($\Delta L_{cav} > 0$) that allow the longitudinally advanced radiation pulse to be delayed. As in this case we assume that the reflectivity cannot be reduced, we keep the reflectivity constant over all passes and we de-tune the cavity by ΔL_{cav} to reduce the net gain in the steady-state regime. The detuning and the reflectivity are two complementary knobs. The larger the reflectivity difference $\Delta R = R_{set} - R_{equil}$ is, the longer the detuning is needed.

In Figure 8a, a cavity detuning is simulated for a range of set reflectivities R_{set} between 11% and 15%. The cavity detuning curve for each reflectivity shows how much the length of the cavity should be shifted to move from the maximum net gain (shown with the vertical arrow), to zero net gain (intersections between the horizontal dashed line and detuning curve). The cavity detuning for maximum power gain is independent of the total reflectivity as expected, as it depends on the total slippage per pass, which is in turn dependent on the wavelength, the periods of the modulator and the group velocity of the field. Taking again the example of $R_{set} = 14\%$, in Figure 7a we need 46 passes to reach the desired in-cavity peak power level with the optimum detuning of $\Delta L_{cav} = 2.7\,\mu m$, and from Figure 8b we see that a detuning of $\Delta L_{cav} = -14.1\,\mu m$ keeps the in-cavity peak power level constant. The result is shown in Figure 8b, where the cavity length is shifted by 16.8 µm and equilibrium is reached and maintained.

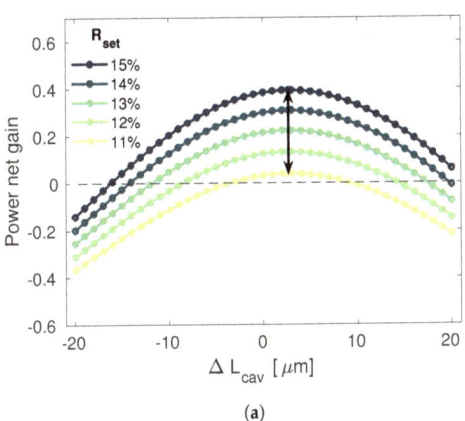 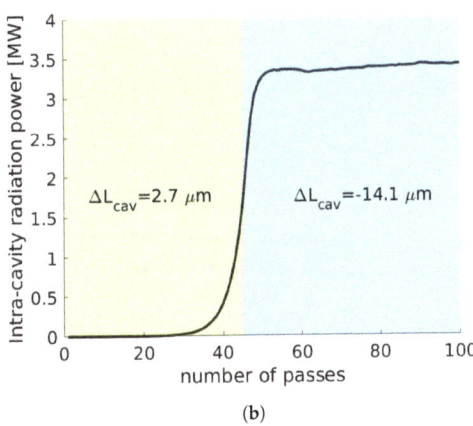

Figure 8. (a) Detuning curves for a 300 fs flat-top electron beam. The optimum detuning length is at $\Delta \lambda = 2.7\,\mu m$, for all set reflectivities, as shown with the vertical arrow. The zero net gain point shown with the horizontal dashed line, shows the detuning that needs to be applied to reach equilibrium for each total reflectivity R_{set}. Keeping the reflectivity constant and changing the cavity length can transition the system from positive to zero net gain. We remind the readers that the power net gain has no units as it is the difference between the peak power at the beginning of pass n + 1 and at pass n, divided by the peak power at pass n. (b) With an oscillator starting from the random fluctuation of the electron beam distribution, a transition between amplification of the power and maintenance of the peak power is achieved by detuning the cavity length from $\Delta L_{cav} = 2.7\,\mu m$ to $\Delta L_{cav} = -14.1\,\mu m$. For all passes the reflectivity is $R_{set} = 14\%$.

For the implementation of this technique there are different options that can be considered. When detuning the cavity length, the position of one or more mirrors needs to be adjusted within µm and with a MHz repetition rate. This depends heavily on the mirror choice and mirror size and weight. As an alternative solution, in the past a similar dynamic cavity desynchronization was considered for FELIX [51] in order to control the growth rate and the final power at saturation and the fluctuations in power [52,53]. It was proposed that instead of mechanically adjusting the mirrors, it is preferable to ramp the electron bunch repetition rate frequency by Δf_{rep} to achieve a cavity detuning of $\Delta L_{cav} = L\Delta f_{rep}/f_{rep}$ [53]. In this case, a dynamic desynchronization along the bunch train is important.

As a final remark, it is important to point out that the cavity detuning results in a change in the temporal and spectral distribution of the stored FEL pulse. This has been extensively discussed in FEL oscillators in the past [54–56]. The consequences on the properties of the output FEL should be carefully considered before applying this method for power gain control.

4.3. Optical Klystron

Another well-established method of gain control in FELs is the use of an Optical Klystron (OK), first introduced in [57]. It was originally introduced for gain control in oscillator FELs [58], but its application has been expanded. It has been used as a method to speed up the FEL process in SASE operation, when the total amplifier length is not sufficient for a given wavelength [59–61]. In addition, it is used in a seeding scheme when the seed laser peak power is not sufficient to increase the energy modulation required in seeding [17]. The simplest configuration of an optical klystron consists of two undulators tuned at the same resonant wavelength and a dispersive section in between them. The electron beam travels in the first undulator starting from some initial conditions (noise, or external seed) and a relatively weak energy modulation is induced. Then, the dispersive element modifies the electron beam phase space. This way, the bunching at this fundamental wavelength is increased, and the bunched electron beam generates coherent emission in the second undulator with increased gain. The dependence of the power gain on the longitudinal dispersion is a useful knob for our setup.

In an oscillator, the two modulator sections separated by the dispersive section are in the resonator as shown in Figure 9. A 1D theory of optical klystron is discussed in [61] and a recent revision can be found in [62]. The optimum longitudinal dispersion depends on the energy spread and in our case can be estimated as

$$R_{56,1} = \frac{\lambda_{res}}{2\pi\delta}, \tag{8}$$

where δ is the relative energy spread. With the studied parameter space, the optimum longitudinal dispersion is predicted as $R_{56,1} = 89\ \mu m$. Note that the sum of the length of modulator 1 and modulator 2 in Figure 9 is equal to the length of the modulator in Figure 1, so the power gain increase is introduced by chicane 1 only, and not by increasing the length of the modulator.

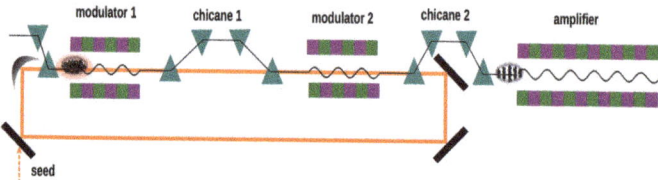

Figure 9. In an oscillator-based HGHG scheme, an optical klystron can be employed. To do so, the cavity contains two modulators separated by a chicane. This way this chicane can be tuned to control the gain per pass.

In order to transition to the zero net gain regime, the $R_{56,1}$ should initially be set to a value close to the optimal, and later on tuned to another value which would reduce the gain in the second modulator. In Figure 10a, we show the net gain achieved for different reflectivities and $R_{56,1}$. The $R_{56,1}$ at the steady state is determined by the intersection of the curves and the horizontal dashed line, which shows the zero net gain. We are interested in the range $R_{56,1} < 75\ \mu m$, because a too large $R_{56,1}$ would cause an over-rotation of the longitudinal phase space which is not useful, as we still need to increase the bunching at a harmonic of the seed wavelength with the $R_{56,2}$. The optimum longitudinal dispersion appears at around $R_{56,1} = 73\ \mu m$, which is approximately in agreement with Equation (8). Note, here, that the reflectivities required with the optical klystron are dramatically reduced, by more than an order of magnitude, when we compare to Figure 8a. As an example, with a reflectivity $R_{set} = 0.38\%$, we can build-up the peak power needed for seeding with $R_{56,1} = 42.5\ \mu m$, and after 19 passes change the longitudinal dispersion of the first chicane to $R_{56,1} = 30\ \mu m$ to achieve zero net gain, and stable peak power of the radiation field per pass as shown in Figure 10b. Note, here, that the input peak power is considerably lower in the order of 120 kW compared to the roughly 3.5 MW needed in all other gain-control methods presented already, to achieve the same energy modulation $A = 7$. In addition, the reflectivity required, $R_{set} = 0.38\%$, which considerably relaxes the requirements on the mirror specifications.

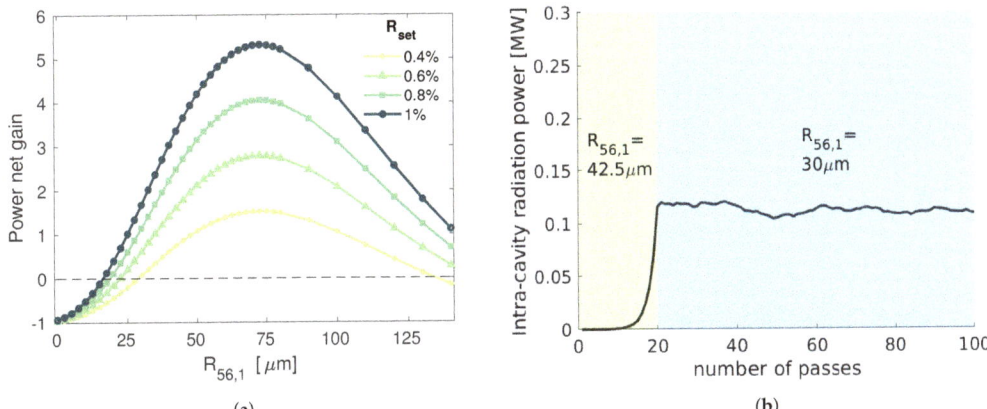

Figure 10. (**a**) Changing the $R_{56,1}$ of the chicane affects drastically the gain in power. Here we show the net power gain for selected set reflectivities R_{set}, between 0.4% and 1%. The horizontal line shows the zero net gain. (**b**) With a reflectivity $R_{set} = 0.38\%$, it is possible to transition from positive gain to zero gain by adjusting the longitudinal dispersion of chicane1 as shown in Figure 8, from $R_{56,1} = 42.5\,\mu\text{m}$ to $R_{56,1} = 30\,\mu\text{m}$, respectively.

The optical klystron has many advantages. As already explained, the first one is that it makes the transition from positive to zero net gain possible. In addition, it increases the gain both in the positive gain regime and in the zero net gain regime as $R_{56,1} \neq 0$ as well. This relaxes significantly the requirements in mirror reflectivity in the XUV range. Moreover, the optical klystron could be used as an active tuning tool to adjust the gain per pass and absorb different sources of jitter which contribute to gain changes. Concerning technical requirements, a chicane consisting of fast kickers for this purpose should be able to change the R_{56} by several µm and with a MHz repetition rate. Stripline fast kickers are already standard technology and are, for instance, used at the European XFEL for extracting individual electron bunches with up to 4.5 MHz repetition rate [63,64]. Let us assume that a change of 10 µm is sufficient to transition from positive net gain to zero net gain. The longitudinal dispersion of the chicane is approximately $R_{56} \approx L\theta^2$, where L is the distance between the first and second dipole of a chicane and θ is the bending angle of the first dipole. A kicker adds an angle

$$\Delta\theta[\mu\text{rad}] = L_{kicker}[\text{cm}] B_{kicker}[\text{Gauss}] / E_b[\text{GeV}],$$

with L_{kicker} and B_{kicker} being the length and field of the kicker and E_b the electron beam energy. With these kickers, a kick angle of 0.6 mrad can be achieved with $E_b = 1$ GeV and the change of R_{56} shown in Figure 10b would be possible within 1 µs. It is important to ensure that implementing this change in R_{56} will not affect the stability of the system. Using the kickers only in the build-up regime would ensure stability during the steady-state regime. For the build-up regime, the stability is not so important, as long as the peak power is reached, since during these passes no seeded radiation is generated.

5. Comparison of Simulation Results

Until now, we have only discussed about the process in the modulator and resonator. In this section, we compare simulation results at a final wavelength of 4.167 nm, reached with different schemes and this time we show the final FEL pulses generated at the amplifier. For the HGHG simulations, this wavelength is the 12th harmonic of a 50 nm resonant modulator. We consider the following four cases:

- A SASE setup, starting from shot noise and without changing any electron beam parameters. The FEL pulse is extracted at the same position as the seeding simulations.
- A single-pass standard HGHG setup, starting with an ideal Gaussian seed laser pulse instead.
- An HGHG seeded oscillator-amplifier starting with a low repetition rate seed laser. This scheme was discussed in detail in [22]. For the first electron bunch an external seed laser pulse is injected, and then the seed pulse is stored in the cavity.
- An HGHG seeded oscillator-amplifier system starting from shot noise. This was described in detail in Section 4. A reflectivity change from $R_{build-up} = 14\%$ to $R_{equil} = 10.6\%$ was used to transition from positive to zero net gain.

In Table 2, we have summarized the main simulation results for the four different cases, and in Figure 11 we show the final spectra for the four different cases with the same final wavelength of 4.167 nm. In addition, for completeness, we have added the pulse properties of the output FEL at 2 nm with the EEHG simulations discussed in Section 2.1.2. The output FEL is shown in Figure 4. Note that the peak power is comparable for all HGHG seeded pulses as expected; however, as the resulting pulse duration differs, the bandwidth cannot be directly compared. It is important to emphasize that a single-spike spectrum was generated in all seeded schemes. The power spectral density in the multi-pass HGHG starting with a seed laser, and in the standard single-pass HGHG are almost identical, while the multi-pass HGHG starting from shot noise seems to have almost an order of magnitude higher spectral density as shown in Figure 11d. In this case, we have used a monochromator with an rms bandwidth of $\Delta\lambda/\lambda = 2.5 \times 10^{-4}$ in the resonator, which stretches the radiation pulses and filters the radiation in the frequency domain. Because of this, the result in Figure 11d deviates compared to the other two HGHG cases.

Table 2. Simulation results for final FEL pulse at the same position along amplifier. For the multi-pass simulations, we examine the FEL pulse after 100 passes. For the SASE, we calculate based on the average over 50 simulations with different shot noise. For EEHG, we consider the simulation results of a 2 nm output FEL shown in Figure 4.

	Peak Power	$\Delta\lambda_{FWHM}/\lambda$	rms Pulse Duration
SASE	3 MW	2×10^{-3}	75 fs
Standard HGHG	1.2 GW	1.6×10^{-4}	20 fs
multi-pass HGHG (seed)	1.2 GW	2×10^{-4}	27 fs
multi-pass HGHG (shot-noise)	1.1 GW	5×10^{-5}	60.6 fs
single-pass EEHG	0.18 GW	1.6×10^{-4}	11.35 fs

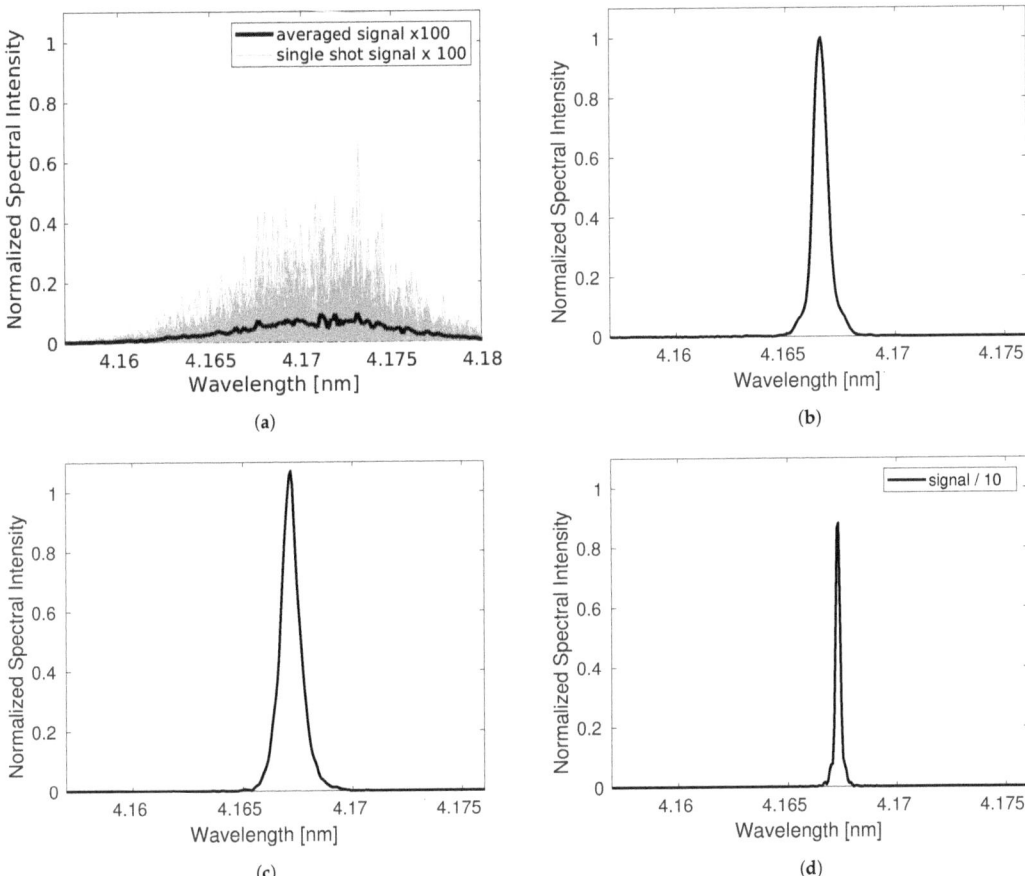

Figure 11. Spectra of final FEL pulse at the same position at the amplifier and with the same electron beam parameters shown at Table 1. The spectral intensity is normalized to the peak intensity calculated at the standard single-pass HGHG simulation. (**a**) SASE. Please notice the extended horizontal axis. The average SASE spectrum over 50 shots is shown with the black line. (**b**) Standard HGHG in a single-pass. (**c**) Oscillator-FEL starting with an external seed laser pulse. (**d**) Oscillator-FEL starting from shot-noise.

6. Discussion

In this paper, we described different seeding schemes that can benefit by employing an oscillator setup to increase the repetition rate of a seeded FEL. We presented an overview of simulations and requirements for its implementation. We developed a simple model to estimate the amplification and modulation process in the modulator. This gave an insight into the design of the resonator in terms of modulator length, resonator requirements, and feasibility of the implementation of this scheme. Then, we focused on simulation results of an HGHG scheme. We showed that there is a number of methods that could be used to dynamically control the power gain in the resonator when the process starts from shot-noise and we compared the performance of a single pass HGHG, a multi-pass HGHG starting with a low repetition rate seed laser and of SASE, which is to be considered as our background.

Where so far the wavelength range mentioned here could only be reached with an EEHG scheme, the use of a resonator now would make it possible to reach the same wavelength with an HGHG scheme. Alternatively, starting with a shorter wavelength in an EEHG scheme, the use of the resonator could push the minimum wavelength beyond the water window and transition metals, making seeding in this important wavelength range possible. These options will be studied in future studies.

In addition, there are still a number of considerations that need to be addressed as we are moving towards more detailed studies for the realization of this scheme. Even though first stability studies were presented in [22], it is still crucial to study the stability of this scheme over several passes with a non-ideal electron beam, including imperfections and energy chirp effects. In addition, there are other important questions related to its implementation, such as how the repetition rate can be adjusted when experiments need a lower repetition rate, the space constraints to insert mirrors when the longitudinal dispersion required for seeding at short wavelengths is small, the requirements in terms of diagnostics for the recirculating radiation field, and realizing wavelength tunability. These are expected to be addressed in future work.

Author Contributions: Conceptualization, B.F.; data curation, G.P. and F.P.; validation, G.P., B.F. and G.G.; formal analysis, G.P.; writing—Original draft preparation, G.P.; writing—Review and editing, G.P., S.A., B.F., G.G., T.L., F.P., L.S. and J.Z.; project administration, G.P. and G.G. All authors have read and agreed to the published version of the manuscript.

Funding: This work was supported by the Impuls- und Vernetzungsfond der Helmholtz-Gemeinschaft e.V. within the CAS-Helmholtz International Laboratory on Free-Electron Laser Science and Technology (CHILFEL), grant number InterLabs-0002.

Institutional Review Board Statement: Not applicable.

Informed Consent Statement: Not applicable.

Data Availability Statement: Not applicable.

Acknowledgments: The authors would like to thank Fred Bijkerk for consultation regarding mirrors in the EUV, Frank Obier for information on kickers, Enrico Allaria and Pardis Niknejadi for useful discussions, and the Maxwell computational resources operated at Deutsches Elektronen-Synchrotron (DESY), Hamburg, Germany. Finally the authors thank Chao Feng, and Elke Ploenjes-Palm for a careful proofreading of the manuscript.

Conflicts of Interest: The authors declare no conflict of interest.

References

1. Saldin, E.L.; Schneidmiller, E.A.; Yurkov, M.V. *The Physics of Free Electron Lasers*; Springer: Berlin/Heidelberg, Germany, 2000.
2. Saldin, E.; Schneidmiller, E.; Yurkov, M. Statistical Properties of Radiation from VUV and X-ray Free Electron Laser. *Opt. Commun.* **1998**, *148*, 383–403. [CrossRef]
3. Amann, J.; Berg, W.; Blank, V.; Decker, F.J.; Ding, Y.; Emma, P.; Feng, Y.; Frisch, J.; Fritz, D.; Hastings, J.; et al. Demonstration of self-seeding in a hard-X-ray free-electron laser. *Nat. Photonics* **2012**, *6*, 693–698. [CrossRef]
4. Geloni, G.; Kocharyan, V.; Saldin, E. A novel self-seeding scheme for hard X-ray FELs. *J. Mod. Opt.* **2011**, *58*, 1391–1403. [CrossRef]
5. Rosenzweig, J.; Alesini, D.; Andonian, G.; Boscolo, M.; Dunning, M.; Faillace, L.; Ferrario, M.; Fukusawa, A.; Giannessi, L.; Hemsing, E.; et al. Generation of ultra-short, high brightness electron beams for single-spike SASE FEL operation. *Nucl. Instrum. Methods Phys. Res. Sect. Accel. Spectrometers Detect. Assoc. Equip.* **2008**, *593*, 39–44. [CrossRef]
6. Marinelli, A.; MacArthur, J.; Emma, P.; Guetg, M.; Field, C.; Kharakh, D.; Lutman, A.; Ding, Y.; Huang, Z. Experimental demonstration of a single-spike hard-X-ray free-electron laser starting from noise. *Appl. Phys. Lett.* **2017**, *111*, 151101. [CrossRef]
7. Prince, K.; Allaria, E.; Callegari, C.; Cucini, R.; Giovanni, D.N.; Di Mitri, S.; Diviacco, B.; Ferrari, E.; Finetti, P.; Gauthier, D.; et al. Coherent control with a short-wavelength Free Electron Laser. *Nat. Photonics* **2016**, *10*, 176–179. [CrossRef]
8. Gauthier, D.; Ribič, P.R.; De Ninno, G.; Allaria, E.; Cinquegrana, P.; Danailov, M.B.; Demidovich, A.; Ferrari, E.; Giannessi, L. Generation of Phase-Locked Pulses from a Seeded Free-Electron Laser. *Phys. Rev. Lett.* **2016**, *116*, 024801. [CrossRef] [PubMed]
9. Gauthier, D.; Allaria, E.; Coreno, M.; Cudin, I.; Dacasa, H.; Danailov, M.; Demidovich, A.; Di Mitri, S.; Diviacco, B.; Ferrari, E.; et al. Chirped pulse amplification in an extreme-ultraviolet free-electron laser. *Nat. Commun.* **2016**, *7*, 13688. [CrossRef] [PubMed]
10. Gorobtsov, O.; Mercurio, G.; Capotondi, F.; Skopintsev, P.; Lazarev, S.; Zaluzhnyy, I.; Danailov, M.; Dell'Angela, M.; Manfredda, M.; Pedersoli, E.; et al. Seeded X-ray free-electron laser generating radiation with laser statistical properties. *Nat. Commun.* **2018**, *9*, 4498. [CrossRef]
11. Yu, L.H.; Babzien, M.; Ben-Zvi, I.; DiMauro, L.F.; Doyuran, A.; Graves, W.; Johnson, E.; Krinsky, S.; Malone, R.; Pogorelsky, I.; et al. High-Gain Harmonic-Generation Free-Electron Laser. *Science* **2000**, *289*, 932–934. [CrossRef]

12. Allaria, E.; Cinquegrana, P.; Cleva, S.; Cocco, D.; Cornacchia, M.; Craievich, P.; Cudin, I.; D'Auria, G.; Dal Forno, M.; Danailov, M.; et al. Highly coherent and stable pulses from the FERMI seeded free-electron laser in the extreme ultraviolet. *Nat. Photonics* **2012**, *6*, 699–704. [CrossRef]
13. Xiang, D.; Stupakov, G. Echo-enabled harmonic generation free electron laser. *Phys. Rev. ST Accel. Beams* **2009**, *12*, 030702. [CrossRef]
14. Feng, C.; Deng, H.; Zhang, M.; Wang, X.; Chen, S.; Liu, T.; Zhou, K.; Gu, D.; Wang, Z.; Jiang, Z.; et al. Coherent extreme ultraviolet free-electron laser with echo-enabled harmonic generation. *Phys. Rev. Accel. Beams* **2019**, *22*, 050703. [CrossRef]
15. Ribič, P.; Abrami, A.; Badano, L.; Bossi, M.; Braun, H.H.; Bruchon, N.; Capotondi, F.; Castronovo, D.; Cautero, M.; Cinquegrana, P.; et al. Coherent soft X-ray pulses from an echo-enabled harmonic generation free-electron laser. *Nat. Photonics* **2019**, *13*, 1–7. [CrossRef]
16. Lechner, C.; Ackermann, S.; Azima, A.; Aßmann, R.; Biss, H.; Drescher, M.; Faatz, B.; Grattoni, V.; Hartl, I.; Hartwell, S.; et al. Seeding R&D at sFLASH. In Proceedings of the FEL'19, Geneva, Switzerland, 26–30 August 2019; Number 39 in Free Electron Laser Conference; pp. 230–233. [CrossRef]
17. Yan, J.; Gao, Z.; Qi, Z.; Zhang, K.; Zhou, K.; Liu, T.; Chen, S.; Feng, C.; Li, C.; Feng, L.; et al. Self-Amplification of Coherent Energy Modulation in Seeded Free-Electron Lasers. *Phys. Rev. Lett.* **2021**, *126*, 084801. [CrossRef] [PubMed]
18. Wang, X.; Feng, C.; Faatz, B.; Zhang, W.; Zhao, Z. Direct-Amplification Enabled Harmonic Generation for Seeding a High-Repetition-Rate Free-Electron Laser. 2021. Available online: http://xxx.lanl.gov/abs/2103.11971 (accessed on 10 May 2021).
19. Ackermann, S.; Faatz, B.; Grattoni, V.; Lechner, C.; Paraskaki, G.; Geloni, G.; Serkez, S.; Tanikawa, T.; Hillert, W. High-Repetition-Rate Seeding Schemes Using a Resonator-Amplifier Setup. In Proceedings of the International Free Electron Laser Conference (FEL'19), Hamburg, Germany, 26–30 August 2019; Number 39 in International Free Electron Laser Conference; JACoW: Geneva, Switzerland, 2019; [CrossRef]
20. Paraskaki, G.; Ackermann, S.; Faatz, B.; Grattoni, V.; Lechner, C.; Mehrjoo, M.; Geloni, G.; Serkez, S.; Tanikawa, T.; Hillert, W. Study of a Seeded Oscillator-Amplifier FEL. In Proceedings of the International Free Electron Laser Conference (FEL'19), Hamburg, Germany, 26–30 August 2019; Number 39 in International Free Electron Laser Conference; JACoW: Geneva, Switzerland, 2019; [CrossRef]
21. Ackermann, S.; Faatz, B.; Grattoni, V.; Kazemi, M.M.; Lang, T.; Lechner, C.; Paraskaki, G.; Zemella, J.; Geloni, G.; Serkez, S.; et al. Novel method for the generation of stable radiation from free-electron lasers at high repetition rates. *Phys. Rev. Accel. Beams* **2020**, *23*, 071302. [CrossRef]
22. Paraskaki, G.; Grattoni, V.; Lang, T.; Zemella, J.; Faatz, B.; Hillert, W. Optimization and stability of a high-gain harmonic generation seeded oscillator amplifier. *Phys. Rev. Accel. Beams* **2021**, *24*, 034801. [CrossRef]
23. Dattoli, G.; Giannessi, L.; Ottaviani, P.; Torre, A. Dynamical behavior of a free-electron laser operating with a prebunched electron beam. *Phys. Rev. E Stat. Phys. Plasmas Fluids Relat. Interdiscip. Top.* **1994**, *49*, 5668–5678. [CrossRef]
24. Dattoli, G.; Faatz, B.; Giannessi, L.; Ottaviani, P.L. The tandem FEL dynamic behavior. *IEEE J. Quantum Electron.* **1995**, *31*, 1584–1590. [CrossRef]
25. Dattoli, G.; Giannessi, L.; Ottaviani, P. Oscillator-amplifier free electron laser devices with stable output power. *J. Appl. Phys.* **2004**, *95*, 3211. [CrossRef]
26. Kim, K.J.; Shvyd'ko, Y.; Reiche, S. A Proposal for an X-Ray Free-Electron Laser Oscillator with an Energy-Recovery Linac. *Phys. Rev. Lett.* **2008**, *100*, 244802. [CrossRef]
27. Nguyen, D.C.; Sheffield, R.L.; Fortgang, C.M.; Goldstein, J.C.; Kinross-Wright, J.M.; Ebrahim, N.A. First lasing of the regenerative amplifier FEL. *Nucl. Instrum. Methods Phys. Res. A* **1999**, *429*, 125–130. [CrossRef]
28. Faatz, B.; Feldhaus, J.; Krzywinski, J.; Saldin, E.; Schneidmiller, E.; Yurkov, M. Regenerative FEL amplifier at the TESLA test facility at DESY. *Nucl. Instrum. Methods Phys. Res. Sect. A Accel. Spectrometers Detect. Assoc. Equip.* **1999**, *429*, 424–428. [CrossRef]
29. Huang, Z.; Ruth, R.D. Fully Coherent X-ray Pulses from a Regenerative-Amplifier Free-Electron Laser. *Phys. Rev. Lett.* **2006**, *96*, 144801. [CrossRef]
30. Freund, H.P.; van der Slot, P.J.M.; Shvyd'ko, Y. An X-ray regenerative amplifier free-electron laser using diamond pinhole mirrors. *New J. Phys.* **2019**, *21*, 093028. [CrossRef]
31. Trovò, M.; Clarke, J.; Couprie, M.; Dattoli, G.; Garzella, D.; Gatto, A.; Giannessi, L.; Günster, S.; Kaiser, N.; Marsi, M.; et al. Operation of the European storage ring FEL at ELETTRA down to 190 nm. *Nucl. Instrum. Methods Phys. Res. Sect. A Accel. Spectrometers Detect. Assoc. Equip.* **2002**, *483*, 157–161. [CrossRef]
32. Gandhi, P.; Penn, G.; Reinsch, M.; Wurtele, J.; Fawley, W. Oscillator seeding of a high gain harmonic generation free electron laser in a radiator-first configuration. *Phys. Rev. Spec. Top. Accel. Beams* **2013**, *16*, 020703. [CrossRef]
33. Li, K.; Yan, J.; Feng, C.; Zhang, M.; Deng, H. High brightness fully coherent x-ray amplifier seeded by a free-electron laser oscillator. *Phys. Rev. Accel. Beams* **2018**, *21*, 040702. [CrossRef]
34. Petrillo, V.; Bacci, A.; Rossi, A.R.; Serafini, L.; Drebot, I.; Conti, M.R.; Ruijter, M.; Opromolla, M.; Samsam, S.; Broggi, F.; et al. Coherent, high repetition rate tender X-ray Free-Electron Laser seeded by an Extreme Ultra-Violet Free-Electron Laser Oscillator. *New J. Phys.* **2020**, *22*, 073058. [CrossRef]
35. Mirian, N.; Opromolla, M.; Rossi, G.; Serafini, L.; Petrillo, V. High-repetition rate and coherent free-electron laser in the tender x rays based on the echo-enabled harmonic generation of an ultraviolet oscillator pulse. *Phys. Rev. Accel. Beams* **2021**, accepted.

36. Newnam, B.E. Extreme ultraviolet free-electron laser-based projection lithography systems. *Opt. Eng.* **1991**, *30*, 1100–1108. [CrossRef]
37. Penco, G.; Perosa, G.; Allaria, E.; Di Mitri, S.; Ferrari, E.; Giannessi, L.; Spampinati, S.; Spezzani, C.; Veronese, M. Enhanced seeded free electron laser performance with a "cold" electron beam. *Phys. Rev. Accel. Beams* **2020**, *23*, 120704. [CrossRef]
38. Beye, M. *FLASH2020+: Making FLASH Brighter, Faster and More Flexible : Conceptual Design Report*; Verlag Deutsches Elektronen-Synchrotron: Hamburg, Germany, 2020; pp. 1–126. [CrossRef]
39. Reiche, S. GENESIS 1.3: A fully 3D time-dependent FEL simulation code. *Nucl. Instrum. Methods Phys. Res. Sect. A Accel. Spectrometers Detect. Assoc. Equip.* **1999**, *429*, 243–248. [CrossRef]
40. Faatz, B.; Plönjes, E.; Ackermann, S.; Agababyan, A.; Asgekar, V.; Ayvazyan, V.; Baark, S.; Baboi, N.; Balandin, V.; von Bargen, N.; et al. Simultaneous operation of two soft x-ray free-electron lasers driven by one linear accelerator. *New J. Phys.* **2016**, *18*, 062002. [CrossRef]
41. Rossbach, J.; Schneider, J.R.; Wurth, W. 10 years of pioneering X-ray science at the Free-Electron Laser FLASH at DESY. *Phys. Rep.* **2019**, *808*, 1–74. [CrossRef]
42. Nölle, D. FEL Operation at the European XFEL Facility. In Proceedings of the International Free Electron Laser Conference (FEL'19), Hamburg, Germany, 26–30 August 2019; Number 39 in International Free Electron Laser Conference; JACoW: Geneva, Switzerland, 2019; [CrossRef]
43. Liu, T.; Dong, X.; Feng, C. Start-to-end Simulations of the Reflection Hard X-Ray Self-Seeding at the SHINE Project. In Proceedings of the FEL'19, Geneva, Switzerland, 26–30 August 2019; Number 39 in Free Electron Laser Conference; pp. 254–257. [CrossRef]
44. Hemsing, E.; Marcus, G.; Fawley, W.M.; Schoenlein, R.W.; Coffee, R.; Dakovski, G.; Hastings, J.; Huang, Z.; Ratner, D.; Raubenheimer, T.; et al. Soft X-ray seeding studies for the SLAC Linac Coherent Light Source II. *Phys. Rev. Accel. Beams* **2019**, *22*, 110701. [CrossRef]
45. Reiche, S. Overview of Seeding Methods for FELs. In Proceedings of the 4th International Particle Accelerator Conference, Shanghai, China, 12–17 May 2013.
46. Xie, M. Design optimization for an X-ray free electron laser driven by SLAC LINAC. *Conf. Proc.* **1996**, *C950501*, 183–185. [CrossRef]
47. Hemsing, E.; Stupakov, G.; Xiang, D.; Zholents, A. Beam by design: Laser manipulation of electrons in modern accelerators. *Rev. Mod. Phys.* **2014**, *86*, 897–941. [CrossRef]
48. Guenster, S.; Ristau, D.; Gatto, A.; Kaiser, N.; Trovo, M.; Danailov, M.; Sarto, F. VUV Optics Development for the Elettra Storage Ring FEL. In Proceedings of the 26th International Free Electron Laser Conference & 11th FEL Users Workshop, Trieste, Italy, 29 August–3 September 2004.
49. Henke, B.; Gullikson, E.; Davis, J. X-ray Interactions: Photoabsorption, Scattering, Transmission, and Reflection at E = 50-30,000 eV, Z = 1-92. *At. Data Nucl. Data Tables* **1993**, *54*, 181–342. Available online: https://henke.lbl.gov/optical_constants/mirror2.html (accessed on 10 May 2021). [CrossRef]
50. Agapov, I.; Geloni, G.; Tomin, S.; Zagorodnov, I. OCELOT: A software framework for synchrotron light source and FEL studies. *Nucl. Instrum. Methods Phys. Res. A* **2014**, *768*, 151–156. [CrossRef]
51. Oepts, D.; van der Meer, A.; van Amersfoort, P. The Free-Electron-Laser user facility FELIX. *Infrared Phys. Technol.* **1995**, *36*, 297–308. [CrossRef]
52. Jaroszynski, D.; Oepts, D.; Van Der Meer, A.; Van Amersfoort, P.; Colson, W. Consequences of short electron-beam pulses in the FELIX project. *Nucl. Instrum. Methods Phys. Res. Sect. A Accel. Spectrometers Detect. Assoc. Equip.* **1990**, *296*, 480–484. [CrossRef]
53. Knippels, G.M.H.; Bakker, R.J.; van der Meer, A.F.G.; Jaroszynski, D.A.; Oepts, D.; van Amersfoort, P.W.; Hovenier, J.N. Dynamic cavity desynchronisation in FELIX. *Nucl. Instrum. Methods Phys. Res. A* **1994**, *341*, ABS26–ABS27. [CrossRef]
54. MacLeod, A.M.; Yan, X.; Gillespie, W.A.; Knippels, G.M.H.; Oepts, D.; van der Meer, A.F.G.; Rella, C.W.; Smith, T.I.; Schwettman, H.A. Formation of low time-bandwidth product, single-sided exponential optical pulses in free-electron laser oscillators. *Phys. Rev. E* **2000**, *62*, 4216–4220. [CrossRef]
55. Zhao, Z.Y.; Li, H.T.; Jia, Q.K. Effect of cavity length detuning on the output characteristics for the middle infrared FEL oscillator of FELiChEM. *Chin. Phys. C* **2017**, *41*, 108101. [CrossRef]
56. Kiessling, R.; Colson, W.B.; Gewinner, S.; Schöllkopf, W.; Wolf, M.; Paarmann, A. Femtosecond single-shot timing and direct observation of subpulse formation in an infrared free-electron laser. *Phys. Rev. Accel. Beams* **2018**, *21*, 080702. [CrossRef]
57. Vinokurov, N.A.; Skrinsky, A.N. *About the Maximum Power of an Optical Klystron on a Storage Ring*; Report No. BINP 77-67; Budker Institute for Nuclear Physics: Novossibirsk, Russia, 1977.
58. Dattoli, G.; Giannessi, L.; Ottaviani, P. MOPA optical klystron FELs and coherent harmonic generation. *Nucl. Instrum. Methods Phys. Res. Sect. A Accel. Spectrometers Detect. Assoc. Equip.* **2003**, *507*, 26–30. [CrossRef]
59. Penco, G.; Allaria, E.; Ninno, G.D.; Ferrari, E.; Giannessi, L. Experimental Demonstration of Enhanced Self-Amplified Spontaneous Emission by an Optical Klystron. *Phys. Rev. Lett.* **2015**, *114*, 013901. [CrossRef]
60. Penco, G.; Allaria, E.; De Ninno, G.; Ferrari, E.; Giannessi, L.; Roussel, E.; Spampinati, S. Optical Klystron Enhancement to Self Amplified Spontaneous Emission at FERMI. *Photonics* **2017**, *4*, 15. [CrossRef]
61. Ding, Y.; Emma, P.; Huang, Z.; Kumar, V. Optical klystron enhancement to self-amplified spontaneous emission free electron lasers. *Phys. Rev. ST Accel. Beams* **2006**, *9*, 070702; Erratum in **2020**, *23*, 019901. [CrossRef]

62. Geloni, G.; Guetg, M.; Serkez, S.; Schneidmiller, E. A Revision of Optical Klystron Enhancement Effects in SASE FELs. *Phys. Rev. Accel. Beams.* **2021**, submitted.
63. Keil, B.; Baldinger, R.; Ditter, R.; Gloor, M.; Koprek, W.; Marcellini, F.; Marinkovic, G.; Roggli, M.; Rohrer, M.; Stadler, M.; et al. Status of The European XFEL Transverse Intra Bunch Train Feedback System. In Proceedings of the International Beam Instrumentation Conference (IBIC2015), Melbourne, Australia, 13–17 September 2015; Number 4 in International Beam Instrumentation Conference; JACoW: Geneva, Switzerland, 2016; pp. 492–496. [CrossRef]
64. Obier, F.; Decking, W.; Hüning, M.; Wortmann, J. Fast Kicker System for European XFEL Beam Distribution. In Proceedings of the 39th International Free-Electron Laser Conference, Hamburg, Germany, 26–30 August 2019; JACoW Publishing: Geneva, Switzerland, 2019; p. 4. [CrossRef]

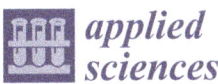

Article

High Repetition Rate and Coherent Free-Electron Laser Oscillator in the Tender X-ray Range Tailored for Linear Spectroscopy

Michele Opromolla [1,2,*], Alberto Bacci [2], Marcello Rossetti Conti [2], Andrea Renato Rossi [2], Giorgio Rossi [1], Luca Serafini [2], Alberto Tagliaferri [3] and Vittoria Petrillo [1,2]

[1] Dipartimento di Fisica, Universitá degli Studi di Milano, Via Celoria, 16 20133 Milano, Italy; giorgio.rossi2@unimi.it (G.R.); vittoria.petrillo@mi.infn.it (V.P.)
[2] INFN-Sezione di Milano, Via Celoria 16, 20133 Milano, Italy; alberto.bacci@mi.infn.it (A.B.); marcello.rossetticonti@mi.infn.it (M.R.C.); andrea.rossi@mi.infn.it (A.R.R.); luca.serafini@mi.infn.it (L.S.)
[3] Politecnico di Milano, P.zza Leonardo da Vinci, 20133 Milano, Italy; alberto.tagliaferri@polimi.it
* Correspondence: michele.opromolla@mi.infn.it

Abstract: Fine time-resolved analysis of matter—that is, spectroscopy and photon scattering—in the linear response regime requires fs-scale pulsed, high repetition rate, fully coherent X-ray sources. A seeded Free-Electron Laser, driven by a linac based on Super Conducting cavities, generating 10^8–10^{10} coherent photons at 2–5 keV with 0.2–1 MHz of repetition rate, can address this need. The scheme proposed is a Free-Electron Laser Oscillator at 3 keV, working with a cavity based on X-ray mirrors. The whole chain of the X-ray generation is here described by means of start-to-end simulations.

Keywords: free-electron lasers; X-rays; regenerative amplifiers

1. Introduction

Synchrotron radiation (SR) sources based on low-emittance electron storage rings, as well as Free Electron Lasers (FELs) driven by linear electron accelerators (Linacs), allow the fine analysis of matter, with applications extending from life sciences to material physics. Most FELs worldwide operate in the Self-Amplified Spontaneous Emission (SASE) mode [1–8], providing extremely brilliant and short pulses with more than 10^{12} photons per pulse, and shot-to-shot time and intensity jitters determined by the intrinsic fluctuations of the emission process. These Ultra-Violet (UV) or X-ray flashes are used to probe matter in highly excited states, to study nonlinear processes or to test before destroying individual objects such as macromolecules constituting proteins, thus replacing crystallography with single object imaging. In order to remain below the linear response threshold and to collect adequate statistics in a short time, spectroscopic probes, as well as pump–probe photoemission experiments in advanced atomic, molecular, nano- and solid- state physics, instead require ultra-short photon pulses (order 10 fs), MHz-class repetition rates and moderate fluxes of photons/pulse. Currently available FEL sources produce a number of photons per pulse exceeding by 2–4 orders of magnitude the linear response level: severe attenuation of the pulses, with a huge waste of energy, is therefore required in photoemission or X-ray absorption spectroscopy. The pulses' repetition rate is determined by the acceleration technology, and is much higher in Super-Conducting facilities, exceeding the 10–100 Hz range of Warm Linacs up to MHz-class [4,5]. Moreover, spectroscopic applications with X-ray FELs are severely limited by SASE fluctuations and full seeding, successfully conducted at FERMI (Free-Electron laser for Multidisciplinary Investigations) in the XUV-soft X-ray range [9], should ideally be extended to X-ray energies.

There is therefore a scientific need, and ample room, for a novel type of source that is able to provide 10 fs coherent pulses of 10^7–10^8 photons at 0.5–2 MHz in the tender X ray range, bridging the gap between the most advanced SR and the current FEL sources.

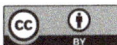

These demanding requests about structure, intensity, repetition rate, reduced jitters and true coherence of the pulses are addressed by conceiving a tailored seeded or self-seeded FEL driven by a linac based on Super Conducting cavities, providing 10^7–10^{10} coherent photons at 2–5 keV, at 1 MHz of repetition rate.

In the seeded amplifier FEL configuration, the pulses' stability and coherence is strongly increased by an external coherent source imprinting its temporal phase on the electron beam at the undulator entrance, thus enabling us to reach a high degree of temporal coherence within a short distance. The direct seeding [10] implementation is limited by the lack of high-power coherent seeds in the Vacuum-UV regime and below. High Gain Harmonic Generation (HGHG) multistage cascades [11], seeded with harmonics of an IR laser generated in crystals [11–13], were studied in the optical-UV range [14–16] and were demonstrated at FERMI up to a few nm wavelengths [9]. The implementation and reliability of this scheme in the tender/hard X-ray spectral range is highly demanding and has ye to be proven. In perspective, the X-ray range could be reached with the technique of the Echo Enabled Harmonic Generation (EEHG) [17–20], in which two coherent radiation pulses seed the electron beam in two sequential modulators interspersed by a strong dispersive section. Both cascaded schemes allow us to reach the boundary between Extreme Ultra-Violet and soft X-ray frequencies, and may be seeded by laser harmonics generated in gases or UV oscillators [21–24]. A major limit of all seeding schemes based on lasers is created by the achievable repetition rate, which is typically below tens of kHz, and their extension to higher repetition rates has so far only been studied theoretically [25–27].

The single spike SASE operation [28–30], as well as self-seeding processes [31,32], are able to achieve only partial longitudinal coherence. Another FEL configuration capable of producing stable radiation pulses is the FEL Oscillator (FELO), in which the radiation process builds up via multiple passes of a stable and high repetition rate pulse train of electron bunches through an undulator embedded in a low-loss optical cavity [23,33–37]. The lower gain required in such systems relaxes the requirements on peak current and electron beam quality. Thanks to the technological advancements in the field of optics and mirrors fabrication [38], FEL oscillators (XFELO) [37,39] and regenerative amplifiers (RAFEL) based on X-ray cavities [40–44] have been proposed as a direct source of coherent X-rays [36,37,40,45], or as seed for subsequent cascades [24,25,46]. However, limit cycle oscillations have been observed and studied in FELOs [47]: these fluctuations, depending on the cavity specifics and working point, can even be comparable to the fluctuations found in SASE FELs. Among all the methods for producing coherent X-ray radiation, we analyze here the case of a tender X-ray FEL Oscillator, driven by a moderate energy electron beam and based on a short period undulator. Diamond mirrors and beam splitters, foreseen at about 3 keV, constitute a ring cavity where the radiation pulses are synchronized with the electron bunches. In this paper, we show the operation of such a source. The electron beam is supposed to be generated by the accelerator of the MariX project (Multi-disciplinary Advanced Research Infrastructure for the generation and application of X-rays) [48], based on superconducting cavities and equipped with an arc compressor. The compact footprint (with a total dimension of less than 500 m) of the infrastructure and the contained costs should permit its construction in medium-sized research infrastructures or within university campuses. Hereafter, we will discuss the nominal parameters and start-to-end simulations of the system. Final comments will be presented in the conclusions.

2. Materials and Methods

Our analyses rely on the electron beam foreseen by the accelerator of the MariX project [48]. MariX is based on the innovative and compact design of a two-pass, two-way superconducting linear electron accelerator equipped with an arc compressor [49–51], to be operated in CW mode at 1 MHz. The characteristics of the electron beam, as evaluated after start-to-end simulations [52], are listed in Table 1. A short period, planar undulator can allow the production of radiation pulses in the desired wavelength range (5–2 Å, or in energy 2–5 keV), starting from the moderate electron energy provided by the MariX accelerator (at a maximum of 3.8 GeV). From the resonance relation,

$$\lambda = \frac{\lambda_w}{2\gamma^2}(1+a_w^2),\qquad(1)$$

where $a_w = 0.657\lambda_w(\text{cm})B(\text{T})$ is the undulator parameter and γ the electron Lorentz factor for an electron beam energy of 2.4 GeV, we can deduce that an undulator period $\lambda_w = 1.2$ cm, corresponding to a peak on-axis magnetic field of $B = 0.93$ T, is suitable for emitting at 3 keV. Both the structure and length of the undulator depend on the seeding scheme: the XFELO requires a single short undulator module, equipped with a sequence of X-ray crystal mirrors.

Table 1. Electron beam for MariX FEL.

Property	Unit	Value	Property	Unit	Value
Energy	GeV	1.6–3.8	Current	kA	1.6
Charge	pC	8–50	Bunch duration	fs	2.5–16
rms relative energy spread	10^{-4}	5–3	slice energy spread	10^{-4}	4–2
rms normalized emittance	mm mrad	0.3–0.5	slice normalized emittance	mm mrad	0.3–0.5

FEL simulations have been performed with the three-dimensional code GENESIS 1.3 [53] in time-dependent mode. The SASE radiation at 4.16 Angstrom is described for reference in Figure 1.

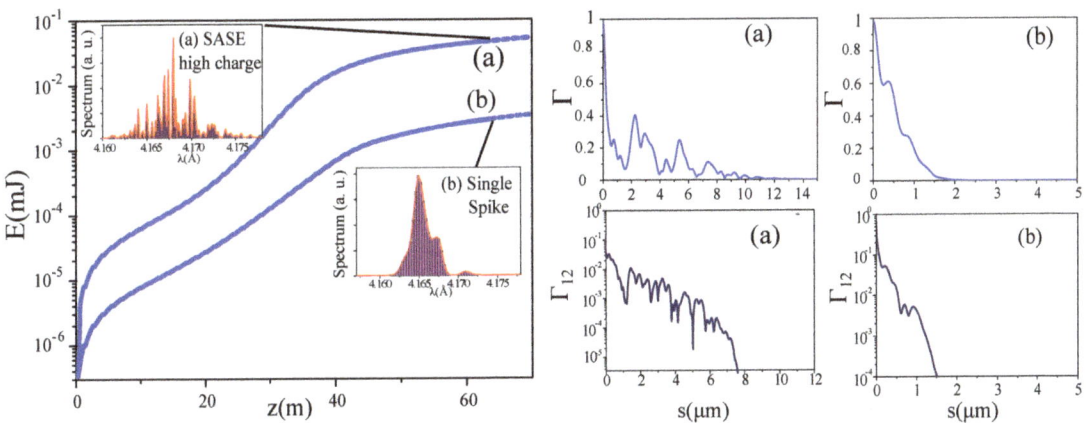

Figure 1. *Left plot*: SASE energy growth for the high (**a**) and low (**b**) charge working points and corresponding spectral profiles at saturation (inner boxes). *Right windows*: self (Γ, upper row) and mutual ($\Gamma_{1,2}$, lower row) coherence degrees vs. $s = c\tau$ for the two analyzed working points (**a**) and (**b**).

On the left, the growth along the undulator is presented for (a) high (50 pC) and (b) low (8 pC) charge cases. Saturation is reached in about 50 m with a level of (a) 8×10^{11} and (b) 4×10^9 photons/pulse, respectively. The spectral profiles are reported in the inner boxes, showing the SASE fluctuations in the high charge case (a) and the single spike mode in the low charge one (b). The coherence degree, evaluated from the correlation,

$$\Gamma_{n,m}(\tau) = \left|\frac{\int dt\, E_n(t) E_m(t-\tau)}{\sqrt{\int dt\, |E_n|^2}\sqrt{\int dt\, |E_m|^2}}\right|,\qquad(2)$$

between two different generic pulses or for one single pulse ($\Gamma = \Gamma_{1,1}$), is shown in the windows on the right part of Figure 1. In expression (2), E_n and E_m are the complex electric fields of the pulses as a function of time. In the SASE mode (case (a)), phase coherence on one single pulse and shot-to-shot stability are poor, with a coherence length less than 1 µm over a 10 µm long pulse and an equal time coherence degree ($\Gamma_{1,2}(0)$) of about 4×10^2. In the single spike mode (case (b)), the coherence length coincides with the pulse's, but the shot-to-shot stability is low, with $\Gamma_{1,2}(0) = 2 \times 10^1$. The characteristics of the SASE radiation are summarized in Table 2, in the third (high charge working point) and fourth (single spike mode) columns. The patterns of the SASE power (a) and spectral distribution (b) are shown in Figure 2 as a function of the number of shots. From this graph, the modest size of the coherence areas and the poor stability of the SASE process are evident.

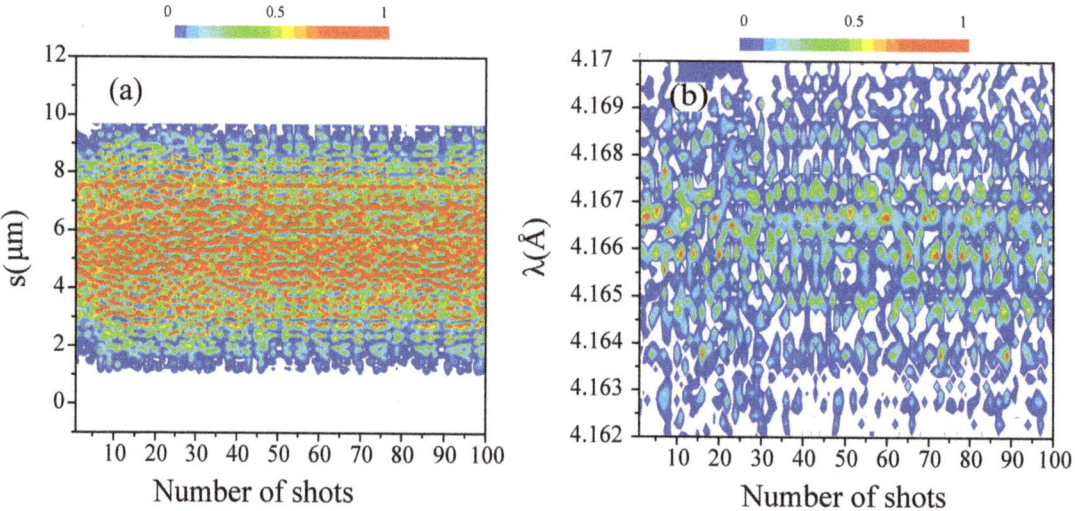

Figure 2. SASE (**a**) power vs. $s = c\tau$ and (**b**) spectrum vs. λ as a function of the number of shots. Logarithmic scale.

The XFELO operation has been numerically studied by extracting the radiation simulated by GENESIS 1.3 from the oscillator undulator, driving it through the optical line and superimposing it on the successive electron bunches. In order to simulate the electron bunch train fluctuations, the microscopic distribution of the electron beam is changed shot-to-shot in the simulations. The transport inside the cavity is done by using the Huygens integral [54]

$$E(\underline{x}',t') = \frac{i}{B\lambda_0} \int d\underline{x} E(\underline{x},t) e^{-\frac{i\pi}{\lambda B}(Ar^2 - 2(xx'+yy') + Dr'^2)}, \qquad (3)$$

where $\underline{x} = (x;y)$, $r^2 = x^2 + y^2$ and $r'^2 = x'^2 + y'^2$. Here, the electric field is the output of the FEL simulation (performed with about 2048 particles and 7000 slices), which is extracted at the end of the undulator over a three-dimensional grid (grid dimensions: transverse ~ 2 µm, longitudinal ~ 1.6 nm). In the first step, the Huygens integral is extended from the end of the undulator up to the first mirror. A, B, C and D are the elements of a 2×2 matrix describing the optical path and depending on the drift length and on the focal length of the mirror. The effect of the mirror is modelled with a transfer function, taking into account its reflectivity and spectral selectivity. Its action is evaluated by computing the convolution between the electric field at the mirror position and the Fourier anti-transform T of the mirror transfer function,

$$E(\underline{x}, t') = \frac{1}{\sqrt{2\pi}} \int dt T(t - t') E(\underline{x}, t). \quad (4)$$

The process is reiterated for each drift and cavity mirror up to the beginning of the undulator in the next step. The electric field, calculated in this way, is superimposed to the successive electron bunches after each cavity round trip. The mirror and beam splitter reflectivities have been simulated with the XOP (X-ray Oriented Programs) code [55].

3. Results

Figure 3 shows the scheme of the coherent source, constituted by a short (about 7–10 m long) undulator module with period λ_w = 1.2 cm, embedded within a ring cavity.

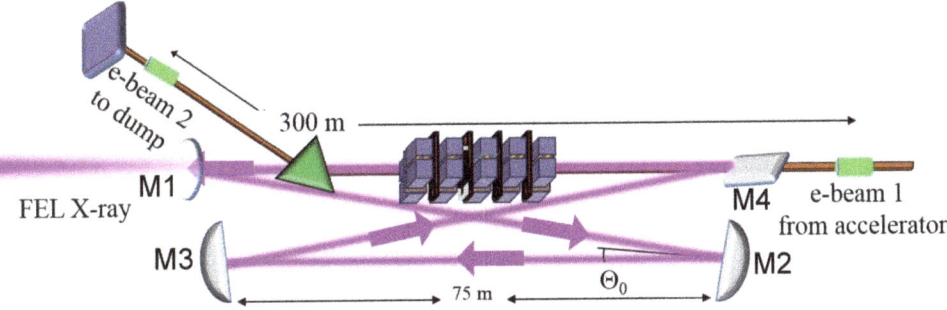

Figure 3. Scheme of the X-ray FEL Oscillator: λ_w = 1.2 cm undulator module within a ring cavity made of three Diamond mirrors (M_2, M_3 and M_4) and one beam splitter (M_1, outcoupling the radiation). The X-ray radiation is emitted from right to left. Θ_0 is the incidence angle on the cavity mirrors with respect to the normal. The distance $M_{1,4}$–$M_{3,2}$ between two mirrors is 75 m, giving a cavity round trip length of 300 m, equal to the distance between two successive electron bunches.

For an electron beam repetition rate of 1 MHz, the round trip of the cavity must be 300 m. The sequence of the accelerated beam packets entering the undulator is synchronized with the radiation reflected and recirculated by hard X-ray mirrors. Three Diamond mirrors and one beam splitter, made by Zincblend perfect single crystals (lattice parameters: $a = b = c = 3.566$ Å, $\alpha = \beta = \gamma = 90$) operating in the range of about 3.0–3.5 keV, namely 3.6–4 Å(with an incidence angle θ < 30 from normal), have been considered. At least two of the mirrors are assumed to be bent and focusing.

Figure 4 presents the transfer function T of the total optical line as a function of the energy of the photons for a central energy of 3.015 keV and a quasi-orthogonal reflection (incidence angle Θ_0 = 3), compared with the natural SASE spectral line.

The mirror transfer function is narrower than the natural FEL spectral line and the spectral filtering of the mirrors is the dominant effect in the reduction of the spectral width. The angular filtering is instead absolutely inefficient, since the angular width of the transfer function is about 2 mrad, to be compared to the much smaller SASE divergence of 25 µrad. FEL simulations were performed for a 50 pC electron beam. Figure 5 shows the intracavity radiation energy as a function of the number of round trips. The saturation is reached in about 50 cycles, with an intracavity energy level of about 20 µJ. Due to the short undulator and wavelength, the slippage is very low: the simulated time window (12 µm) is thus adjusted to the electron beam and reported in the inner boxes of Figure 5.

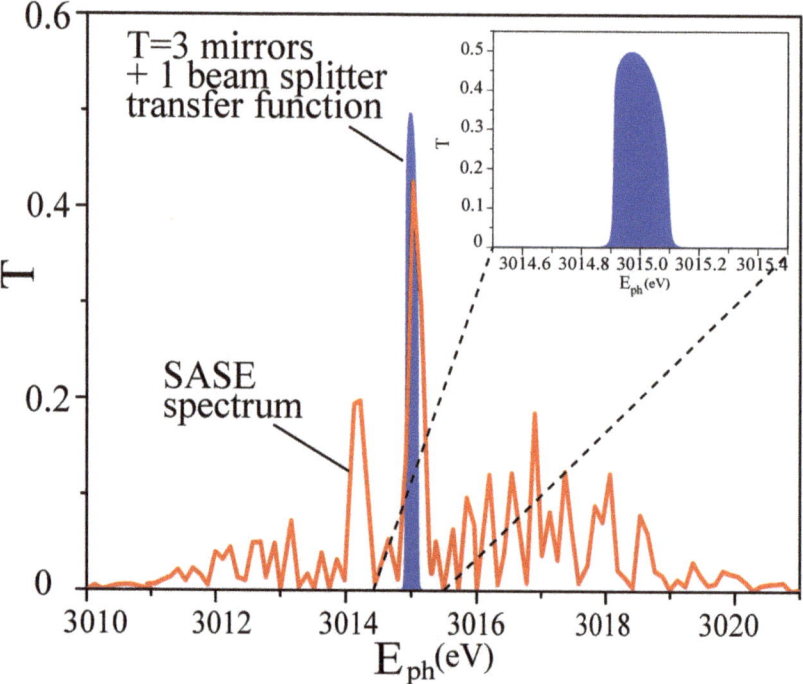

Figure 4. Transfer function T of an optical line made by three diamond mirrors and one beam splitter (in blue) vs. the photon energy for an incidence angle Θ_0 of 3 with respect to the normal. SASE spectrum (in red) in arbitrary units. The reflectivities are simulated with the XOP code [55].

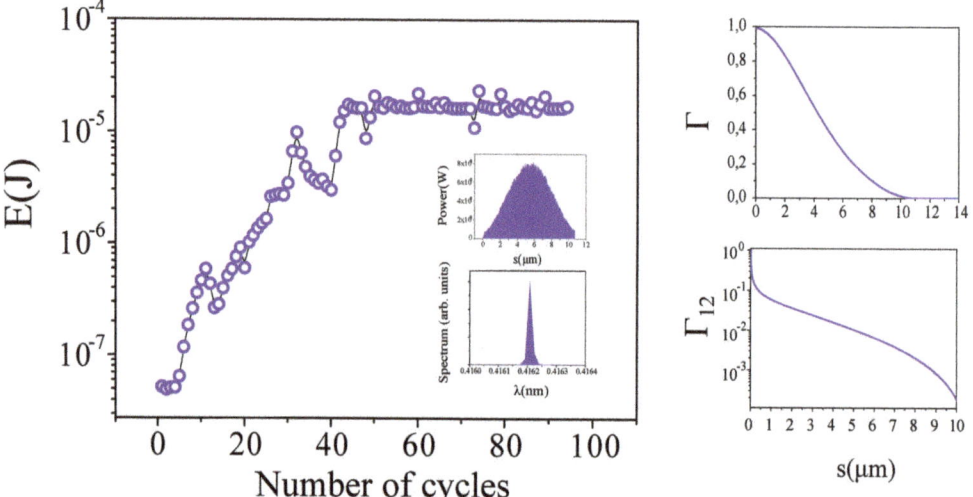

Figure 5. FEL Oscillator. **Left window**: intracavity energy growth as a function of the number of round trips. Inner boxes: temporal and spectral distributions at saturation. **Right windows**: auto (Γ) and mutual ($\Gamma_{1,2}$) coherence degrees vs. $s = c\tau$.

Jitters occur due to the different microscopic structures of the successive electron bunches. In the inner boxes, the temporal and spectral distributions at saturation are presented. The right windows of Figure 5 show the auto (Γ) and mutual ($\Gamma_{1,2}$) coherence degrees of the XFEL-Oscillator, pointing out its enhanced coherence and stability with respect to the SASE's reported in Figure 1.

The longitudinal distributions along $s = c\tau$ of the power (a) and the spectral amplitude structure (b) are shown in Figure 6 as a function of the round trip number in the X-ray cavity. The output radiation is much more stable and quasi monochromatic if compared to the analogous patterns of the SASE radiation already shown in Figure 2. The studied X-FEL Oscillator results in an almost fully coherent pulse, characterized by a very small spectral bandwidth. Table 2 summarizes the main properties of SASE (third and fourth columns) and XFELO (fifth column) radiation. Despite the lower number of photons produced by the XFELO with respect to the SASE case, its pulses' stability, directionality and brilliance are higher.

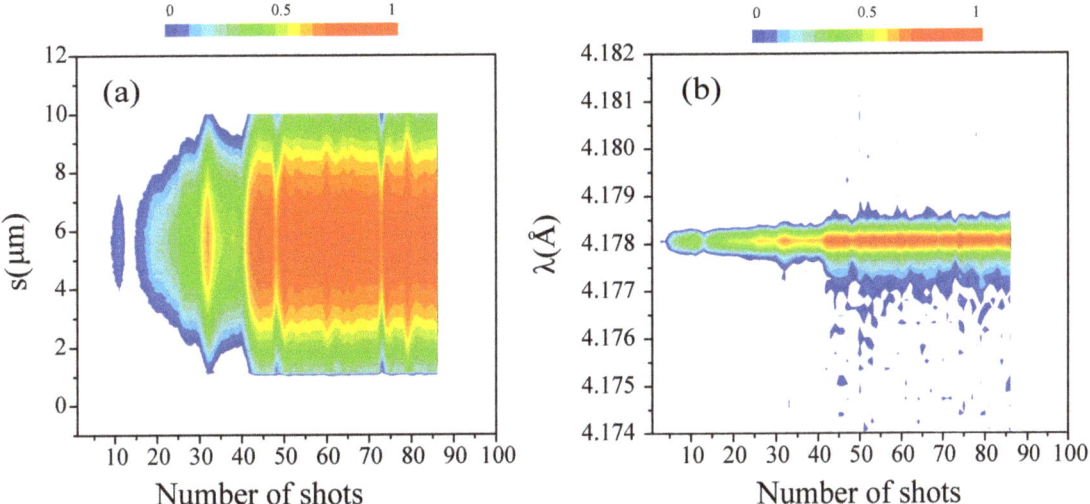

Figure 6. Intracavity power vs. s and spectrum vs. λ as a function of the round trip number in logarithmic scale. XFELO (**a**) intra-cavity power vs $s = c\tau$ and (**b**) spectrum vs λ as function of the round trip number. Logarithmic scale.

Table 2. The repetition rate of the source is 1 MHz. $=Photons/s/mm^2/mrad^2/bw(‰).

Radiation Mode		SASE	Single Spike	XFELO
Electron charge	pC	50	8	50
Photon energy	keV	3	3	3
Radiation wavelength	Å	4.16	4.16	4.16
Photon/shot	10^{10}	80	0.36	4.4
Bandwidth	0.1%	2.1	0.7	4
Pulse length	fs	10	3	16
Pulse divergence	μrad	25	45	14
Pulse size	μm	130	140	35
Radiation energy	μJ	55	1.7	21
Photon/s	10^{16}	80	0.36	4.4
Peak brilliance	$10^{30}$$	3.6	0.043	3.8
Average brilliance	$10^{22}$$	3.6	0.013	4

4. Conclusions

The MariX facility is dedicated to and optimized for ultrafast coherent-X-ray spectroscopy and inelastic photon scattering, and for highly penetrating X-ray imaging of mesoscopic and macroscopic samples. In the range of wavelengths between 2 and 5 Å, MariX provides 10^{10}–10^{11} photons per shot with a repetition rate of 1 MHz in SASE mode. The studied X-ray FEL Oscillator configuration based on diamond mirrors produces 10^7–10^{10} coherent photons per shot at 3–3.5 keV at 1 MHz. These estimations do not take into account degradations due to errors, misalignments or jitters, and exceed by one or more orders of magnitude the target values set by the scientific case. MariX will therefore be capable of satisfying the expected FEL photon beam parameters, considering also a safety margin dealing with the losses in delivering the photon beams to the experimental hutch. Higher repetition rates could relax the cavity length requirements. The novel source will create absolutely novel conditions for experiments that cannot be performed satisfactorily at the present and foreseen sources based on storage rings or SASE-FEL.

Author Contributions: Conceptualization V.P., L.S., A.T. and M.O.; Definition of the scientific case G.R.; Methodology V.P., M.O., A.T.; Software and data curation M.O., M.R.C. and A.B.; Writing—original draft preparation V.P. and M.O.; writing—review and editing V.P., M.O.; Supervision V.P., L.S. and G.R.; Funding acquisition A.R.R., L.S. All authors have read and agreed to the published version of the manuscript.

Funding: This research received no external funding.

Institutional Review Board Statement: Not applicable.

Informed Consent Statement: Not applicable.

Conflicts of Interest: The authors declare no conflict of interest.

References

1. Faatz, B.; Schreiber, S. First Lasing of FLASH2 at DESY Synch. *Rad. News* **2014**, *27*, 6.
2. Emma, P.; Akre, R.; Arthur, J.; Bionta, R.; Bostedt, C.; Bozek, J.; Brachmann, A.; Bucksbaum, P.; Coffee, R.; Decker, F.-J.; et al. First lasing and operation of an Angstrom-wavelength free-electron laser. *Nat. Phot.* **2010**, *4*, 641. [CrossRef]
3. Pile, D. First light from SACLA. *Nat. Phot.* **2011**, *5*, 456. [CrossRef]
4. Weise, H.; Decking, W. Commissioning and First Lasing of the European XFEL. In Proceedings of the FEL2017, MOC03, Santa Fe, NM, USA, 20–25 August 2017.
5. Gruenbein, M.L.; Bielecki, J.; Gorel; A.; Stricker, M.; Bean, R.; Cammarata, M.; Doerner, K.; Froehlich, L.; Hartmann, E. Megahertz data collection from protein microcrystals at an X-ray free-electron laser. *Nat. Comm.* **2018**, *9*, 3487. [CrossRef]

6. SwissFEL at Paul Scherrer Institute (PSI) Website. Available online: https://www.psi.ch/en/swissfel/about-swissfel (accessed on 1 June 2021).
7. Ko, I.S.; Kang, H.; Heo, H.; Kim, C.; Kim, G.; Min, C.K.; Yang, H.; Baek, S.Y.; Choi, H.; Mun, G.; et al. Construction and commissioning of PAL-XFEL facility. *Appl. Sci.* **2017**, *7*, 479. [CrossRef]
8. Wang, D.; SXFEL team. Soft X-ray Free-Electron Laser at SINAP. In Proceedings of the IPAC2016, TUZA01, Busan, Korea, 8–13 May 2016.
9. Allaria, E.; Appio, R.; Badano, L.; Barletta, W.A.; Bassanese, S.; Biedron, S.G.; Borga, A.; Busetto, E.; Castronovo, D.; Cinquegrana, P.; et al. Highly coherent and stable pulses from the FERMI seeded free-electron laser in the extreme ultraviolet. *Nat. Phot.* **2012**, *6*, 699. [CrossRef]
10. Giannessi, L.; Artioli, M.; Bellaveglia, M.; Briquez, F.; Chiadroni, E.; Cianchi, A.; Couprie, M.E.; Dattoli, G.; Di Palma, E.; Di Pirro, G.; et al. High-Order-Harmonic Generation and Superradiance in a Seeded Free-Electron Laser. *Phys. Rev. Lett.* **2012**, *108*, 164801. [CrossRef] [PubMed]
11. Yu, L.H.; Babzien, M.; Ben-Zvi, I.; DiMauro, L.F.; Doyuran, A.; Graves,W.; Johnson, E.; Krinsky, S.; Malone, R.; Pogorelsky, I.; et al. High-gain harmonic-generation free-electron laser. *Science* **2000**, *289*, 932. [CrossRef]
12. Doyuran, A.; Di Mauro, L.; Graves, W.S.; Johnson, E.D.; Heese, R.; Krinsky, S.; Loos, H. Characterization of a high-gain harmonic-generation free-electron laser at saturation. *Phys. Rev. Lett.* **2001**, *86*, 5902. [CrossRef] [PubMed]
13. Takahashi, E.J.; Nabekawa, Y.; Mashiko, H.; Hasegawa, H.; Suda, A.; Midorikawa, K. Generation of strong optical field in soft X-ray region by using high-order harmonics. *IEEE J. Quant. Electr.* **2004**, *10*, 6. [CrossRef]
14. Yu, L.H.; DiMauro, L.; Doyuran, A.; Graves,W.S.; Johnson, E.D.; Heese, R; Krinsky, S.; Loos, H.; Murphy, J.B.; Rakowsky, G.; et al. First Ultraviolet High-Gain Harmonic-Generation Free-Electron Laser. *Phys. Rev. Lett.* **2003**, *91*, 074801. [CrossRef]
15. Togashi, T.; Takahashi, E.J.; Midorikawa, K.; Aoyama, M.; Yamakawa, K.; Sato, T.; Iwasaki, A.; Owada, S.; Yamanouchi, K.; Hara, T. Extreme ultraviolet free electron laser seeded with high-order harmonic of Ti:sapphire laser. *Opt. Exp.* **2011**, *19*, 317 . [CrossRef] [PubMed]
16. Giannessi, L.; Bellaveglia, M.; Chiadroni, E.; Cianchi, A.; Couprie, M.E.; DelFranco, M.; Di Pirro, G.; Ferrario, M.; Gatti, G.; Labat, M.; et al. Superradiant Cascade in a Seeded Free-Electron Laser. *Phys. Rev. Lett.* **2013**, *110*, 04480. [CrossRef]
17. Xiang, D.; Stupakov, G. Echo-enabled harmonic generation free electron laser. *Phys. Rev. Accel. Beams* **2009**, *12*, 030702. [CrossRef]
18. Hemsing, E.; Dunning, M.; Garcia, B.; Hast, C.; Raubenheimer, T.; Stupakov, G.; Xiang, D. Echo- enabled harmonics up to the 75th order from precisely tailored electron beams. *Nat. Phot.* **2016**, *10*, 512. [CrossRef]
19. Feng, C.; Deng, H.; Zhang, M.; Wang, X.; Chen, S.; Liu, T.; Zhou, K.; Gu, D.; Wang, Z.; Jiang, Z.; et al. Coherent extreme ultraviolet free-electron laser with echo-enabled harmonic generation. *Phys. Rev. Accel. Beams* **2019**, *22*, 050703. [CrossRef]
20. Rebernik Ribič, P.; Abrami, A.; Badano, L.; Bossi, M.; Braun, H.H.; Bruchon, N.; Capotondi, F.; Castronovo, D.; Cautero, M.; Cinquegrana, P.; et al. Coherent soft X-ray pulses from an echo-enabled harmonic generation free-electron laser nature research. *Nat. Phot.* **2019**, *13*, 1–7. [CrossRef]
21. Lambert, G.; Gautier, J.; Hauri, C.P.; Zeitoun, P.; Valentin, C.; Marchenko, T.; Tissandier, F.; Goddet, J.P.; Ribière, M.; Rey, G.; et al. An optimized kHz two-colour high harmonic source for seeding free-electron lasers and plasma-based soft X-ray lasers. *New J. Phys.* **2009**, *11*, 083033. [CrossRef]
22. Labat, M.; Bellaveglia, M.; Bougeard, M.; Carré, B.; Ciocci, F.; Chiadroni, E.; Cianchi, A.; Couprie, M.E.; Cultrera, L.; Del Franco, M.; et al. High-Gain Harmonic-Generation Free-Electron Laser Seeded by Harmonics Generated in Gas. *Phys. Rev. Lett.* **2011**, *107*, 224801. [CrossRef] [PubMed]
23. Petrillo, V.; Opromolla, M.; Bacci, A.; Drebot, I.; Ghiringhelli, G.; Petralia, A.; Puppin. E.; Rossetti Conti, M.; Rossi, A.R.; Tagliaferri, A.; et al. High repetition rate and coherent Free-Electron Laser in the X-rays range tailored for linear spectroscopy. *Instruments* **2019**, *3*, 47. [CrossRef]
24. Wurtele, J.; Gandhi, P.; Gu, W.X. Tunable soft X-ray oscillators. In Proceedings of the FEL2010, Malmö, Sweden, 23–27 August 2010.
25. Petrillo, V.; Opromolla, M.; Bacci, A.; Broggi, F.; Drebot, I.; Ghiringhelli, G.; Puppin, E.; Rossetti Conti, M.; Rossi, A.R.; Ruijter, M.; et al. Coherent, high repetition rate tender X-ray Free-Electron Laser seeded by an Extreme Ultra-Violet Free-Electron Laser Oscillator. *New J. Phys.* **2020**, *22*, 073058. [CrossRef]
26. Mirian, N.S.; Opromolla, M.; Rossi, G.; Serafini, L.; Petrillo, V. High repetition rate and coherent Free-Electron Laser in the tender X-rays based on the Echo-Enabled Harmonic Generation of an Ultra-Violet Oscillator pulse. *Phys. Rev. Accel. Beams* **2021**, *24*, 050702. [CrossRef]
27. Ackermann, S.; Faatz, B.; Grattoni, V.; Kazemi, M.-M.; Lang, T.; Leclmer, C.; Paraskaki, G.; Zemella, J. Novel method for the generation of stable radiation from free-electron lasers at high repetition rates. *Phys. Rev. Accel. Beams* **2020**, *23*, 071302. [CrossRef]
28. Rosenzweig, J.; Alesini, D.; Andonian, G.; Boscolo, M.; Dunning, M.; Faillace, L.; Ferrario, M.; Fukusawa, A.; Giannessi, L. Generation of ultra-short, high brightness electron beams for single-spike SAS FEL operation. *Nucl. Instr. Meth. Phys. Res. Sect. A* **2008**, *593*, 39. [CrossRef]
29. Marinelli, A.; MacArthur, J.; Emma, P.; Guetg, M.; Field, C.; Kharakh, D.; Lutman, A.A.; Ding, Y.; Huang, Z. Experimental demonstration of a single-spike hard-X-ray free-electron laser starting from noise. *Appl. Phys. Lett.* **2017**, *111*, 151101. [CrossRef]

30. Villa, F.; Anania, M.P.; Artioli, M.; Bacci, A.; Bellaveglia, M.; Bisesto, M.G.; Biagioni, A.; Carpanese, M.; Cardelli, F.; Castorin, G. Generation and characterization of ultra-short electron beams for single spike infrared FEL radiation at SPARC_LAB. *Nucl. Instr. Meth. Phys. Res. Sect. A* **2017**, *865*, 43–46. [CrossRef]
31. Geloni, G.; Kocharyan, V.; Saldin, E. '=A novel self-seeding scheme for hard X-ray FELs. *J. Mod. Opt.* **2011**, *58*, 1391–1403. [CrossRef]
32. Amann, J.; Berg, W.; Blank, V.; Decker, F.-J.; Ding, Y.; Emma, P.; Feng, Y.; Frisch, J.; Fritz, D.; Hastings, J.; et al. Demonstration of self-seeding in a hard-X-ray free-electron laser. *Nat. Phot.* **2012**, *6*, 693–698. [CrossRef]
33. Dattoli, G.; Palma, E.D.; Petralia, A. Free-electron laser oscillator efficiency. *Opt. Comm.* **2018**, *425*, 29.
34. Ciocci, F.; Dattoli, G.; De Angelis, A.; Faatz, B.; Garosi, F.; Giannessi, L.; Ottaviani, P.L.; Torre, A. Design considerations on a high-power VUV FEL. *IEEE J. Quant. Electr.* **1995**, *31*, 1242–1252. [CrossRef]
35. der Slot, P.J.M.V.; Freund, H.P.; Miner, W.W., Jr.; Benson, S.V.; Schinn, M.; Boller K.-J. Time-dependent Three dimensional simulation of free-electron laser oscillators. *Phys. Rev. Lett.* 2009, 102, 244802. [CrossRef] [PubMed]
36. Kim, K.-J.; Shvyd'ko, Y. Tunable optical cavity for an X-ray Free-Electron Laser Oscillator. *Phys. Rev. Accel. Beams* **2009**, *12*, 030703. [CrossRef]
37. Kim, K.-J.; Shvyd'ko, Y.; Reiche, S. A proposal for an X-ray oscillator with an Energy recovery Linac. *Phys. Rev. Lett.* **2008**, *100*, 244802. [CrossRef]
38. Shvyd'ko, Y.; Stoupin, S.; Cunsolo, A.; Said, A.H.; Huang, X. High-reflectivity high-resolution X-ray crystal optics with diamonds. *Nat. Phys.* **2010**, *6*, 196. [CrossRef]
39. Qin, W.; Huang, S.; Liu, K.X.; Kim, K.-J.; Lindberg, R.R.; Ding, Y.; Huang, Z.; Maxwell, T.; Bane, K.; Marcus, G. Start-to-end simulations for an X-ray FEL oscillator at the LCLS-II and LCLS-HE. In Proceedings of the FEL2017, Santa Fe, NM, USA, 20–25 August 2017.
40. Huang, Z.; Ruth, R.D. Fully Coherent X-Ray Pulses from a Regenerative-Amplifier Free-Electron Laser. *Phys. Rev. Lett.* **2006**, *96*, 144801. [CrossRef]
41. McNeil, B.W.J.; Thompson, N.R.; Dunning, D.J.; Karssenberg, J.G.; van der Slot, P.J.M.; Boller, K.-J. A design for the generation of temporally-coherent radiation pulses in the VUV and beyond by a seld-seeded high gain free electron laser amplifier. *New J. Phys.* **2007**, *9*, 239. [CrossRef]
42. Li, K.; Deng, H. Systematic design and three-dimensional simulation of X-ray FEL oscillator for Shanghai Coherent Light Facility. *Nucl. Instr. Meth. Phys. Res. Sect. A* **2018**, *895*, 40–47. [CrossRef]
43. Marcus, G.; Ding, Y.; Feng, Y.; Halavanau, A.; Huang, Z.; Krzywinski, J.; MacArthur, J.; Margraf, R.; Raubenheimer T.; Zhu, D.; et al. Regenerative amplification for a hard-X ray Free-Electron laser. In Proceedings of the FEL 2019, TUP032, Hamburg, Germany, 26–30 August 2019.
44. Marcus, G.; Decker, F.-J. Cavity-based Free-Electron Laser research and development: A Joint Argonne National Laboratory and SLAC National Laboratory collaboration. In Proceedings of the FEL 2019, TUD04, Hamburg, Germany, 6–30 August 2 2019.
45. Freund, H.P. ; Slot, P.J.M.v.; Shvydko, Y. An X-ray Regenerative Amplifier Free-Electron Laser Using Diamond Pinhole Mirrors. *New J. Phys.* **2019**, *21*, 093028. [CrossRef]
46. Li, A.K.; Yan, J.; Feng, C.; Zhang, M.; Deng, H. High brightness fully coherent X-ray amplifier seeded by a free-electron laser oscillator. *Phys. Rev. Accel. Beams* **2018**, *21*, 040702. [CrossRef]
47. Freund, H.P.; Nguyen, D.C.; Sprangle, P.A.; Slot, P.J.M.V. Three-dimensional, time-dependent simulation of a regenerative amplifier free-electron laser. *Phys. Rev. Accel. Beams* **2013**, *16*, 010707. [CrossRef]
48. Serafini, L.; Bacci, A.; Bellandi, A.; Bertucci, M.; Bolognesi, M.; Bosotti, A.; Broggi, F.; Calandrino, R.; Camera, F.; Canella, F.; et al. MariX, an advancedMHz-class repetition rate X-ray source for linear regime time-resolved spectroscopy and photon scattering. *Nucl. Instr. Meth. Phys. Res. Sect. A* **2019**, *930*, 167–172. [CrossRef]
49. Mitri, S.D.; Cornacchia, M. Transverse emittance-preserving arc compressor for highbrightness electron beam-based light sources and colliders. *Europhys. Lett.* **2015**, *109*, 62002. [CrossRef]
50. Mitri, S.D. Feasibility study of a periodic arc compressor in the presence of coherent synchrotron radiation. *Nucl. Instr. Meth. Phys. Res. Sect. A* **2016**, *806*, 184. [CrossRef]
51. Placidi, M.; Di Mitri, S.; Pellegrini, C.; Penn, G. Compact FEL-driven inverse compton scattering gamma-ray source. *Nucl. Instr. Meth. Phys. Res. Sect. A* **2017**, *855*, 55–60. [CrossRef]
52. Bacci, A.; Rossetti Conti, M.; Bosotti, A.; Cialdi, S.; Di Mitri, S.; Drebot, I.; Faillace, L.; Ghiringhelli, G.; Michelato, P.; Monaco, L.; et al. Two-pass two-way acceleration in a Super-Conducting CW linac to drive low jitters X-ray FELs. *Phys. Rev. Accel. Beams* **2019**, *22*, 111304. [CrossRef]
53. Reiche, S. GENESIS 1.3: A fully 3D time-dependent FEL simulation code. *Nucl. Instr. Meth. Phys. Res. Sect. A* **1999**, *429*, 243. [CrossRef]
54. Belanger, P.A. Beam propagation and the ABCD ray matrices. *Opt. Lett.* **1991**, *16*, 196. [CrossRef] [PubMed]
55. Software XOP, Download from European Synchrotron Radiation Facility Website. Available online: https://www.esrf.fr/Instrumentation/software/data-analysis/xop2.4 (accessed on 1 May 2020).

Article

Two-Beam Free-Electron Lasers and Self-Injected Nonlinear Harmonic Generation

Elio Sabia *, Emanuele Di Palma and Giuseppe Dattoli

ENEA—Frascati Research Center, Via Enrico Fermi 45, 00044 Rome, Italy; emanuele.dipalma@enea.it (E.D.P.); pinodattoli@libero.it (G.D.)
* Correspondence: elio.sabia@gmail.com

Abstract: The possibility of extending the tunability of Free-Electron Lasers towards short wavelengths has been explored through the design of devices conceived to enhance the mechanisms of nonlinear harmonic generation. In this respect, different schemes of operation have been suggested in the past, such as harmonic seeding, bi-harmonic undulators, and two-beam self-seeding devices. In this paper, we discuss how these methods can be merged into a tool, extending the performance of FEL devices.

Keywords: free-electron laser; electron accelerators; undulators; two harmonic undulators; seeding

1. Introduction

Nonlinear harmonic generation (NLHG) is one of the key mechanisms adopted to extend the spectral tunability range of Free-Electron Laser (FEL) [1–5]. Harmonic seeding [6,7] and NLHG have been widely exploited in the past to push the FEL and its application towards shorter wavelengths. Other suggestions, although promising, have been carefully studied, but have not found specific applications so far.

In this article, we discuss the possibility of combining two different proposals, developed in the past, concerning the use of devices exploiting NLHG in high-gain FEL devices [4,8]. We deal with the harmonically coupled two-beam self-injection [9] and bi-harmonic undulators [10,11], conceived to enhance the FEL coherent harmonic content emission and extend the capabilities of the device itself.

(a) *Nonlinear Harmonic Generation*

Although the mechanism of nonlinear harmonic generation occurs in a FEL device operating with linearly and helically polarized undulators, here we treat the linear case only and consider undulators with on-axis field vector

$$\vec{B}_u \equiv B_0[0, \sin(k_u z), 0]. \tag{1}$$

The pattern to the higher harmonic emission is an intrigued interplay between all the processes underlying the FEL lasing and involving energy modulation, bunching, coherent emission, higher-order bunching, and saturation [7]. The relevant study is afforded by exploiting a generalization of the FEL pendulum equations, including the evolution of the fields of the individual harmonics, namely [1]

$$\frac{d^2}{d\tau^2}\zeta = \sum_{n=0}^{\infty} |a_n| \cos(\psi_n), \quad \psi_n = n\zeta + \phi_n,$$

$$a_n = |a_n|e^{i\phi_n}, \tag{2}$$

$$\frac{d}{d\tau}a_n = -j_n \langle e^{-in\zeta} \rangle.$$

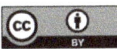

where n refers to the order of the harmonic, (a, j) are the Colson's dimensionless amplitude and current respectively, ζ is the dimensionless electron phase, finally the brackets $\langle \ldots \rangle$ denote averages on the initial phase distribution. The modulus of a is linked to the field intensity (power density) I by the identities

$$|a|^2 = 8\pi^2 \frac{I}{I_s},$$
$$I_s = \frac{c}{8\pi}\left(\frac{m_e c^2}{e}\right)^2 \left(\frac{\gamma}{N}\right)^4 \left(\lambda_u \frac{K}{\sqrt{2}} f_b\right)^{-2}. \quad (3)$$

The quantity I_s denotes the FEL saturation intensity, a key quantity either in FEL and conventional lasers. It controls the onset of saturation, which starts playing a role when the FEL intensity is close to I_s [12].

The physical content of the previous set of equations can be summarized as follows. The fundamental harmonic ($n = 1$) drives the bunching, which allows the growth of the different harmonics if the corresponding dimensionless currents j_n are nonvanishing. In the case of FEL devices operating with linear undulators, this is automatically ensured by the on-axis coupling to odd harmonics.

An example of nonlinear harmonic generation intensity growth is given in Figure 1, drawn using the analytical formulae summarized in Equation (4). The relevant agreement with numerical computation has been benchmarked with the Prometeo code [13], as discussed below.

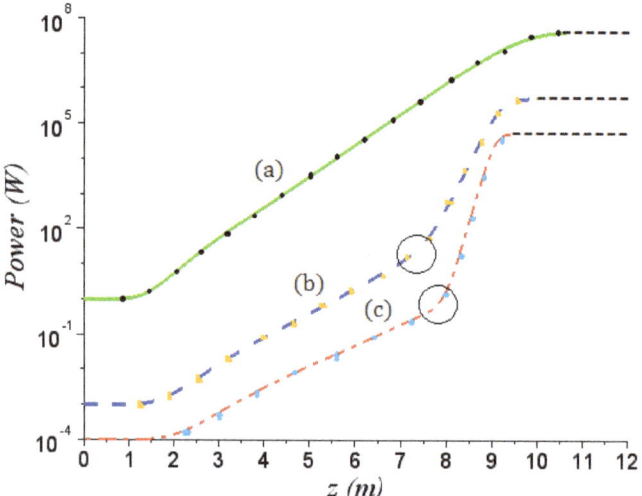

Figure 1. Harmonic power growth vs. the undulator length in m; (**a**) First Harmonic (green) (**b**) Third harmonic (blue) (**c**) Fifth harmonic (red). The encircled region around the inflection points, where the transition to the NLHG regime occurs, is not well reproduced by the analytical formulae. Linear and NLHG contributions are indeed summed incoherently, namely through the sum of two intensities ($\Lambda_n(z)$ and $\Pi_n(z)$), without including the respective phases determining at that point an insignificant oscillation.

The process consists of two distinct parts. In the first, the fundamental ($n = 1$) and higher-order harmonics (3,5) grows independently, till the bunching at higher harmonics, induced by the fundamental, triggers the nonlinear harmonic generation mechanisms.

The analytical procedure developed in the past [14] yields a fairly straightforward description of the different evolution steps. The model equations are reported below, and we have denoted with $\Lambda_n(z)$ and $\Pi_n(z)$ the terms accounting for the small-signal and nonlinear harmonic generation parts respectively

$$P_1 = P_1(z) = P_0 \frac{A(z)}{1 + \frac{P_0}{P_{F,1}}[A(z) - 1]},$$

$$A(z) = \frac{1}{9}\left[3 + 2\cosh\left(\frac{z}{L_{g,1}}\right) + 4\cos\left(\frac{\sqrt{3}}{2}\frac{z}{L_{g,1}}\right)\cosh\left(\frac{z}{2L_{g,1}}\right)\right],$$

$$P_n(z) = \Lambda_n(z) + \Pi_n(z), \quad n = 3, 5... \quad \Lambda_n(z) = P_{0,n} A_n(z).$$

For the case with $n > 1$ the gain length should be replaced by

$$L_{g,n}^* = \frac{\lambda_u}{4\pi\sqrt{3}\rho_n^*} = n^{-1/3} L_{g,n}, \quad \rho_n^* = n^{1/3}\rho_n, \quad P_{0,n} \text{ input seed power}, \qquad (4)$$

$\rho_n \equiv n-$th harmonic Pierce parameter,

$$\rho_n = \left(\frac{f_{b,n}}{f_{b,1}}\right)^{2/3} \rho_1,$$

$$f_{b,n} = J_{\frac{n-1}{2}}(n\xi) - J_{\frac{n+1}{2}}(n\xi), \quad \xi = \frac{1}{4}\frac{K^2}{1+\frac{K^2}{2}},$$

$$\rho_1 \cong \frac{8.63 \times 10^{-3}}{\gamma}\left[J(\lambda_u K f_{b,1})^2\right]^{1/3}.$$

The formula for the Pierce parameter of the harmonic (ρ_1) is expressed in a practical form, where J is given in A/m^2 and λ_u in m. The NLHG contributions are specified by the formulae

$$\Pi_n(z) = \Pi_{0,n}\frac{\exp\left(\frac{nz}{L_{g,1}}\right)}{1 + \frac{\Pi_{0,n}}{\Pi_{F,n}}\left[\exp\left(\frac{nz}{L_{g,1}}\right) - 1\right]}, \quad \Pi_{0,n} = c_n\left(\frac{P_0}{9\rho_1 P_E}\right)^n \Pi_{F,n}, \quad c_3 = 8, \quad c_5 = 116, \qquad (5)$$

$$\Pi_{F,n} = \sqrt{n}\left(\frac{\rho_n}{n\rho_1}\right)^3 P_{F,1} = \frac{1}{\sqrt{n}}\left(\frac{f_{b,n}}{nf_{b,1}}\right)^2 P_{F,1},$$

where the saturated power $P_{F,1}$ reads

$$P_{F,1} = \sqrt{2}\rho_1 P_E \qquad (6)$$

and P_E is the e-beam power.

We note therefore that

1. The first harmonic power grows initially by exhibiting the lethargic phase followed by the exponential behavior, characterized by the gain length $L_{g,1}$.
2. The same occurs for the higher-order harmonics (with gain length $L_{g,n}^*$), till the bunching effects trigger the mechanism of nonlinear harmonic generation.
3. This last phase is characterized by a sudden change in the growth rate followed by a kind of saturation. The characteristic gain length is a fraction of that of the fundamental (namely $L_n^{(NH)} = \frac{L_{g,1}}{n}$).

The inflexion point (before the change in the intensity growth derivative) occurs at $z = z*$, where the $\Lambda_n(z)$ and $\Pi_n(z)$ contributions balance. The dots refer to a numerical benchmark with the code Prometeo, for a set of specific parameters. After the saturation the figure exhibits a flat top, without displaying the characteristic power oscillations. This is an artefact of the analytical approximations. It should be noted that, although not significant for the present discussion, these oscillations can be included in the analytical scheme as shown in refs. [15,16].

(b) Bi-Harmonic undulator

The use of bi-harmonic undulators [10,11] has been suggested in the past as a device allowing the enhancement of the nonlinear harmonic generation in high-gain FEL devices.

In the case of an undulator exhibiting a field with linear orthogonal polarization, specified by the vector

$$\vec{B}_u \equiv [3 B_0 \sin(3 k_u z), B_0 \sin(k_u z), 0], \tag{7}$$

The corresponding FEL pendulum equation can be written by extending those reported in (2) and reads

$$\begin{aligned}
\frac{\partial^2 \zeta_{x,1}}{\partial \tau^2} &= |a_{x,1}| \cos(\zeta_{x,1} + \varphi_{x,1}), \\
\frac{\partial a_{x,3}}{\partial \tau} &= -j_{x,3} \langle e^{-i\zeta_{x,3}} \rangle, \\
\frac{\partial a_{x,1}}{\partial \tau} &= -j_{x,1} \langle e^{-i\zeta_{x,1}} \rangle, \\
\frac{\partial a_y}{\partial \tau} &= -j_y \langle e^{-i\zeta_y} \rangle; \ \zeta_{x,3} = \zeta_y = 3\zeta_{x,1}.
\end{aligned} \tag{8}$$

The relevant physical meaning is not dissimilar from that discussed as a comment to Equation (2). In this case, we have considered 1st and 3rd harmonics only, with the significant difference that two "third" harmonics, with orthogonal polarization, are driven by the fundamental. The third harmonics bears both vertical and linear polarization components and the relevant dimensionless amplitude are defined as

$$|a_\sigma|^2 = 0.8 \pi^4 \frac{I_\sigma}{I_{s,\sigma}}, \tag{9}$$

where $\sigma = x, y$ and I_s is the associated saturation intensity

$$I_{s,\sigma} \left[\frac{MW}{cm^2}\right] = \frac{6.9 \times 10^2 \left(\frac{\gamma}{N_\sigma}\right)^4}{[\lambda_{u,\sigma}[cm] K f_{b,\sigma}(\xi)]^2}. \tag{10}$$

Please note that $N_x = 3N_y$, $\lambda_{u,x} = \lambda_{u,y}/3$.

The corresponding Bessel factors are specified below (the wavelength of the first harmonic is $\lambda_1 = (\lambda_u/2\gamma^2)(1+K^2)$. Further comments are provided in Section 3)

$$\begin{aligned}
f_{b,1x} &= {}^{(3)}J_0\left(\xi, \frac{\xi}{3}\right) - {}^{(3)}J_1\left(\xi, \frac{\xi}{3}\right), \\
f_{b,3x} &= -{}^{(3)}J_1(3\xi, \xi) + {}^{(3)}J_2(3\xi, \xi), \\
f_{b,3y} &= {}^{(3)}J_0(3\xi, \xi) - {}^{(3)}J_2(3\xi, \xi), \\
\xi &= \frac{1}{4}\frac{K^2}{1+K^2},
\end{aligned} \tag{11}$$

and $^{(m)}J_n(x, y)$ are generalized Bessel functions defined through the generating function

$$\sum_{n=-\infty}^{+\infty} t^n \left[{}^{(m)}J_n(x, y) \right] = e^{\frac{x}{2}\left(t - \frac{1}{t}\right) + \frac{y}{2}\left(t^m - \frac{1}{t^m}\right)}, \tag{12}$$

and the series expansions (for further comments see ref. [17])

$${}^{(m)}J_n(x, y) = \sum_{l=-\infty}^{+\infty} J_l(x) J_{n-ml}(y). \tag{13}$$

In Figure 2 an example is given of bi-harmonic power growth. The 1-D simulation displays the already anticipated behavior: along with the fundamental "two" third harmonics, with radial and vertical components, are generated through the nonlinear mechanism.

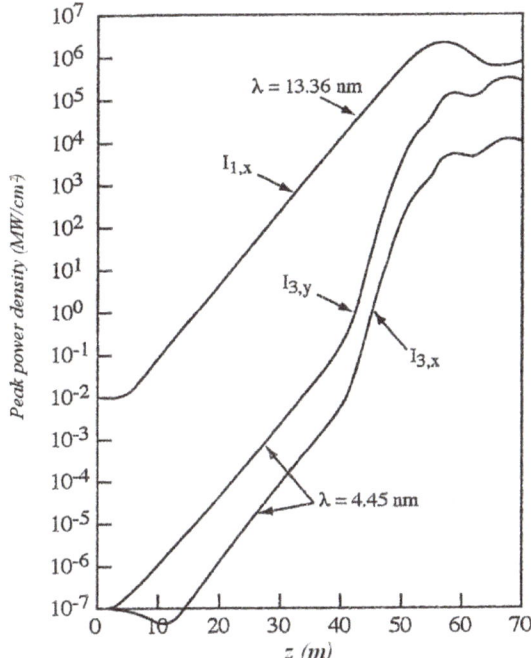

Figure 2. Power growth of main and third harmonics for a bi-harmonic undulator with, $E = 1078$ Mev, $\lambda_u = 6$ cm, $K = 0.99$, $\rho = 1.258 \times 10^{-3}$ (numerical simulation PROMETEO).

The physical content of the figure is not different from what we have already discussed when we commented Figure 1 and is worded as reported below. The first harmonic grows and induces, via NLHG, two third harmonics with distinct orthogonal polarizations. The signature for the nonlinear growth is specified by the abrupt change of the growth rate. The two phases of the growth are characterized by the respective gain lengths, namely

$$L^*_{g,3_x} = \frac{1}{3^{1/3}} \frac{\lambda_u}{4\pi\sqrt{3}\rho_{3_x}},$$

$$L^*_{g,y} = \frac{\lambda_u}{4\pi\sqrt{3}3^{1/3}\rho_y}, \tag{14}$$

and

$$L_g^{(NH)} = \frac{L_{g,1_x}}{3}, \tag{15}$$

where

$$\rho_{1_x} \cong \tfrac{8.63\times 10^{-3}}{\gamma}\left[J\left(\lambda_u K f_{b,1_x}\right)^2\right]^{1/3},$$

$$\rho_{3_x} = \rho_{1_x}\left(\frac{f_{b,3_x}}{f_{b,1_x}}\right)^{\frac{3}{2}}, \qquad (16)$$

$$\rho_y = \rho_{1_x}\left(\frac{1}{3}\frac{f_{b,3_y}}{f_{b,1_x}}\right)^{\frac{3}{2}}.$$

The y-polarized component is significantly larger than its x-counterpart and grows almost at the level of the first.

This is an interesting result since, for the single harmonic undulator, the third exhibits a power of two orders of magnitude below that of the fundamental.

The proposal, the design and construction of this type of undulator traces back to more than three decades ago [18,19]. Although exploited in Storage Ring (SR) sources, they did not find any specific application in the development of FEL, although they have been extensively discussed in the literature [20].

It is certainly true that such a structure is not easy to design, to measure and to handle. Possible alternatives are ensured by segmented undulators, consisting of two undulator sections with emission frequency of the second a sub-multiple of the first [21–23]. Such a solution, more manageable from the technical point of view, preserves some of the features of the whole device and will be commented on in the concluding section.

A further possibility, suggested by McNeil, Robb and Poole [24] is that of the harmonically coupled 2-beam FEL (HCB). In their proposal, it is foreseen the use of two beams operating at different energies, passing through a linearly polarized undulator, to run an FEL operating at different harmonics. The relativistic factor of the higher energy beam is chosen in such a way that $\gamma_2 = \sqrt{n}\gamma_1$.

In loose terms, the mechanism of growth of the FEL signal can be described as reported below. The first beam induces the bunching conditions to trigger the third harmonics, if $n = 3$, which eventually seeds the first harmonic emitted by the higher energy beam.

In the forthcoming section we model the dynamics of the harmonically coupled beams FEL, using the already quoted semi-analytical procedure [14].

2. Harmonically Coupled Two Beams and High-Gain FELs

As already underlined the HBC scheme foresees two beams with energies γ_1 and $\gamma_2 = \sqrt{n}\gamma_1$, both injected in a linearly polarized undulator. Instabilities of two-stream nature, spoiling the FEL dynamics do not play any role because of the (large) beam energies.

The condition on the energies of beams (1) and (2), ensures that the first harmonic, radiated by the beam (2), coincides with one of the higher-order harmonics of the first (1).

As already established, the two beams radiate independently and give rise to two distinct FEL process, until the n-th harmonic, of the beam with lower energy, seeds that emitted by the beam with larger energy.

The Pierce parameter associated with the two beams are

$$\rho^{(1)} \cong \sqrt[3]{J^{(1)}}\, U(\lambda_u, K),$$

$$\rho^{(2)} \cong \tfrac{1}{\sqrt{n}}\sqrt[3]{J^{(2)}}\, U(\lambda_u, K), \qquad (17)$$

$$U(\lambda_u, K) = \tfrac{8.36\times 10^{-3}}{\gamma_1}[\lambda_u K f_b(K)]^{\frac{2}{3}},$$

The Pierce parameters are therefore linked by

$$\frac{\rho^{(2)}}{\rho^{(1)}} = \frac{1}{\sqrt{n}}\sqrt[3]{\frac{J^{(2)}}{J^{(1)}}}. \qquad (18)$$

If we assume that the two beams have the same current density, we obtain that the Pierce parameter associated with the beam at higher energy is lower by a factor $n^{-1/2}$.

The two fields grow inside the undulator independently. If $E_2/E_1 = \sqrt{3}$, the wavelength radiated by the beam (2) is the same of the third harmonic associated with the emission process of the beam (1). The intensities of the fields (1,2) grow independently, until NLHG occurs, when the third harmonics of the beam (1) seeds that from (2) (see Figure 3).

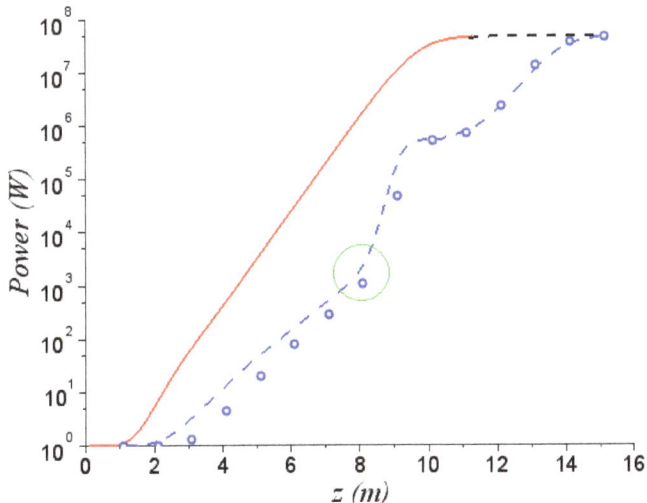

Figure 3. Intensity associated with the FEL action of the low energy beam (continuous red), and of the higher energy beam (dashed blue). The green circle stresses the same comment regarding Figure 1. The small blue circles refer to numerical benchmark with PROMETEO.

The nonlinear harmonic growth is superimposed to the emission of the beam 2 and after the plateau of the nonlinear harmonic generation, eventually reaches the saturation which follows an exponential growth with the same gain length of the initial phase (lethargic and exponential) $L_{g,1}^{(2)} = \sqrt{3} L_{g,1}^{(1)}$.

The last step, including saturation, can be figured out as a straightforward exponential growth, namely

$$P^{(2)}(z) = \Pi_{n,F} \frac{\exp\left[\frac{(z-z*)}{L_g^{(2)}}\right]}{1 + \frac{\Pi_{n,F}}{P_F^{(2)}}\left[\exp\left[\frac{(z-z*)}{L_g^{(2)}}\right] - 1\right]},$$

$$P_F^{(2)} \cong \sqrt{2} \rho^{(2)} P_E^{(2)}, \tag{19}$$

$P_E^{(2)} \equiv$ power of the higher energy beam,

$$L_g^{(2)} \equiv \frac{\lambda_u}{4\pi\sqrt{3}\rho^{(2)}} = \sqrt{n} L_g^{(1)}.$$

If the two beams bear the same peak current (this is our assumption), the saturated power of the two laser beams is, approximately, the same.

Regarding the high energy part, the length of the undulator section necessary to reach the saturation, from the first plateau, is simply given by

$$\Pi_{n,F} \exp\left[\frac{\Delta_u}{\sqrt{n} L_g^{(1)}}\right] \cong P_F^{(2)}, \qquad (20)$$

which yields

$$\Delta_U \cong \sqrt{n} \ln\left(\frac{P_F^{(2)}}{\Pi_{n,F}}\right) L_{g,1}^{(1)} = \sqrt{n} \left(\frac{5}{2} \ln(n) + 2 \ln\left(\frac{f_{b,1}}{f_{b,n}}\right)\right) L_{g,1}^{(1)}. \qquad (21)$$

It is evident that we have considered a fairly idealized case. We have also assumed that the two beams have identical current densities. This means that if the beams bear the same current and are supposed to be round the following condition should be satisfied

$$\beta^{(1)} \varepsilon^{(1)} = \beta^{(2)} \varepsilon^{(2)}, \qquad (22)$$

where $\beta^{(1,2)}$ are the associated Twiss parameters and $\varepsilon^{(1,2)}$ the e-beam emittances. Furthermore, including the usual scaling of the emittance with energy, we may also conjecture that $\beta^{(2)} \cong \frac{\beta^{(1)}}{\sqrt{3}}$. These are qualitative statements, to be better framed within a specific design context of the electron beams transport channel, which will be discussed elsewhere.

The presence of a non-negligible energy spread might be sources of troubles. The Pierce parameter associated with the second beam is indeed lower by a factor $\sqrt{3}$, therefore the relative energy spread $\sigma_\varepsilon^{(2)} < \frac{2}{\sqrt{3}} \rho^{(1)}$, which is a condition not hard to achieve since the relative energy spread scales with the inverse of the energy.

The original result by McNeil, Robb and Poole is reported in Figure 4, which provides the evolution of the first and third harmonic, according to the previously discussed patterns. The analytical method reproduces the growth of the first harmonic till the onset of the saturation (the after saturation is just replaced by the dot line superimposed to the figure). The red and green dots denote the predictions with the semi-analytical model. We underscore therefore the reliability of our procedure, benchmarked against an independent numerical treatment.

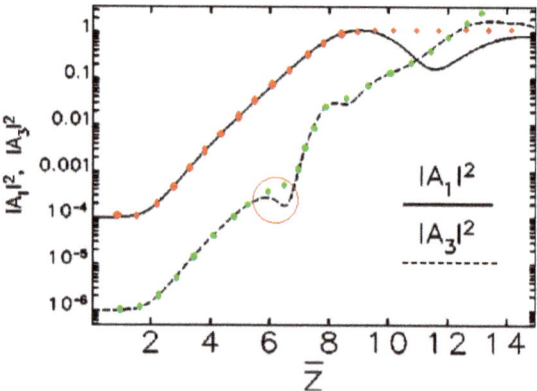

Figure 4. Growth of the first harmonic and of the higher-order self-injected contributions (courtesy of McNeil, Robb and Poole). $\bar{z}$ and $|A|^2$ are normalized longitudinal coordinate and field intensity respectively, the subscript 1,3 denote the harmonic order. The encircled region marks the transition between linear and NLHG, with a characteristic oscillation. The red and green dots refer to the semi-analytical benchmark.

Apart from the assumption that the initial seeds are different, the analytical picture we have exploited captures well the physics of the process, as previously described. The numerical analysis of ref. [9] has been accomplished using an ad-hoc developed numerical code, the model developed in this article has been benchmarked with PROMETEO [13].

We have illustrated two different concepts, both based on the NLHG mechanism. At first glance, they might be viewed as equivalent, but this is not true. The two harmonic undulator uses one beam only and the effect of the FEL induced energy spread determines the saturation of the fundamental and of the higher harmonics. On the other side in the HCB scheme the second beam is fresh, while the first is not completely burnt.

The two schemes are complementary and in the forthcoming section we will see how the two mechanisms can be combined to obtain a device offering further flexibilities for new FEL architectures.

3. FEL Operating with HCB and Bi-Harmonic Undulators

In the present section, we show how HCB and bi-harmonic undulators can be combined to obtain a laser beam with different harmonics and polarizations.

The idea we would like to present is that of two beams with different energies injected in an undulator displaying the following on-axis magnetic field

$$\vec{B}_u \equiv [d\, B_0 \sin(h\, k_u z), B_0 \sin(k_u z), 0], \quad (23)$$

where h is an integer and d is a numerical factor, smaller or larger than unit and not necessarily an integer.

The spectral content of the on-axis emitted radiation is fairly rich [25] and the order of the harmonics depend on the polarization of the emitted harmonics, we have indeed

$$\lambda_{n,x} = \frac{\lambda_u}{2n\gamma^2}\left[1 + \frac{K^2}{2}\left(1 + \frac{d^2}{h^2}\right)\right],$$

$$\lambda_{n,y} = \frac{\lambda_u}{2(hn)\gamma^2}\left[1 + \frac{K^2}{2}\left(1 + \frac{d^2}{h^2}\right)\right]. \quad (24)$$

The derivation of the FEL evolution equations involves a rather awkward algebra, partially alleviated by the use of multi-variable Bessel functions, which become an efficient tool to evaluate the associated Pierce parameter.

The advantage of the bi-harmonic undulator is that we are not obliged to consider odd harmonics of the fundamental only. If we keep $h = 2$ in Equation (23) we expect higher harmonics of even order. According to Equation (24) $\lambda_{1,y}$ is the second harmonic of the fundamental, with y polarization.

The general expression of the Bessel factor terms reads

$$f_{b,n_x} = (-1)^{\frac{n-1}{2}}\left[{}^{(h)}J_{\frac{n-1}{2}}\left(n\xi, (-1)^{h+1}\frac{d^2}{h^2}\left(\frac{n\xi}{h}\right)\right) - {}^{(h)}J_{\frac{n+1}{2}}\left(n\xi, (-1)^{h+1}\frac{d^2}{h^2}\left(\frac{n\xi}{h}\right)\right)\right],$$

$$f_{b,(hn)_y} = \frac{d}{h}(-1)^{\frac{(n-1)h}{2}}\left[{}^{(h)}J_{\frac{h(n-1)}{2}}\left(hn\xi, (-1)^{h+1}\frac{d^2}{h^2}n\xi\right) + (-1)^{h(h)}J_{\frac{h(n+1)}{2}}\left(hn\xi, (-1)^{h+1}\frac{d^2}{h^2}n\xi\right)\right], \quad (25)$$

$$\xi = \frac{1}{4}\frac{K^2}{1+\frac{K^2}{2}\left(1+\left(\frac{h}{d}\right)^2\right)}.$$

Regarding therefore $h = 2, d = 2$ we obtain for the Bessel factors

$$f_{b,1_x} = \left[{}^{(2)}J_0\left(\xi, -\frac{\xi}{2}\right) - {}^{(2)}J_1\left(\xi, -\frac{\xi}{2}\right)\right],$$

$$f_{b,2_y} = \left[{}^{(2)}J_0(2\,\xi, -\xi) + {}^{(2)}J_2(2\,\xi, -\xi)\right], \quad (26)$$

$$f_{b,3_x} = -\left[{}^{(2)}J_1\left(3\,\xi, -\left(\frac{3\xi}{2}\right)\right) - {}^{(2)}J_2\left(3\,\xi, -\left(\frac{3\xi}{2}\right)\right)\right]$$

and for the Pierce parameters

$$\rho_{3_x} = \left(\frac{f_{b,3_x}}{f_{b,1_x}}\right)^{\frac{2}{3}} \rho_{1_x},$$

$$\rho_y = \left(\frac{f_{b,2_y}}{2f_{b,1_x}}\right)^{\frac{2}{3}} \rho_{1_x}, \quad (27)$$

$$\rho_{1_x} = U(\lambda_u, K) \sqrt[3]{J} \left(f_{b,1_x}(K)\right)^{\frac{2}{3}},$$

$$U(\lambda_u, K) = \frac{8.36 \times 10^{-3}}{\gamma} [\lambda_u K]^{\frac{2}{3}}.$$

We consider the same parameter in Figure 2 which for $h = 2$ yields three harmonics at saturation, with wavelengths 13.36 nm (x-pol), 6.68 nm (y-pol) and 4.43 (x-pol).

In Figure 5 we have reported the behavior of the Pierce parameters vs. K and in Figure 6 the growth of the three harmonics vs. the undulator length for $E_2/E_1 = \sqrt{3}$. The second harmonic (with y-polarization) grows at the same level of the first and the third, seeds (with x-polarization) the first associated with the higher energy beam.

We have so far shown that the mechanism of two harmonic undulators and of harmonically coupled beams, works, at least in principle. In the forthcoming section we will add further elements, stressing the prospective usefulness of these concepts.

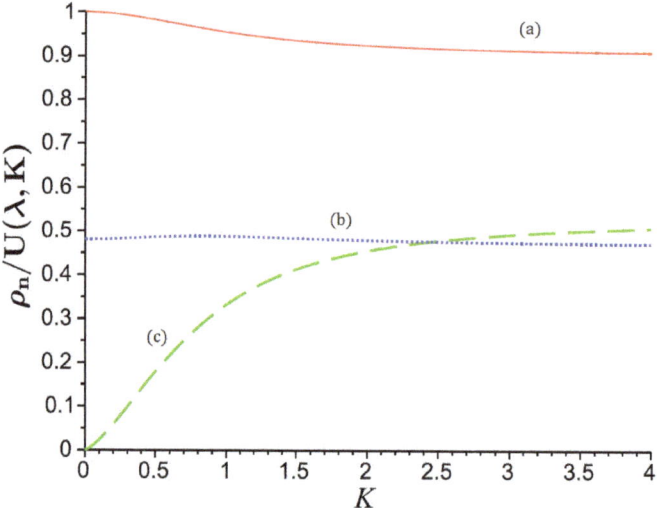

Figure 5. Pierce parameter ($\frac{\rho_n}{U(\lambda,K)}$) vs. K; (**a**) $(1)_x$ continuous line (**b**) $(2)_y$ dot line (**c**) $(3)_x$ dash line.

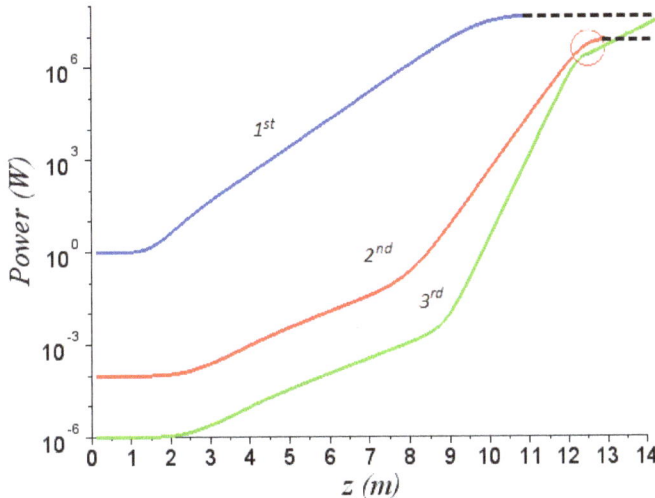

Figure 6. Evolution of the first, second and third harmonics. The third harmonic is further amplified by the second beam at higher energy and brought at the same level of the first.

4. Final Comments

In the previous section we have discussed the possibility of merging two concepts, regarding FEL devices, which can operate with "harmonic" beams and undulators. The concepts we have developed can be framed within analogous efforts discussed in the past involving the use of undulators with orthogonal polarizations [20,26,27] and segmented undulators [28], as well.

Regarding this last point, we note that FELs operating with segmented undulators in the SASE mode employ two (or more) undulator sections, tuned at a sub-harmonic of the preceding one.

$$P_n(z) = P_{b,n}^L F_n^L(z) + P_{b,n}^B \frac{F_n^B(z)}{1 + \frac{P_{b,n}^B}{\Pi_{F,n}} F_n^B(z)}, \quad n = 3,5$$

$$P_{b,3}^L = \frac{9}{2}|b_{3,0}|^2, \quad P_{b,5}^L = \frac{5}{2}|b_{5,0}|^2, \quad P_{b,n}^B = |b_{n,0}|^2 \Pi_{F,n}, \quad (28)$$

$$F(z) = 2\left[\cosh\left(\frac{z}{L_{g,1}}\right) - \cos\left(\frac{z}{2L_{g,1}}\right)\cosh\left(\frac{z}{2L_{g,1}}\right)\right],$$

where $F_n^L(z)$ and $F_n^B(z)$ are given by $F(z)$ with $L_{g,1}$ substituted by $L_{g,n}^*$ and $L_{g,1}/n$ respectively. An idea how the segments can be arranged is given in Figure 7. The figure reports the evolution of the laser power in three different undulator sections. The first harmonic grows till a certain point, where the undulator is cut. In the second section the field growth is dominated by the induced bunching. The same happens if the cut occurs further in the longitudinal coordinate.

The third harmonic behaves in a similar way. In the last section it grows, according to the mechanism discussed in the previous sections, to the levels fixed by $\Pi_{F,n}$.

If the undulator is cut at $z = 8$ m and the missing section, from 8 to 12 m, is replaced by an undulator tuned at the third harmonic of the first it would act as a radiator, with an emission pattern similar to the green line (dot and continuous) reported in Figure 7. The solid lines in the figure follow from the numerical computation, the superimposed dashed line is the result of the analytical approximation, which regarding the last part dominated by the bunching yields a qualitative agreement only.

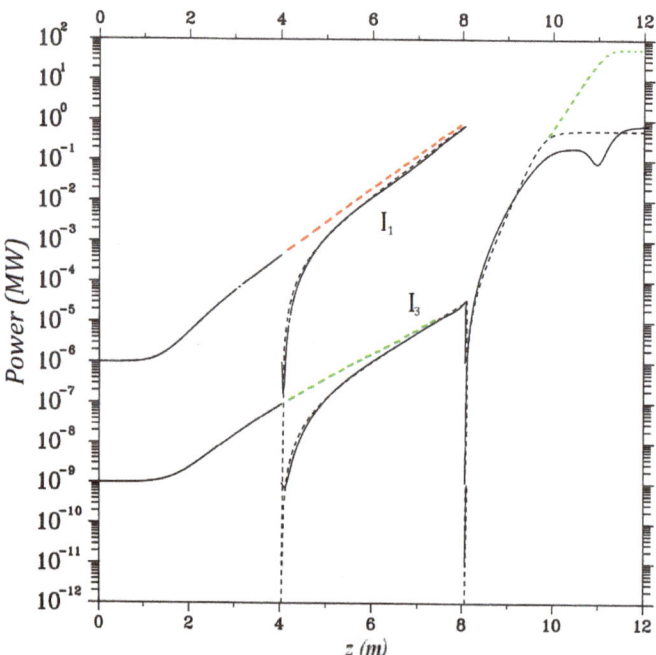

Figure 7. First and third harmonic evolution, in a segmented undulator. At each undulator segment (4 and 8 m) the field growth is dominated by the bunching acquired during the interaction inside the undulator segment. The red and green lines represent the growth with the inclusion of the intensity (considered to be a kind of seeding). The final section, where nonlinear harmonic generation occurs, is dominated by the bunching, when the second beam is superimposed the power intensity grows according to the usual pattern.

The saturated power can however be increased by injecting a second beam according to the prescription reported below.

The power emitted in the last section can be enhanced using a second beam not necessarily harmonically coupled to the first or with larger energy.

We consider indeed a FEL operating in the SASE regime with a first undulator section with $\lambda_u^{(1)} \cong 2.8$ cm, $K^{(1)} \cong 2.133$, a first beam energy of $E^{(1)} \cong 346$ MeV, an associated resonant wavelength $\lambda^{(1)} \cong 100$ nm and the remaining parameters arranged to have a Pierce parameter $\rho^{(1)} \cong 2.64 \times 10^{-3}$.

A second undulator section is foreseen to have a period $\lambda_u^{(2)} \cong 1.4$ cm, $K^{(2)} \cong 1$, the energy of the second beam is supposed to be $E^{(2)} \cong 288$ MeV and therefore the wavelength emitted in the second part is tuned at the third harmonic of the first.

If the first undulator is cut at the onset of the saturation induced at the third harmonic of the first section ($Z \cong 10$ m) and if the parameters are arranged in such a way that $\rho^{(1)} \cong \rho^{(2)}$ the FEL power at 33 nm, seeded by the maximum field in the first section, reaches the same power level of the field at 100 nm (as already noted we have managed to have equal Pierce parameters in the two sections this means current of the order of hundreds of Amperes and beam power ranging around 10^4 MW).

It is evident that such a configuration is not too much realistic for an actual FEL operation; however, it shows that sophisticated FEL architectures using multi-beam configuration can be exploited, which may also involve oscillator FEL devices.

The use of two-beam oscillator FELs has not been explored so far, in a forthcoming investigation we will discuss the possible advantages offered by a solution of this type.

As a matter of facts, FEL is a device of pivotal importance in applied sciences. The extreme versatility in terms of tunability, pulse duration, peak and average power... of fourth generation synchrotron radiation X-ray sources is the reason of their spectacular success in materials science, chemistry and biology [29].

Following the successful operation of Flash [30] and LCLS [31] and justified by their unique achievements, further XFEL facilities have been operated or are under construction around the world with different peculiarities of operation modes [32–38].

The elements of discussion outlined in this article suggest the use of pulses at different colors, with different polarizations. These additional elements foresee the assembling of hybrid FEL architectures, with characteristics useful for users, interested in applications demanding for polarization control of the laser light and/or in spectrally resolved pump and probe experiments. In these studies, a chemical reaction, an excitation or a structural change on the surface of a solid, is triggered by a first pulse with a fixed frequency and, after a delay, a second pulse, at a different frequency, records the previous event. In this way, following its time evolution, information on pathways, barriers and transition states of the phenomenon can be accessed.

X-ray FEL beams, consisting of colored (not necessarily harmonics) pair pulses, are suited to conduct experiments on structural dynamics, designed to probe the ultrafast evolution of atomic, electronic and magnetic structures [39–41]. The control of the polarization offers a further degree of freedom for selective excitation of species.

The use of two-color laser pulses, with orthogonal polarizations of comparable intensities, allows the selective excitation of the molecular fluorescence and opens the possibility of controlling the internal organization and space orientation of molecules, thus providing a significant improvement of techniques based on fluorescence anisotropy and dichroism [42,43].

FEL schemes capable of producing dual frequency beams have been tested in the past [44–50]. Other interesting proposals to generate two-color FEL emission in the X-ray region have been discussed in the literature [51–53].

Along with these efforts, further research work has been focused on the study of X-FEL beams with tunable polarization [26,54–57]. Within this respect different schemes have been proposed and developed, they include crossed-planar undulators [26,54] and elliptical permanent undulators in after-burner [55,56].

The drawback of the first scheme is associated with the relatively low degree of polarization, the elliptical undulators, on the other side, produce FEL pulses with well-defined polarizations.

This is indeed the case of the Delta-like undulator, installed at LCLS and at SPARC [58]. Experiments have shown that the radiation from the Delta undulator exhibits an extremely high degree of circular polarization compared to crossed-planar undulators. Even though the switching of the polarization at KHz rate appears problematic.

We have mentioned that the schemes we have proposed are by no means straightforward regarding either the electron beam (s) handling and the undulator construction. The effective implementation of a bi-harmonic device is not straightforward, cheap and the relevant magnetic characterization is by no means an easy task, but largely within the present technology.

The same comment applies to the production and use of beams with different energies. The proposal of high repetition rate X-ray FELs driven by superconducting Linacs, and the significant improvements of fast kickers and pulses timing open the possibility of designing systems producing "bunch-to-bunch energy-changed beams". The proposal of multi-beam energy operation [59] at SHINE [60] is extremely promising. Without commenting on the relevant specific issues, we report the sketch of Figure 8. It exhibits an achromatic and isochronous delay system, inserted before the last accelerating section. Consequently, the arrival time of the electron beam at the last accelerating section is changed, which means a different accelerating phase and eventually beams with different energies. This device combined with undulators of bi-orthogonal type can produce high repetition rate multicolor/variable polarization pulses.

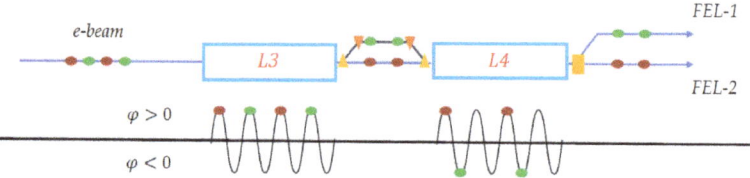

Figure 8. Sketch of multi-beam energy device proposed at SHINE ($\varphi \equiv$ accelerating phase).

Author Contributions: Conceptualization, E.D.P., E.S., G.D.; methodology, E.D.P., E.S., G.D.; software, E.D.P., E.S., G.D.; validation, E.D.P., E.S., G.D.; formal analysis, E.D.P., E.S., G.D.; data curation, E.D.P., E.S., G.D.; writing original draft preparation, E.D.P., E.S., G.D.; writing review and editing, E.D.P., E.S., G.D.; visualization, E.D.P., E.S., G.D.; supervision, E.D.P., E.S., G.D.; project administration, E.D.P., E.S., G.D. All authors have read and agreed to the published version of the manuscript.

Funding: This research received no external funding.

Institutional Review Board Statement: Not applicable.

Informed Consent Statement: Not applicable.

Data Availability Statement: Not applicable.

Conflicts of Interest: The authors declare no conflict of interest.

References

1. Colson, W.B. The nonlinear wave equation for higher harmonics in free-electron lasers. *IEEE J. Quantum Electron.* **1981**, *17*, 1417–1427. [CrossRef]
2. Colson, W.B. Free-electron lasers operating in higher harmonics. *Phys. Rev. A* **1981**, *24*, 639–641. [CrossRef]
3. Colson, W.B.; Dattoli, G.; Ciocci, F. Angular-gain spectrum of free electron lasers. *Phys. Rev. A* **1985**, *31*, 828–842. [CrossRef] [PubMed]
4. Freund, H.P.; Biedron, S.G.; Milton, S.V. Non Linear Harmonic Generation in Free Electron Lasers. *IEEE J. Quantum Elelectron.* **2000**, *36*, 275–281. [CrossRef]
5. Geloni, G.; Saldin, E.; Schneidmiller, E.; Yurkov, M. Theory of Harmonic Generation in Free Electron Lasers with helical wigglers. *Nucl. Instr. Meth. A* **2007**, *581*, 856–865. [CrossRef]
6. Giannessi, L. *Seeding and Harmonic Generation in Free Electron Laser, in Synchrotron Light Sources and Free-Electron Lasers*; Jaeschke, E.J., Khan, S., Schneider, J.R., Hastings, J.B., Eds.; Springer Nature Switzerland AG: Cham, Switzerland, 2020; pp. 119–147.
7. Ciocci, F.; Dattoli, G.; Torre, A.; Renieri, A. *Insertion Devices for Synchrotron Radiation and Free Electron Lasers*; World Scientific: Singapore, 2000
8. Dattoli, G.; Ottaviani, P.L.; Pagnutti, S. Non Linear Harmonic Generation in high gain Free Electron Lasers. *J. Appl. Phys.* **2005**, *97*, 113102. [CrossRef]
9. McNeil, B.W.J.; Poole, M.W.; Robb, G.R.M. Two-beam free-electron laser. *Phys. Rev. E* **2004**, *70*, 035501. [CrossRef] [PubMed]
10. Dattoli, G.; Giannessi, L.; Ottaviani, P.L.; Freund, H.P.; Biedron, S.G.; Milton, S. Two harmonic undulators and harmonic generation in high gain free electron lasers. *Nucl. Instruments Methods Phys. Res. Sect. A* **2002**, *495*, 48–57. [CrossRef]
11. Dattoli, G.; Doria, A.; Giannessi, L.; Ottaviani, P.L. Bunching and exotic undulator configurations in SASE FELs. *Nucl. Instr. Meth. Phys. Res. A* **2003**, *507*, 388–391. [CrossRef]
12. Dattoli, G.; Renieri, A.; Torre, A. *Lectures on the Free Electron Laser Theory and Related Topics*; World Scientific: Singapore, 1993. [CrossRef]
13. Dattoli, G.; Ottaviani, P.L.; Pagnutti, S. The PROMETEO Code: A flexible tool for Free Electron Laser study. *Il Nuovo Cimento* **2009**, *32*, 283–287.
14. Dattoli, G.; Ottaviani, P.L.; Pagnutti, S. Booklet for FEL Design: A Collection of Practical Formulae, ENEA Report RT/2007/40/FIM (2007). Available online: https://www.fel.enea.it/booklet/pdf/Booklet_for_FEL_design.pdf (accessed on 12 July 2021).
15. Dattoli, G.; Ottaviani, P.L.; Pagnutti, S. High gain amplifiers: Power oscillations and harmonic generation. *J. Appl. Phys.* **2007**, *102*, 033103. [CrossRef]
16. Hemsing, E. Simple model for the nonlinear radiation field of a free electron laser. *Phys. Rev. Accel. Beams* **2020**, *23*, 120703. [CrossRef]

17. Dattoli, G.; Di Palma, E.; Licciardi, S.; Sabia, E. Generalized Bessel Functions and Their Use in Bremsstrahlung and Multi-Photon Processes. *Symmetry* **2021**, *13*, 159. [CrossRef]
18. Schmidt, M.J.; Elliott, C.J. The effects of harmonic wiggler field components on free-electron laser operation. *IEEE J. Quant. Electron.* **1987**, *23*, 1552. [CrossRef]
19. Asakawa, M.; Mima, K.; Nakai, S.; Imasaki, K.; Yamanaka, C. Higher harmonic generation in a modified wiggler magnetic field. *Nucl. Instr. Meth. A* **1992**, *318*, 538–545. [CrossRef]
20. Mirian, N.S. Harmonic Generation in Two Orthogonal Undulators. In Proceedings of the FEL2015, Daejeon, Korea, 23–28 August 2015.
21. Schneidmiller, E.; Yurkov, M. Harmonic Lasing in X-ray Free Electron Laser. *Phys. Rev.* **2012**, *15*, 080702. [CrossRef]
22. Schneidmiller, E.; Yurkov, M. *First operation of a Harmonic Lasing Self-Seeded FEL*; ICFA Workshop: Arcidosso, Italy, 2017.
23. Ciocci, F.; Anania, M.P.; Artioli, M.; Bellaveglia, M.; Carpanese, M.; Chiadroni, E.; Villa, F. *Segmented Undulator Operation at the SPARC-FEL Test Facility, Advances in X-ray Free-Electron Lasers Instrumentation III*; Biedron, S.G., Ed.; SPIE: Bellingham, WA, USA, 2015; Volume 9512, p. 951203. [CrossRef]
24. McNeil, B.W.; Robb, G.R.M. The Harmonically Coupled 2-beam FEL. In Proceedings of the 2004 FEL Conference, Trieste, Italy, 29 August–3 September 2004; pp. 598–601.
25. Dattoli, G.; Voykov, G.K. Spectral properties of two-harmonic undulator radiation. *Phys. Rev.* **1993**, *48*, 3030–3039. [CrossRef] [PubMed]
26. Dattoli, G.; Mirian, N.S.; Di Palma, E.; Petrillo, V. Two-color free-electron laser with two orthogonal undulators. *PRSTAB* **2014**, *17*, 050702. [CrossRef]
27. McNeil, B. First light from hard X-ray laser. *Nat. Photon.* **2009**, *3*, 375–377. [CrossRef]
28. Dattoli, G.; Mezi, L.; Ottaviani, P.L.; Pagnutti, S. Theory of high gain free-electron lasers operating with segmented undulators. *J. Appl. Phys.* **2006**, *99*, 044907. [CrossRef]
29. Huang, N.; Deng, H.; Liu, B.; Wang, D.; Zhao, Z. Features and Futures of Free Electron Lasers. *Cellpress Partn. J. Innov.* **2021**. [CrossRef]
30. Ackermann, W.A.; Asova, G.; Ayvazyan, V.; Azima, A.; Baboi, N.; Bähr, J.; Winter, A. Operation of a free-electron laser from the extreme ultraviolet to the water window. *Nat. Photon.* **2007**, *1*, 336–342. [CrossRef]
31. Emma, P.; Akre, R.; Arthur, J.; Bionta, R.; Bostedt, C.; Bozek, J.; Brachmann, A.; Bucksbaum, P.; Coffee, R.; Decker, F.J.; et al. First lasing and operation of an Ångstrom wavelength free-electron laser. *Nat. Photon.* **2020**, *4*, 641–647. [CrossRef]
32. Ishikawa, T.; Aoyagi, H.; Asaka, T.; Asano, Y.; Azumi, N.; Bizen, T.; Ego, H.; Fukami, K.; Fukui, T.; Furukawa, Y.; et al. A compact X-ray free-electron laser emitting in the sub-Ångström region. *Nat. Photon.* **2012**, *6*, 540–544. [CrossRef]
33. Kang, H.S.; Min, C.K.; Heo, H.; Kim, C.; Yang, H.; Kim, G.; Nam, I.; Baek, S.Y.; Choi, H.J.; Mun, G.; et al. Hard X-ray free-electron laser with femto-second-scale timing jitter. *Nat. Photon.* **2017**, *11*, 708–713. [CrossRef]
34. Prat, E.; Abela, R.; Aiba, M.; Alarcon, A.; Alex, J.; Arbelo, Y.; Zimoch, E. A compact and cost-effective hard X-ray free-electron laser driven by a high-brightness and low-energy electron beam. *Nat. Photon.* **2020**, *14*, 748–754. [CrossRef]
35. Allaria, E.; Appio, R.; Badano, L.; Barletta, W.A.; Bassanese, S.; Biedron, S.G.; Zangrando, M. Highly coherent and stable pulses from the FERMI seeded free-electron laser in the extreme ultraviolet. *Nat. Photon.* **2012**, *6*, 699–704. [CrossRef]
36. Zhao, Z.; Wang, D.; Gu, Q.; Yin, L.; Fang, G.; Gu, M.; Jiang, H. SXFEL: A soft X-ray free electron laser in China. *Synchrotron Radiat. News* **2017**, *30*, 29–33. [CrossRef]
37. Galayda, J. The Linac Coherent Light Source-II Project. In Proceedings of the 5th International Particle Accelerator Conference (IPAC'14), Geneva, Switzerland, 15–20 June 2014; JACoW: Dresden, Germany, 2014.
38. Decking, W.; Abeghyan, S.; Abramian, P.; Abramsky, A.; Aguirre, A.; Albrecht, C.; Alou, P.; Altarelli, M.; Altmann, P.; Amyan, K.; et al. A MHz-repetition-rate hard X-ray free-electron laser driven by a superconducting linear accelerator. *Nat. Photon.* **2020**, *14*, 391–397. [CrossRef]
39. Tavella, F.; Stojanovic, N.; Geloni, G.; Gensch, M. Few-femtosecond timing at fourth-generation X-ray light sources. *Nat. Photon.* **2011**, *5*, 162. [CrossRef]
40. Ding, Y.; Decker, F.J.; Emma, P.; Feng, C.; Field, C.; Frisch, J.; Huang, Z.; Krzywinski, J.; Loos, H.; Welch, J.; et al. Femtosecond X-ray Pulse Characterization in Free-Electron Lasers Using a Cross-Correlation Technique. *Phys. Rev. Lett.* **2012**, *109*, 254802. [CrossRef] [PubMed]
41. Finetti, P. Optical-EUV pump and probe experiments with variable polarization on the newly open LDM beamline of FERMI@Elettra. In Proceedings of the FEL Conference 2013, New York, NY, USA, 26–30 August 2013.
42. Lakowicz, J.R. *Principles of Fluorescence Spectroscopy*, 3rd ed.; Chapter 10–12 Deal with Fluorescence Polarization Spectroscopy; Springer: Berlin/Heidelberg, Germany, 2006.
43. Kazansky, A.K.; Grigorieva, A.V.; Kabachnik, N.M. Dichroism in short-pulse two-color XUV plus IR multiphoton ionization of atoms. *Phys. Rev. A* **2012**, *85*, 053409. [CrossRef]
44. Lutman, A.A.; Coffee, R.; Ding, Y.; Huang, Z.; Krzywinski, J.; Maxwell, T.; Messerschmidt, M.; Nuhn, H.D. Experimental Demonstration of Femtosecond Two-Color X-ray Free-Electron Lasers. *Phys. Rev. Lett.* **2013**, *110*, 134801. [CrossRef] [PubMed]
45. Petrillo, V.; Anania, M.P.; Artioli, M.; Bacci, A.; Bellaveglia, M.; Chiadroni, E.; Cianchi, A.; Ciocci, F.; Dattoli, G.; Di Giovenale, D.; et al. Observation of Time-Domain Modulation of Free-Electron-Laser Pulses by Multipeaked Electron-Energy-Spectrum. *Phys. Rev. Lett.* **2013**, *111*, 114802. [CrossRef]

46. Allaria, E.; Bencivenga, F.; Borghes, R.; Capotondi, F.; Castronovo, D.; Charalambous, P.; Cinquegrana, P.; Danailov, M.B.; De Ninno, G.; Demidovich, A.; et al. Two-colour pump-probe experiments with a twin-pulse-seed extreme ultraviolet free-electron laser. *Nat. Commun.* **2013**, *4*, 2476. [CrossRef] [PubMed]
47. Mahieu, B.; Allaria, E.; Castronovo, D.; Danailov, M.B.; Demidovich, A.; De Ninno, G.; Di Mitri, S.; Fawley, W.M.; Ferrari, E.; Fröhlich, L.; et al. Two-colour generation in a chirped seeded free-electron laser: A close look. *Opt. Express* **2013**, *21*, 22728. [CrossRef]
48. Marinelli, A.; Lutman, A.A.; Wu, J.; Ratner, D.; Gilevich, S.; Decker, F.J.; Turner, J.; Loos, H.; Ding, Y.; Krzywinski, J.; et al. Two-Color Schemes at LCLS. In Proceedings of the FEL Conference 2013, New York, NY, USA, 26–30 August 2013.
49. Ronsivalle, C.; Anania, M.P.; Bacci, A.; Bellaveglia, M.; Chiadroni, E.; Cianchi, A.; Ciocci, F.; Dattoli, G.; Di Giovenale, D.; Di Pirro, G.; et al. Large-bandwidth two-color free-electron laser driven by a comb-like electron beam. *New J. Phys.* **2014**, *16*, 033018. [CrossRef]
50. Chiadroni, E.; Anania, M.P.; Artioli, M.; Bacci, A.; Bellaveglia, M.; Cianchi, A.; Ciocci, F.; Dattoli, G.; Di Giovenale, D.; Di Pirro, G.; et al. Two Color FEL Driven by a Comb-Like Electron Beam Distribution. *Phys. Procedia* **2014**, *52*, 27–35. [CrossRef]
51. Freund, H.P.; O'Shea, P.G. Two-Color Operation in High-Gain Free-Electron Lasers. *Phys. Rev. Lett.* **2000**, *84*, 2861. [CrossRef]
52. Thompson, N.R.; McNeil, B.W.J. Mode Locking in a Free-Electron Laser Amplifier. *Phys. Rev. Lett.* **2008**, *100*, 203901. [CrossRef]
53. Xiang, D.; Huang, Z.; Stupakov, G. Generation of intense attosecond x-ray pulses using ultraviolet laser induced microbunching in electron beams. *Phys. Rev. ST Accel. Beams* **2009**, *12*, 060701. [CrossRef]
54. Deng, H.; Zhang, T.; Feng, L.; Feng, C.; Liu, B.; Wang, X.; Zhao, Z. Polarization switching demonstration using crossed-planar undulators in a seeded free-electron laser. *Phys. Rev. Accel. Beams* **2014**, *17*, 020704. [CrossRef]
55. Ferrari, E.; Allaria, E.; Buck, J.; De Ninno, G.; Diviacco, B.; Gauthier, D.; Giannessi, L.; Glaser, L.; Huang, Z.; Ilchen, M.; et al. Single shot polarization characterization of XUV FEL pulses from crossed polarized undulators. *Sci. Rep.* **2015**, *5*, 13531. [CrossRef] [PubMed]
56. Allaria, E.; Diviacco, B.; Callegari, C.; Finetti, P.; Mahieu, B.; Viefhaus, J.; Zangr, O.M.; De Ninno, G.; Lambert, G.; Ferrari, E.; et al. Control of the polarization of a vacuum-ultraviolet, high-gain, free-electron laser. *Phys. Rev. X* **2014**, *4*, 041040. [CrossRef]
57. Lutman, A.A.; MacArthur, J.P.; Ilchen, M.; Lindahl, A.O.; Buck, J.; Coffee, R.N.; Dakovski, G.L.; Dammann, L.; Ding, Y.; Dürr, H.A.; et al. Polarization control in an X-ray free-electron laser. *Nat. Photon.* **2016**, *10*, 468–472. [CrossRef]
58. Ciocci, F.; Anania, M.P.; Artioli, M.; Bellaveglia, M.; Carpanese, M.; Chiadroni, E.; Cianchi, A.; Dattoli, G.; Giovenale, D.D.; Palma, E.D.; et al. Segmented undulator operation at the SPARC-FEL test facility. In Proceedings of the Advances in X-ray Free-Electron Lasers Instrumentation III, 951203, Prague, Czech Republic, 12 May 2015; Volume 951203. [CrossRef]
59. Yan, J.; Deng, H. Multi-beam-energy operation for the continuous-wave X-ray free electron laser. *Phys. Rev. Accel. Beams* **2019**, *22*, 090701. [CrossRef]
60. Zhu, Z.Y.; Zhao, Z.T.; Wang, D.; Liu, Z.; Li, R.X.; Yin, L.X.; Yang, Z.H. SCLF: an 8-GeV CW SCRF Linac-based X-ray FEL Facility in Shangai. In Proceedings of the International Free Electron Laser Conference (FEL'17), Santa Fe, Mexico, 20–25 August 2017; No. 38; JACoW: Geneva, Switzerland, 2018; pp. 182–184.

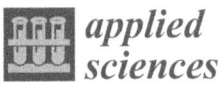

Article

Free Electron Laser High Gain Equation and Harmonic Generation

Giuseppe Dattoli †, Emanuele Di Palma †, Silvia Licciardi *,† and Elio Sabia †

ENEA—Frascati Research Center, Via Enrico Fermi 45, 00044 Rome, Italy; pinodattoli@libero.it (G.D.); emanuele.dipalma@enea.it (E.D.P.); elio.sabia@gmail.com (E.S.)
* Correspondence: silviakant@gmail.com or silvia.licciardi@enea.it; Tel.: +39-06-9400-5421
† These authors contributed equally to this work.

Abstract: The FEL integral equation is reviewed here and is studied under different contexts, accounting for diverse physical regimes. We include higher order harmonics and saturation effects, and explain the origin of scaling relations, widely exploited to describe either FEL dynamics or nonnlinear harmonic generation.

Keywords: free electron laser 78a60; Volterra integral equations (45)D05; non linear harmonic generation laser dynamics; oscillators; amplifiers 81V99

Citation: Dattoli, G.; Di Palma, E.; Licciardi, S.; Sabia, E. Free Electron Laser High Gain Equation and Harmonic Generation. *Appl. Sci.* **2021**, *11*, 85. https://dx.doi.org/10.3390/app11010085

Received: 21 October 2020
Accepted: 17 December 2020
Published: 24 December 2020

Publisher's Note: MDPI stays neutral with regard to jurisdictional claims in published maps and institutional affiliations.

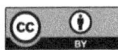

Copyright: © 2020 by the authors. Licensee MDPI, Basel, Switzerland. This article is an open access article distributed under the terms and conditions of the Creative Commons Attribution (CC BY) license (https://creativecommons.org/licenses/by/4.0/).

1. Introduction

This article describes an important mechanism associated with the physics of the free electron laser (FEL) regarding the nonlinear harmonic generation. The topic will be discussed by entering deeply into the mathematical aspects of what is currently referred as the high gain FEL equation.

A FEL is a laser device employing a beam of relativistic electrons injected into an undulator magnet, where it undergoes transverse oscillations and emits bremsstrahlung radiation, inversely proportional to the electrons energy square [1]. The FEL devices can be operated in the oscillator configuration by storing the emitted radiation in an optical cavity (whenever appropriate mirrors to confine the "light" are available). The radiation moves back and forth inside the resonator and interacts, at each entrance inside the undulator, with a freshly injected e-beam, thereby becoming amplified. The intracavity intensity grows, round trip after round trip; it is amplified by the process of stimulated bremsstrahlung emission and exhibits the same pattern of conventional laser oscillators; it undergoes exponential growth, and eventually saturation occurs, when the gain is reduced by the nonlinear contributions to the level of the cavity losses.

In the region of the spectrum where efficient mirrors are not available, cavity-less operation is an obliged step. In this regime, the gain of the system should be sufficiently large to bring the device to saturation in one undulator passage. These FEL devices, nowadays devoted to the production of intense X-ray beams, require long undulators (hundreds of meters) and high energy (up to tens of GeV)/high brightness electron beams (namely, beams with high intensity peak current, low energy, angular and transverse spatial dispersions). The "single pass" FEL devices may be operated in the amplifier configuration, when coherent input seeds are available; if not, the system works in the so-called self-amplified spontaneous emission ($SASE$) regime. The electrons emit ordinary synchrotron radiation at the entrance of the undulator, which reinteracts with the electrons, becomes amplified and eventually reaches saturation.

The paradigmatic steps leading the FEL to the generation of coherent laser-like radiation are the beam energy modulation, the bunching, the exponential growth and the saturation.

These phases are common to all other free electron devices (such as gyrotrons and coherent auto-resonance masers), and most of the relevant theoretical and mathematical descriptions can be framed within the same context [2]. Many *FELs* are presently operating and have operated in the past [3]. They are covering the electromagnetic spectrum from *THz* region to X-rays. The last generation of *FEL* sources (sometimes referred as fourth generation synchrotron radiation sources) has opened up unprecedent scenarios in different research fields because of the radiation characteristics, in terms of brightness (ten orders of magnitude above the ordinary sources) and the shortness of the pulses [4–7].

The growth of the *FEL* field is ruled, in the small signal regime (namely, the dynamical conditions, when the field intensity is not large enough to induce nonlinear effects), by an equation known as the *FEL* integral equation; it is derived from the linearization of the pendulum equation, reported below [8–16].

$$\frac{d^2}{d\tau^2}\zeta = |a|\cos(\zeta+\phi), \qquad \frac{d}{d\tau}a = -j\langle e^{-i\zeta}\rangle,$$
$$\tau = \frac{z}{L}, \qquad j = 2\pi g_0, \qquad a = |a|e^{i\phi}, \qquad \nu = \frac{d}{d\tau}\zeta \tag{1}$$

where z is the longitudinal coordinate; L is the undulator length; g_0 is the small signal gain coefficient; and a and j are Colson's dimensionless amplitude and current respectively, ζ, ν the *FEL* longitudinal phase space variables and the brackets, denote the average of the phase space distribution. The use of dimensionless variables has several advantages. They constitute a set of comprehensive quantities such as a and g_0, allowing one to merge all the significant *FEL* parameters into a single variable, providing quantities of interest (such as the gain and saturation intensity; see below) crucial in the descriptions and designs of *FEL* devices. The relevant small signal limit is achieved through the following approximations [17,18].

(a) From the first of Equation (1), we obtain the lowest order (in the field strength) expansion of ζ, namely

$$\zeta \simeq \zeta_0 + \nu_0\tau + \delta\zeta, \qquad \delta\zeta = \int_0^\tau (\tau-\tau')Re\left(a(\tau')e^{i(\zeta_0+\nu_0\tau')}\right)d\tau' \tag{2}$$

where $\nu_0 = 2\pi N\frac{\omega_0-\omega}{\omega_0}$ is the detuning parameter.

(b) Inserting $\delta\zeta$ in the second of Equation (1) and averaging on the electron-field phase ζ_0, we get

$$\frac{d}{d\tau}a = -2\pi g_0 b_1 e^{-i\nu_0\tau} + i\pi g_0 \int_0^\tau (\tau-\tau')a(\tau')e^{-i\nu_0(\tau-\tau')}d\tau' + $$
$$+ i\pi g_0 b_2 \int_0^\tau (\tau-\tau')a^*(\tau')e^{-i\nu_0(\tau+\tau')}d\tau' \tag{3}$$

where the averages have been taken by considering the e-beam mono-energetic and without spatial and angular dispersion, thereby getting

$$\langle \kappa(\zeta_0)\rangle_{\zeta_0} = \frac{1}{2\pi}\int_0^{2\pi} f(\zeta_0)\kappa(\zeta_0)d\zeta_0,$$
$$f(\zeta_0) = \sum_{n=-\infty}^{\infty} b_n e^{in\zeta_0}, \qquad b_n = \langle e^{-in\zeta_0}\rangle_{\zeta_0}. \tag{4}$$

The physical meaning of Equation (3) is transparent; the three terms on the right-hand side account for three different regimes:

(i) Absence of an initial bunching ($f(\zeta_0)$ constant); in this case Equation (3) reduces to

$$\frac{d}{d\tau}a = i\pi g_0 \int_0^\tau (\tau-\tau')a(\tau')e^{-i\nu_0(\tau-\tau')}d\tau'. \tag{5}$$

The underlying physics is that energy modulation and consequent bunching are due to the input coherent seed a_0.

(ii) Nonconstant $f(\zeta_0)$ and emergence of non zero b_n coefficients; the field may grow in a seedless mode, induced by the initial bunching coefficient, as illustrated below.

In order to understand the role of the bunching coefficients during the early stages of the *FEL* interaction, we must treat Equation (5) in terms of a naïve expansion in the small signal gain coefficient, limiting ourselves to the second-order expansion in the small and neglecting b_2; then we find

$$a(\tau) \simeq a_0 + g_0 a_1 + g_0^2 a_2, \qquad a_0(\tau) = 0,$$
$$\frac{d}{d\tau}a_1 = -2\pi b_1 e^{-i v_0 \tau}, \qquad \frac{d}{d\tau}a_2 = i\pi \int_0^\tau (\tau - \tau') a_1(\tau') e^{-i v_0 (\tau - \tau')} d\tau' \qquad (6)$$

and the relevant solution is

$$a(\tau) \simeq -2\pi b_1 g_0 \left(\frac{\sin(\frac{v_0 \tau}{2})}{\frac{v_0}{2}} e^{-i v_0 \frac{\tau}{2}} - \frac{1}{2}\pi g_0 \frac{(i v_0^2 \tau^2 + 4 v_0 \tau - 6i) e^{-i v_0 \tau} + 6i + 2 v_0 \tau}{v_0^4} \right). \qquad (7)$$

According to the previous equation, the field grows initially because of being triggered by the bunching coefficient. It provides a kind of coherent spontaneous emission, which in the second phase is responsible for the onset of the exponential growth regime (see Figure 1), where we have reported the combined effects of bunching and initial seed.

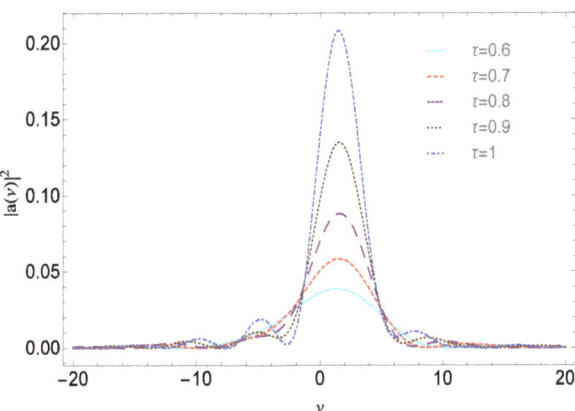

Figure 1. Square modulus of the dimensionless amplitude vs. the detuning parameter for $g_0 = 0.5$ and different values of τ: $(0.5, 0.6, 0.7, 0.8, 0.9, 1)$. The intensity grows with incresing dimensionless time.

The previous results have been obtained using a perturbative expansion, which is not strictly necessary, since the *FEL* integral equation can be reduced to the ordinary differential equation reported below.

$$\left[\hat{D}_\tau^3 + 2 i v_0 \hat{D}_\tau^2 - v_0^2 \hat{D}_\tau \right] a(\tau) = i\pi g_0 \left(a(\tau) + b_2 \, a^*(\tau) e^{-2 i v_0 \tau} \right), \qquad \hat{D}_\tau = \frac{d}{d\tau}, \qquad (8)$$

obtained after noting that integrals of type

$$i\pi g_0 \int_0^\tau (\tau - \tau') a(\tau') e^{-i v_0 (\tau - \tau')} d\tau' = i\pi g_0 e^{-i v_0 \tau} \int_0^\tau \left(\int_0^{\tau'} a(\tau'') e^{i v_0 \tau''} d\tau'' \right) d\tau' \qquad (9)$$

appearing in Equation (6) are double integrals which can be eliminated by keeping two successive derivatives [17,18]. It is evident that, for negligible b_2 (we have checked that the second-order bunching coefficient does not produce any appreciable contribution and can be safely neglected), Equation (8) reduces to a naïve third-order ordinary differential equation, leading to the exponential growth also referred as *FEL* instability, the characteristic of which occurs in any Free Electron device [19–25]. (This type of instability is common to any free electron device (including gyrotrons and cyclotron auto-resonance masers (*CARM*)). This was widely established before the studies developed in the previously quoted references. Some interesting papers within this respect are listed in the bibliography.)

It is worth noting that, even though not explicitly contributing to Equation (8), the bunching coefficient b_1 appears in the initial conditions provided by

$$a(0) = a_0, \qquad \hat{D}_\tau a \mid_{\tau=0} = -2\pi g_0 b_1, \qquad \hat{D}_\tau^2 a \mid_{\tau=0} = 2\pi i \nu_0 g_0 b_1. \qquad (10)$$

We have so far fixed the mathematical formalism to treat the problems associated with the effect of the bunching on the high gain (and not only) *FEL* evolution. The paper outline is reported below.

In Section 2 we discuss solution methods to deal with either the integral and third-order differential equation.

In Section 3 we deal with the extension of the integral equation to the harmonic generation and include effects associated with nonlinear regime.

Section 4 is finally devoted to application of the formalism for the design of *FEL*, exploiting segmented undulator devices.

2. Algorithmic and Analytical Solutions of the *FEL* Integral Equation

The equations we have dealt with in the previous section describe the $1D$ small signal *FEL* dynamics, with the assumption of an ideal, sufficiently long beam such that short pulse effects can be neglected. The last assumption allows one to ignore the possible detrimental effects to the slippage, which will be considered later in this paper.

Within the present context, they are sufficiently general to develop useful considerations on the role of a pre-bunched e-beam on the *FEL* dynamics. We have also noted that Equation (3) can be reduced to a straightforward cubic equation, that analytical solutions are possible and that interesting information is obtained by the use of a perturbative expansion. The analysis has been so far limited (see Equation (7)) to a second-order expansion in terms of the small signal gain coefficient. The perturbative solution of Equation (5) can be obtained by including the higher order terms in g_0, which yields the following recursion:

$$\frac{d}{d\tau} a_n = i\pi \int_0^\tau (\tau - \tau') a_{n-1}(\tau') e^{-i\nu_0(\tau-\tau')} d\tau', \qquad a_n(0) = \delta_{n,0}. \qquad (11)$$

We will go back to perturbative treatments in the forthcoming sections of this article; here we consider the use of the other means based allowing either algorithmic and analytical solutions.

Regarding the first, we consider a method outlined in a paper by F. Ciocci et al. [26]; the procedure will be referred to as the Ciocci algorithm (*CA*). The technique is used via the following steps:

(i) The solution of the cubic equation can be written as

$$a(\tau) = e^{-i\nu_0 \tau} \sum_{j=1}^3 \kappa_j e^{-i\delta\nu_j \tau} \qquad (12)$$

where $\delta\nu_j$ are the roots of the third-degree algebraic equation

$$\delta\nu^2(\nu_0 + \delta\nu) = \pi g_0; \qquad (13)$$

(ii) The amplitudes κ_j are fixed by the initial conditions, as shown below.

$$a(0) = \alpha_0 = \sum_{j=1}^{3} \kappa_j,$$

$$\left.\frac{d}{d\tau}a\right|_{\tau=0} = -i\nu_0\alpha_0 - i\sum_{j=1}^{3} \kappa_j\delta\nu_j = -2\pi g_0 b_1 \rightarrow$$

$$\rightarrow \sum_{j=1}^{3} \kappa_j\delta\nu_j = \alpha_1 = -\nu_0\alpha_0 - 2i\pi g_0 b_1, \quad (14)$$

$$\left.\frac{d^2}{d\tau^2}a\right|_{\tau=0} = -\nu_0^2\alpha_0 - 2i\nu_0\sum_{j=1}^{3} \kappa_j\delta\nu_j - \sum_{j=1}^{3} \kappa_j(\delta\nu_j)^2 \rightarrow$$

$$\rightarrow \sum_{j=1}^{3} \kappa_j(\delta\nu_j)^2 = \alpha_2 = \nu_0^2\alpha_0 + 2i\pi\nu_0 g_0 b_1.$$

(iii) Equation (12) is cast in the more convenient form

$$a(\tau) = e^{-i\nu_0\tau} \sum_{m=0}^{\infty} \frac{(-i)^m}{m!} \alpha_m \tau^m, \qquad \alpha_m = \sum_{j=1}^{3} \kappa_j(\delta\nu_j)^m. \quad (15)$$

(iv) The coefficient α_m is obtained from Equation (13). It can be written as

$$\nu_0(\delta\nu_j)^2 + (\delta\nu_j)^3 = \pi g_0 \quad (16)$$

which after multiplying by κ_j and summing on the index j, yields the recursion

$$\alpha_3 = \pi g_0 \alpha_0 - \nu_0 \alpha_2, \quad (17)$$

and which for the higher order terms ($m > 2$) is generalized as

$$\alpha_m = \pi g_0 \alpha_{m-3} - \nu_0 \alpha_{m-1}, \quad (18)$$

The solution of the cubic equation via CA is easily implemented numerically; it is extremely fast and yields the results contained in Figure 2 reporting the cases of seeded operation and bunching.

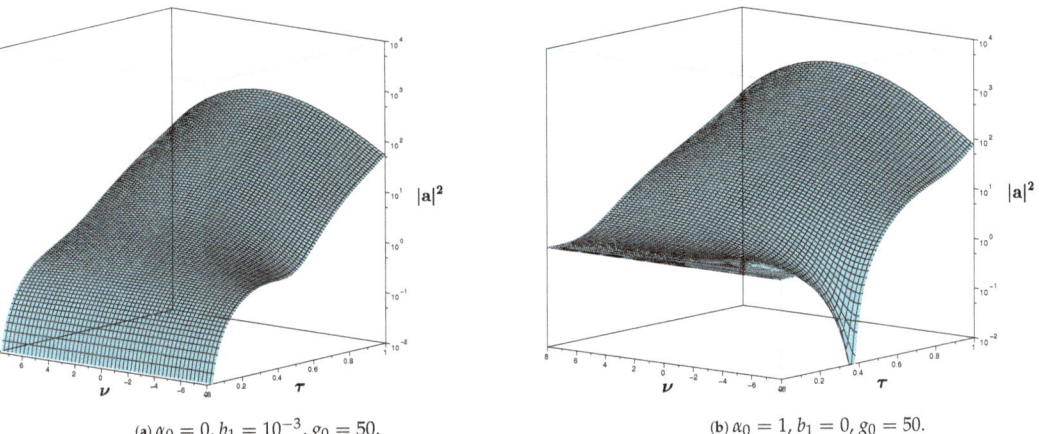

(a) $\alpha_0 = 0, b_1 = 10^{-3}, g_0 = 50$.　　　(b) $\alpha_0 = 1, b_1 = 0, g_0 = 50$.

Figure 2. Intensity vs. detuning ν_0 and dimensionless time τ.

The intensity evolution vs. z for a seedless evolution ($\alpha(0) = 0$, $b_1 \neq 0$) and for the amplifier configuration is reported in Figure 2a,b. The ν_0, τ surfaces yield an idea of the small signal intensity evolution, and further comments will be provided below.

Analytic solutions can be obtained too; they require some algebra, and in particular the use of Cardano's method to get the solution of Equation (13). Putting everything together we find:

(a) The Fang–Torre formula (this Formula appeared in an unpublished manuscript by H. Fang, and was later derived with minor refinements by A. Torre, and reported in [27]) valid for $a_0 \neq 0$, $b_1 = 0$:

$$a(\tau,\nu_0) = \frac{a_0}{3(\nu_0+p+q)} e^{-\frac{2i}{3}\nu_0\tau} \left\{ (-\nu_0+p+q)e^{-\frac{i}{3}(p+q)\tau} + 2(2\nu_0+p+q)e^{\frac{i}{6}(p+q)\tau} \right. $$
$$\left. \cdot \left[\cosh\left(\frac{\sqrt{3}}{6}(p-q)\tau\right) + i\frac{\sqrt{3}\nu_0}{p-q}\sinh\left(\frac{\sqrt{3}}{6}(p-q)\tau\right) \right] \right\}, \quad (19)$$

$$p = \left[\frac{1}{2}(r+\sqrt{d})\right]^{\frac{1}{3}}, \qquad q = \left[\frac{1}{2}(r-\sqrt{d})\right]^{\frac{1}{3}},$$
$$r = 27\pi g_0 - 2\nu_0^3, \qquad d = 27\pi g_0(27\pi g_0 - 4\nu_0^3).$$

The square modulus of $a(\tau,\nu_0)$ yields the intensity growth as a function of the dimensionless time and of the detuning parameter. Regarding Equation (19) we find

$$|a(\tau,\nu_0)|^2 = \frac{|a_0|^2}{9(\nu_0+s_+)^2} \left\{ 4(2\nu_0+s_+)^2 \left[\cosh\left(\frac{\sqrt{3}}{6}s_-\tau\right)^2 + \frac{3\nu_0^2}{s_-^2}\sinh\left(\frac{\sqrt{3}}{6}s_-\tau\right)^2\right] \right.$$
$$+ (-\nu_0+s_+)^2 + 4(-\nu_0+s_+)(2\nu_0+s_+)\left[\cos\left(\frac{s_+}{2}\tau\right)\cosh\left(\frac{\sqrt{3}}{6}s_-\tau\right) \right.$$
$$\left. \left. - \frac{\sqrt{3}\nu_0}{s_-}\sin\left(\frac{s_+}{2}\tau\right)\sinh\left(\frac{\sqrt{3}}{6}s_-\tau\right)\right] \right\}, \quad (20)$$

$$s_\pm = p \pm q.$$

We have very loosely described in introductory remarks the $SASE$ regime or seedless operation. In this case the field grows from a kind of prebunching characterizng the beam itself [28,29].

(b) The field growing from a bunching coefficient associated with the electron distribution and the solution of the evolution problem reads:

$$a(\tau,\nu_0) = \frac{2\pi g_0 b_1}{\Delta} e^{-i\frac{2}{3}\nu_0\tau} \left\{ \mu e^{-\frac{i}{3}(p+q)\tau} + \right.$$
$$\left. - \left(\chi_- \cosh\left[\frac{\sqrt{3}}{6}(p-q)\tau\right] + \chi_+ \sinh\left[\frac{\sqrt{3}}{6}(p-q)\tau\right]\right) e^{\frac{i}{6}(p+q)\tau} \right\}, \quad (21)$$

$$\Delta = \frac{\sqrt{3}}{9}(p^3 - q^3), \qquad \mu = i\frac{\sqrt{3}}{9}[\nu_0 - (p+q)](p-q),$$
$$\chi = \frac{1}{6}\left[\nu_0 + \frac{1}{2}(p+q) - i\frac{\sqrt{3}}{2}(p-q)\right]\left[p+q+i\frac{\sqrt{3}}{3}(p-q)\right], \qquad \chi_\pm = \chi \pm \chi^*.$$

Before proceeding further, we write Equation (21) in a form more appropriate for high gain/$SASE$ FEL operation. To that end, we remind the reader that the small signal gain coefficient and Pierce parameter ρ (see references [8–16]) are linked by the identity

$$\rho = \frac{\sqrt[3]{\pi g_0}}{4\pi N}, \quad (22)$$

where N is the number of undulator periods. The intensity field growth is ruled by the so-called gain length

$$L_g = \frac{\lambda_u}{4\pi\sqrt{3}\rho}, \tag{23}$$

which is the pivotal quantity controlling the small signal high gain dynamics; its inverse defines the growth per unit length. With these remarks in mind, we note that:

(i) Quantities such as ν_0 and τ should be replaced by

$$\nu_0 \to \tilde{\nu}_0 = \frac{\nu_0}{4\pi N\sqrt{3}\rho} = \frac{1}{2\sqrt{3}\rho}\frac{\omega_0 - \omega}{\omega_0}, \qquad \tau \to \tilde{z} = \frac{z}{L_g} \tag{24}$$

and it is worth noting that the number of undulator periods does not appear anymore in the definition of the new dimensionless quantities (see below for further comments);

(ii) Quantities involving the product of p, q and τ, written in the new variables, read

$$p\tau = \sqrt{3}\left(\sqrt[3]{1 + \frac{\sqrt{1 - 4\tilde{\nu}_0^3}}{1 - 2\tilde{\nu}_0^3}}\right)\tilde{z}, \qquad q\tau = \sqrt{3}\left(\sqrt[3]{1 - \frac{\sqrt{1 - 4\tilde{\nu}_0^3}}{1 - 2\tilde{\nu}_0^3}}\right)\tilde{z}. \tag{25}$$

It is finally important to stress that the Colson's dimensionless amplitude in terms of dimensional quantities reads

$$a = 2\sqrt{2}\pi\sqrt{\frac{I}{I_s}} \tag{26}$$

where I is the field intensity (power/surface) and I_s is the saturation intensity [30–33], a quantity which, in the theory of lasers, is exploited as a reference quantity to fix the onset of saturation. Even though its use is more appropriate for FEL operating in the oscillatory configuration, it can be exploited within the context of cavity-less operation too. Its dependence on the FEL parameters is specified by (practical units)

$$I_s\left[\frac{MW}{cm^2}\right] = 6.9312 \cdot 10^2 \left(\frac{\gamma}{N}\right)^4 (\lambda_u[cm]Kf_b(\xi))^{-2}, \qquad \xi = \frac{1}{4}\left(\frac{K^2}{1 + \frac{K^2}{2}}\right). \tag{27}$$

A more appropriate expression for the high gain/$SASE$ regime can be obtained by expressing the second of Equation (1) in the new dimensionless coordinates, thereby finding

$$\frac{d}{d\tilde{z}}\tilde{a} = -\frac{2}{\sqrt{3}}\langle e^{-i\xi}\rangle,$$

$$|\tilde{a}| = 2\sqrt{2}\pi\sqrt{\frac{I}{\tilde{I}_s}}, \qquad \tilde{I}_s\left[\frac{MW}{cm^2}\right] = 6.9312 \cdot 10^2 \frac{(4\pi\gamma\rho)^4}{[\lambda_u[cm]Kf_b(\xi)]^2}. \tag{28}$$

For actual values of the FEL parameters entering in the definition of $\tilde{I}_s$, we obtain for it reference numbers not dissimilar from the FEL saturated power, as discussed later in this paper.

The use of the previous variables allows one to cast the intensity evolution in the dimensional form (valid for $\nu_0 = 0$) [17,18]

$$A(\tilde{z}) = \frac{1}{9}\left[3 + 2\cosh\left(\frac{z}{L_g}\right) + 4\cos\left(\frac{\sqrt{3}}{2}\frac{z}{L_g}\right)\cosh\left(\frac{z}{2L_g}\right)\right],$$

$$I(\tilde{z}) = I_0 A(\tilde{z}), \qquad I_0 = \frac{\tilde{I}_s}{8\pi^2}|a_0|^2. \tag{29}$$

which has been largely exploited in the past [17,18] to describe the small signal *FEL* evolution; early derivations of similar equations trace back to the early eighties of the 20th century [34].

In Figure 3 we have plotted Equation (29) and the mere exponential behavior, which allows the conclusion that the region before the onset of the exponential growth, usually called lethargic region, lasts about two gain lengths, namely,

$$Z_L \simeq 2.1 \, L_g. \tag{30}$$

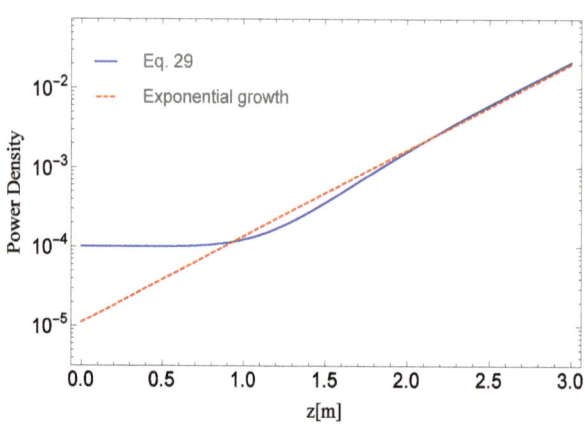

Figure 3. Comparison between Equation (29) and the pure exponential behavior for $L_g = 0.4$.

In any *FEL* device the small signal gain is a crucial parameter; it is naively defined as the relative intensity variation:

$$G = \frac{|\tilde{a}(\tilde{z},\tilde{v}_0)|^2 - |\tilde{a}_0|^2}{|\tilde{a}_0|^2}. \tag{31}$$

In the case of low gain, its maximum value is proportional to the small signal gain coefficient through the well known identity [17,18]

$$G^* = 0.85 \, g_0. \tag{32}$$

Such a quantity measures the amplification of the input seed at the end of the undulator. We can, however, extend the concept by considering the same gain measurement at different points inside the undulator, as shown in Figure 4, after a number of periods

$$N_z = \frac{z}{\lambda_u}. \tag{33}$$

We can therefore write G^* in terms of ρ, z as (see Equation (32))

$$G^* = \frac{0.85}{\pi} \left(\frac{\tilde{z}}{\sqrt{3}} \right)^3. \tag{34}$$

The low gain regime relies on the assumption that the laser amplitude remains constant during the transit inside the undulator. The approximation breaks when higher order terms in g_0 are to be taken into account to specify the maximum gain at a given point in z. These corrections, derived in [35], can be written as

$$G^* = \frac{|\tilde{a}(\tilde{z}, \tilde{v}_0^*)|^2 - |\tilde{a}_0|^2}{|\tilde{a}_0|^2} \simeq$$
$$\simeq \frac{0.85}{\pi}\left(\frac{\tilde{z}}{\sqrt{3}}\right)^3 + \frac{0.19}{\pi^2}\left(\frac{\tilde{z}}{\sqrt{3}}\right)^6 + \frac{4.23 \cdot 10^{-3}}{\pi^3}\left(\frac{\tilde{z}}{\sqrt{3}}\right)^9 + o(\rho^{12}) \quad (35)$$

whose meaning is better explained in Figure 4, where we have also reported the departure of the gain line shape from the anti-symmetric curve, characterizing the early *FEL* experiments [36,37].

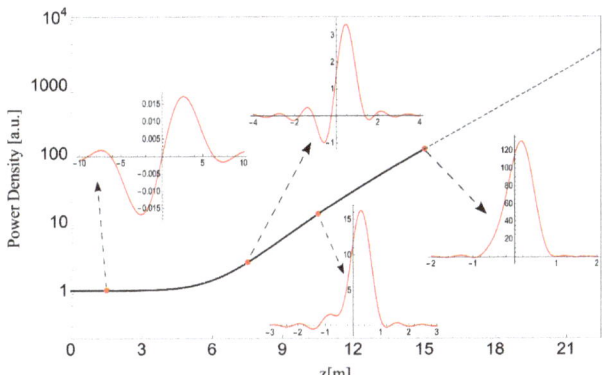

Figure 4. Power density (a.u.) vs. z and gain function "measured" at different points inside the undulator. Above the last point, where the dotted curve starts, the small signal gain is not properly defined because the small signal approximation does not strictly apply. The curves have been derived for the parameters $\rho_0 = 6.8 \cdot 10^{-4}$ and $\lambda_u = 5$ cm. The small signal gain coefficient goes from $5.35 \cdot 10^{-3}$ to 5.35.

In this section we have provided a fairly general analysis describing the solution of the *FEL* high gain small signal equation.

In the forthcoming section we discuss how the technique we have discussed so far can be extended to the treatment of *FEL* induced higher order harmonics.

3. High Gain FEL Equations and Harmonic Generation

In this section we discuss the mechanism of harmonic generation in *FEL* devices, which is a process "naturally" associated with the evolution of the fundemental harmonic. The importance of these further contributions in developing tools extending the capabilities of *FELs* was soon recognized in the community, but the practical implementations took some time.

The pendulum equations, including the higher order harmonics, can be written as (differently from the index n in the perturbative terms discussed in Equation (11); in this case n is just the order of the harmonic) [38]

$$\frac{d^2}{d\tau^2}\zeta = \sum_{n=0}^{\infty} |a_n|\cos(\psi_n), \qquad \psi_n = n\zeta + \phi_n,$$
$$\frac{d}{d\tau}a_n = -j_n\langle e^{-in\zeta}\rangle, \qquad j_n = 2\pi g_{0,n} \quad (36)$$

where $a_n = |a_n| e^{i\phi_n}$ is the dimensionless amplitude of the n-th order harmonics and $g_{0,n}$ is the n-th harmonic small signal gain parameter to be specified later [39].

$$\frac{d}{d\tau}a_n = -2\pi g_0 b_n e^{-i\nu_n \tau} + i\pi n g_n \int_0^\tau (\tau - \tau') a_n(\tau') e^{-i\nu_n(\tau - \tau')} d\tau',$$
$$\nu_n = 2\pi N \frac{n\omega_0 - \omega}{n\omega_0}. \tag{37}$$

It is evident that the same considerations developed for the fundamental harmonic ($n = 1$), hold in the present case too, the only significant difference being that the n-the harmonic Pierce is now specified by

$$\rho_n^* = \sqrt[3]{n}\, \rho_n, \qquad \rho_n = \rho \left(\frac{f_{b,n}}{f_b}\right)^{\frac{2}{3}}, \qquad f_{b,n} = J_{\frac{n-1}{2}}(n\zeta) - J_{\frac{n+1}{2}}(n\zeta), \qquad f_{b,1} = f_b. \tag{38}$$

The gain length determining the harmonic linear growth is

$$L_{g,n}^* = \frac{\lambda_u}{4\pi\sqrt{3}\rho_n^*} = \frac{1}{\sqrt[3]{n}} L_{g,n}. \tag{39}$$

where $L_{g,n}$ is defined in terms of ρ_n as

$$L_{g,n} = \frac{\lambda_u}{4\pi\sqrt{3}\rho_n} \tag{40}$$

The role of $L_{g,n}^*$ in the harmonic generation is clarified below; it is just a consequence of the assumption (summarized in Equation (36), where the electron field phase ψ_n is written as $n\zeta$) that the process is dominated by the bunching induced by the fundamental harmonic.

It is worth noting that the correction term $\sqrt[3]{n}$ in the definition of the harmonic Pierce parameter was initially suggested in references [17,18,39] as a consequence of an accurate analysis of the numerical data from the code PROMETEO [40].

In Figure 5 we have reported the harmonic intensity growth vs. the longitudinal coordinate; the relevant behavior is the same as for $n = 1$, reproduced by equations of the type (29) with $L_{g,n}^*$ in place of L_g.

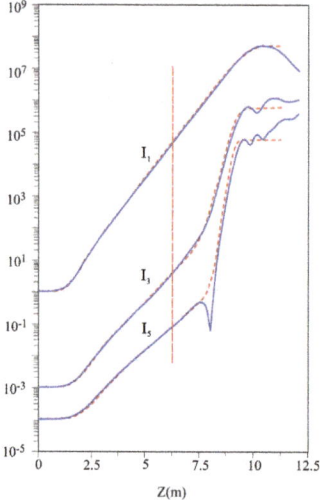

Figure 5. Harmonic evolution and nonlinear harmonic generation which is triggered after the dashed line, where the bunching effects become significant.

However, this is only a part of the story. The harmonic intensities (3,5) follow a growth rate characterized by two different regimes. After the lethargic region, the growth rates is initially specified by the inverse of the harmonic gain length $L_{g,n}^*$ and then by an abrupt increase of the growth ruled by nL_g^{-1}. This behavior is the signature of a complex mechanism underlying the harmonic generation emission.

We have so far considered the harmonic linear dynamics, in which within certain limits (to be discussed in the final section), the evolutions of the associated intensities are independent. It should be noted that harmonics too can be triggered by a bunching coefficient, as implicitly contained in Equation (37). As it is well known, the bunching grows with the intensity itself; the dynamics of each harmonic are the result of intrigued feedback between induced bunching and higher order-bunching (namely, at higher values of n). We crudely describe the process by noting that each harmonic, while the intensity grows, induces further bunching, determining the onset of the sub-harmonics m of the n-th harmonic—namely, the first harmonic indices higher order harmonics and each of them determines a further set of harmonics. In terms of bunching coefficients, we have: The fundamental harmonics ($n = 1$) contributes to the increase of the bunching of order 1 and of other higher order bunching coefficients. The same holds for the higher order harmonics; the third is, e.g., responsible for the bunching of its own harmonics (3, 6, 9, . . . with respect to the fundamental).

The bunching process is not "free," and indeed an energy spread, associated with gain degradation and saturation mechanisms, is produced. This phenomenology is not considered within the present context.

The inclusion of nonlinear terms in our analysis occurs by keeping intensity dependent terms [17,18,41] which allow the following redefinition of the FEL integral equation:

$$\frac{d}{d\tau}a = -2\pi g_0 e^{-i\nu_0\tau} \sum_{m=-\infty}^{\infty} (-i)^m b_{1-m} \frac{J_m(|\Pi|)}{|\Pi|^m} \left(\int_0^\tau (\tau-\tau')a(\tau')e^{i\nu_0\tau'}d\tau'\right)^m, \quad (41)$$

$$\int_0^\tau (\tau-\tau')a(\tau')e^{i\nu_0\tau'}d\tau' = |\Pi|e^{i\psi}$$

where

$$J_m(|\Pi|) = \sum_{r=0}^{\infty} \frac{(-1)^r}{r!(m+r)!}\left(\frac{|\Pi|}{2}\right)^{m+2r}. \quad (42)$$

If we consider a perturbative solution of the above equation in terms of the fundamental intensity, we can write the first three terms as

$$\frac{d}{d\tau}a_l = -2\pi g_0 b_1 e^{-i\nu_0\tau} + i\pi g_0 \int_0^\tau (\tau-\tau')a_l(\tau')e^{-i\nu_0(\tau-\tau')}d\tau',$$

$$\frac{d}{d\tau}a_{nl,2} = -2\pi g_0 e^{-i\nu_0\tau}\frac{b_{-1}}{8}\left(\int_0^\tau (\tau-\tau')a_l(\tau')e^{i\nu_0\tau'}d\tau'\right)^2, \quad (43)$$

$$\frac{d}{d\tau}a_{nl,3} = -2\pi g_0 e^{-i\nu_0\tau}\frac{b_{-2}}{2^3 3!}\left(\int_0^\tau (\tau-\tau')a_0(\tau')e^{i\nu_0\tau'}d\tau'\right)^3$$

which have been derived using the limit $\lim_{|\Pi|\to 0}\frac{J_m(|\Pi|)}{|\Pi|^m} = \frac{1}{m!2^m}$. The subscripts l and nl stand for linear and nonlinear, respectively. The nl-contributions stand for the onset of the nonlinear harmonic generation.

Considering a linearly polarized undulator not providing coupling to even on axis harmonic generation, we obtain from the third Equation (43)

$$a_{nl,3} = -2\pi g_0 \frac{b_{-2}}{2^3 3!} \int_0^\tau e^{-i\nu_0 \tau'} h_3(\nu_0, \tau') d\tau',$$

$$h_3(\nu_0, \tau) = \left(\int_0^\tau (\tau - \tau') a_0(\tau') e^{i\nu_0 \tau'} d\tau' \right)^3. \tag{44}$$

Keeping the fast growing root only and assuming $\nu_0 = 0$, we find a further contribution to the harmonic intensity depending on the power of the fundamental and characterized (as already anticipated) by the gain length

$$L_g^{(nlhg)} = \frac{L_g}{n} \tag{45}$$

where $nlhg$ stands for nonnlinear-harmonic generation.

The conclusion of this discussion is that there are two distinct contributions to the higher order harmonic emission. The first is a kind of lasing on harmonic; this concept was originally introduced in [42] by Colson et al., where the possibility of exploiting this mechanism to sustain higher order harmonics lasing in the oscillator configuration has been discussed. The second provides the well-known nonlinear harmonic generation mechanism; it goes beyond the linear analysis; its characterizing features and scaling relations are further discussed in the final section of this paper.

We have commented on the importance of the harmonic generation mechanism, which has opened the possibility of extending the relevant performances in terms of tunability range and not only.

We want to mention an important application of the harmonic generation in FEL which has determined a significant improvement of the relevant performances. It has already been underscored that running the FEL in the amplifier configuration is feasible if a coherent seed at certain wavelengths is available. This happens with FEL harmonics too, which can be triggered using the seeds from harmonic generation in gas (see references [43,44] for an adequate description). In these devices, the beam of laser (a Ti:sapphire laser, for example), is focused into a xenon gas cell, where high harmonic generation occurs. The output seed beam is then spatially and temporally overlapped to the electron beam moving in an undulator with the period chosen to match the seed frequency. The FEL harmonics then grow according to the mechanisms we have just outlined. The successful implementation of this concept has allowed the possibility of extending the FEL tunability of more than an order of magnitude (for more details, see [43] and references therein). A further idea, concerning the use of segmented undulators, after the beam self induced prebunching, is discussed in the forthcoming section.

4. Inhomogeneous Broadening Partial Amplitudes and High Gain FEL Equation

The high gain integral equation becomes slightly more complicated if the effect of non ideal e-beam qualities is included. The averages in Equation (2) need to be extended to the beam distribution (energy, spatial, angular, etc.). With these premises and limiting ourselves to the effect of the energy spread only, we find [45]

$$\frac{d}{d\tau} a = i\pi g_0 \int_0^\tau a(\tau - \tau') \tau' e^{-i\nu_0 \tau' - \frac{1}{2}(\pi \mu_\varepsilon \tau')^2} d\tau', \qquad \mu_\varepsilon = 4N\sigma_\varepsilon \tag{46}$$

obtained after taking the average of a Gaussian relative energy distribution with r.m.s. σ_ε.

The solution of Equation (46) cannot be obtained in analytical terms; however, the method of partial amplitude expansion pioneered by A. Segreto in references [46,47] yields a fairly useful analytical mean allowing the solution of, e.g., Equation (46) in the form (we use the $\tilde{\nu}_0, \tilde{z}$ variables, more appropriate for the forthcoming discussion)

$$\tilde{a}(\tilde{z},\tilde{v}_0) = \tilde{a}_0 \left(1 + \sum_{k=1}^{\infty} i^k \left(\frac{\tilde{z}}{\sqrt{3}}\right)^{3k} g_k(\tilde{z},\tilde{v}_0,\tilde{\mu}_\varepsilon)\right),$$

$$g_k(\tilde{z},\tilde{v}_0,\tilde{\mu}_\varepsilon) = \frac{M_k \gamma_k}{\Sigma_k} \exp\left[-\frac{(\tilde{\mu}_\varepsilon \tilde{z})^2 (\beta_k + i\xi_k(\tilde{v}_0 \tilde{z})) + 12(i\lambda_k(\tilde{v}_0 \tilde{z}) + (\tilde{v}_0 \tilde{z})^2)}{24 \Sigma_k^2}\right], \qquad (47)$$

$$M_k = \frac{1}{(3k)!}, \quad \gamma_k = (3k+1)\sqrt{\frac{3k+2}{2k(k+1)}}, \quad \Sigma_k = \sqrt{\gamma_k^2 + \frac{1}{12}(\tilde{\mu}_\varepsilon \tilde{z})^2},$$

$$\beta_k = 2\frac{4k+1}{k+1}, \quad \lambda_k = 2(3k+1)\frac{3k+2}{k+1}, \quad \xi_k = 2\frac{(2k+1)(k-1)}{(k+1)(3k+1)}.$$

The previous equation can be profitably used to get information of a practical nature. The low gain expansion ($k = 1$) yields for the intensity growth

$$|\tilde{a}(\tilde{z},\tilde{v}_0)|^2 \simeq |\tilde{a}_0|^2 \left[1 + 2\frac{M_1}{3\sqrt{3}\Sigma_1} \tilde{z}^3 \cdot \exp\left(-\frac{\beta_1 \tilde{\mu}_\varepsilon^2 + \tilde{v}_0^2}{24\Sigma_1^2} \tilde{z}^2\right) \sin\left(\frac{\tilde{v}_0(12\lambda_1 + \xi_1(\tilde{\mu}_\varepsilon \tilde{z})^2)}{24\Sigma_1^2} \tilde{z}\right)\right] \qquad (48)$$

which provides an idea of the interplay between inhomogeneous broadening and the other mechanisms contributing to the laser evolution. In Figure 6 we have reported the analogues of Figure 2b for different values of the inhomogeneous broadening parameter. The plot yields quite a good description of how the intensity growth is diluted by the presence of a non zero energy spread.

Other effects due to angular and spatial distribution of the electron beam can be introduced too. From the conceptual point of view, they do not imply any problem, but for the introduction of a further convolution term in Equation (46). The induced detrimental effects are expressed through appropriate μ-parameters, analogous to those associated with the energy spread. They are listed in [18].

It is important to stress that, from the practical point of view, the effect of non perfect electron beam qualities produces an increase of the gain length, which can be parameterized as [17,18]

$$L_g(\tilde{\mu}_\varepsilon) = \left(1 + 0.185 \frac{\sqrt{3}}{2} \tilde{\mu}_\varepsilon^2\right) L_g \qquad (49)$$

The interest in the method of partial amplitudes stems also for the fact that it can be generalized to more complicated situations, involving, e.g., the pulse propagation contributions.

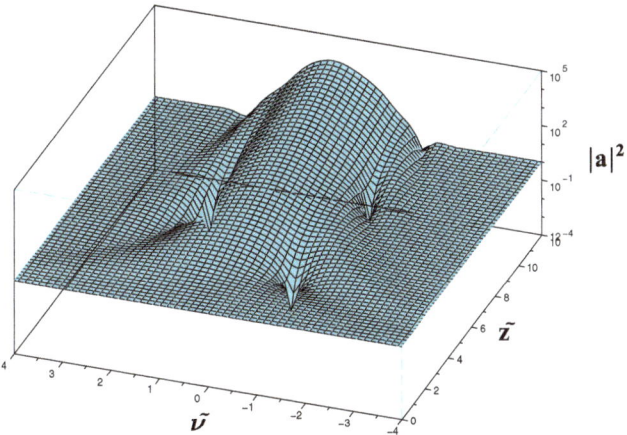

Figure 6. Intensity vs. $\tilde{z}, \tilde{v}$ for inhomogeneous parameters $\tilde{\mu}_\varepsilon = 1$, $g_0 = 100$, $a_0 = 1$.

In the following we make the assumption that the electron bunch is sampled into a series of slices with a longitudinal size of the order of a coherence length [48–50]:

$$\lambda_c = \frac{\lambda}{4\pi\sqrt{3}\rho}. \tag{50}$$

During the interaction the radiation is mismatched with respect to the electron bunch reference by a quantity depending on the slippage length. The computation of this aspect of the problem requires a certain amount of computation which, for the homogeneous case (no energy spread) has been accomplished in [51] and for the present case is summarized below.

According to the aforementioned reference and to the analytical steps outlined in [46,47], the problem is solved, in relatively easy terms, by replacing the detuning parameter with the operator

$$\tilde{v}_0 \to \hat{\tilde{v}}_0 = \tilde{v}_0 + i\frac{\lambda_c}{L_g}\partial_\zeta \tag{51}$$

where ζ is the bunch coordinate. The replacement (51) in the partial amplitudes accounts for the action of the FEL dynamics on the optical packet, expressed by the simple Gaussian (to avoid any misunderstanding, we emphasize that ζ now indicates the optical bunch coordinate and should not be confused with the pendulum coordinate in Equation (1))

$$a_0(\zeta) = \frac{1}{\sqrt[4]{2\pi\sigma_\zeta^2}} e^{-\left(\frac{\zeta}{2\sigma_\zeta}\right)^2}. \tag{52}$$

The action of the partial amplitudes on the initial packet is specified by

$$g_k(\tilde{z}, \hat{\tilde{v}}_0, \tilde{\mu}_\varepsilon)a_0(\zeta) = g_k(\zeta, \tilde{z}, \tilde{v}_0, \tilde{\mu}_\varepsilon)e^{\left(S_k\partial_\zeta + D_k\partial_\zeta^2\right)}a_0(\zeta),$$
$$S_k = \frac{\lambda_c}{2\Sigma_k^2 L_g}\left\{\left[\frac{(\pi\mu_\varepsilon \tilde{z})^2 \tilde{\zeta}_k}{12} + \lambda_k \tilde{z}\right] - i\tilde{v}_0\right\}, \qquad D_k = \frac{1}{2\Sigma_k^2}\left(\frac{\tilde{z}\lambda_c}{L_g}\right)^2. \tag{53}$$

The action of the exponential operator containing the shift (first-order derivative) and diffusive operators (second-order derivative) on the initial packet is provided by

$$e^{\left(S_k\partial_\zeta + D_k\partial_\zeta^2\right)}a_0(\zeta) = \frac{1}{\sqrt[4]{2\pi}}\sqrt{\frac{\sigma_\zeta}{\sigma_\zeta^2 + D_k}}\exp\left[-\frac{1}{4}\frac{\left(\zeta + \zeta_k - i\frac{\tilde{v}_0\lambda_c\tilde{z}}{2\Sigma_k L_g}\right)^2}{\sigma_\zeta^2 + D_k}\right]. \tag{54}$$

A result which allows a few speculations:

(a) The wave packet is shifted back by a quantity

$$\zeta_k = \frac{1}{24\Sigma_k}\left[(\pi\mu_\varepsilon)^2 \tilde{\zeta}_n + 12\lambda_k\right]\frac{\lambda_c}{L_g}. \tag{55}$$

This means that the optical packet is moving back with respect to the bunch frame propagating at velocity c, the associated group velocity is

$$v_{g,k} = \left(1 - \frac{1}{c}\frac{d}{dt}\zeta_k\right)c. \tag{56}$$

The radiation moves slower than c, by the effect of the interaction itself. The gain dilution due to the energy spread counteracts the velocity slow down with respect to the case of negligible energy spread.

The complex refraction index derived from Equation (56) can be written as

$$n_{g,k} \simeq 1 + \frac{1}{c}\frac{d}{dt}\zeta_k .\qquad(57)$$

(b) The optical packed undergoes a longitudinal diffusion specified by

$$\sigma_k = \sqrt{D_k} = \frac{1}{\sqrt{2\Sigma_k}}\left(\frac{\bar{z}\lambda_c}{L_g}\right)\qquad(58)$$

which ensures that in one gain length the additional packet width is essentially a coherence length. This effect has been studied in the theory of mode-locked FEL operation within the context of the oscillator theory; the relevant discussion can be found in [2].

In the forthcoming section we apply the result obtained so far to the slice evolution.

5. Slice Evolution

The concept of slice phase space is a by-product of the $SASE\ FEL$ physics. It is indeed associated with the fact that, in these devices, the combination of mechanisms such as gain, slippage and finite coherence length, determines a local interaction, because the radiation experiences only a portion of the beam, having the longitudinal extension of a coherence length (see Figures 7 and 8). The interaction is therefore sensitive to the slice-brightness, which is characterized by the relevant six dimensional phase space distribution [52–58].

The analysis associated with the transverse phase space and with the relevant electron-beam transport properties has already been accomplished in a number of papers, which have clarified a significant deal of the physical and practical issues regarding the evolution and interplay between slices and FEL power output and performances.

In this section we clarify the effect of longitudinal phase space, by the use of the formalism we outlined in the previous section. We sample the optical bunch as indicated in Figure 7 and characterize each slice with a progressive number [59,60].

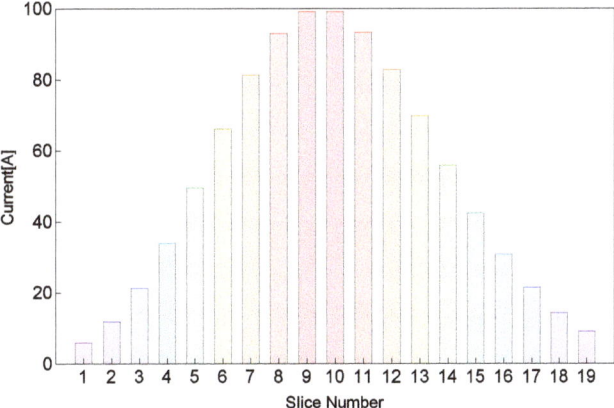

Figure 7. Slice number sampling and shape, using the e-bunch distribution as the reference frame.

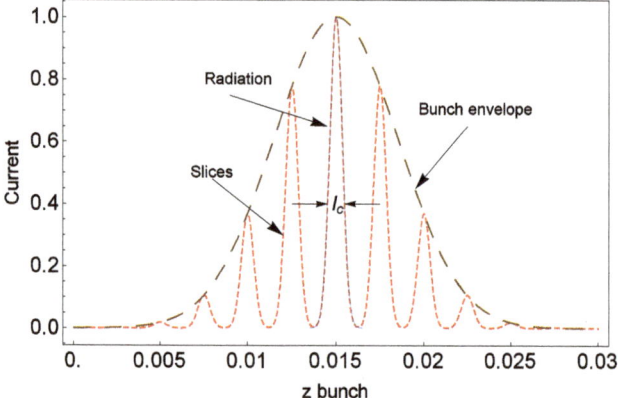

Figure 8. Bunched envelope, associated slices and superimposed radiation.

Each slice is assumed to be Gaussian with an amount of charge Q_s and an associated current

$$I_s = \frac{Q_s}{\sqrt{2\pi}\tau_c}, \qquad \tau_c \simeq \frac{L_c}{c} \equiv coherence-time. \qquad (59)$$

A natural assumption is that the amount of charge follows the Gaussian shape of Figure 8, namely,

$$Q_s = Q_{s^*} e^{-(s-s^*)^2 \delta^2}, \qquad \delta = \frac{2\pi L_c}{\sigma_\zeta} \qquad (60)$$

with δ^{-1} being the number of slices inside the bunch and s^* representing the slice with largest current. With these assumptions we can write the slice Pierce parameter as

$$\rho_s = \rho_{s^*} e^{-\frac{(s-s^*)^2 \delta^2}{3}}. \qquad (61)$$

As we already stressed, each slice carries its own energy spread, and therefore we get a corresponding inhomogeneous parameter specified by

$$\tilde{\mu}_s = \tilde{\mu}_{s^*} e^{-\frac{(s-s^*)^2 \delta^2}{3}}. \qquad (62)$$

The energy spread corresponding to each slice may be completely random and that with largest current may carry the worst spread.

By taking into account these effects, we obtain the results reported in Figures 9 and 10. The first refers to the case in which the slice with maximum current coincides with that at the center of the distribution, and the energy spread of each slice is chosen to be completely random. The second accounts for a configuration in which the maximum current is associated with a slice belonging to the rear part of the bunch.

Further comments including the elements for a more accurate computation of the slice distribution, are discussed in the forthcoming section dedicated to concluding remarks.

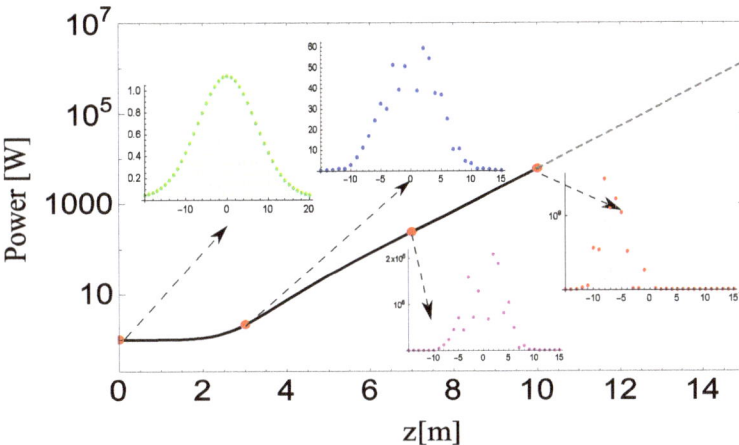

Figure 9. Slice evolution inside the undulator at different Z; the energy spread has been randomly chosen and the current follows the bunch Gaussian distribution with $s* = 0$, $\lambda_u = 0.02$, $\rho_0 = 0.001$, $\mu_\varepsilon = 0.0004$ and $\nu = 0$. The initial distribution $z = 0$ of the slices is the same as in Figure 8. The vertical axis is in log-scale; the insets are plotted in linear scale.

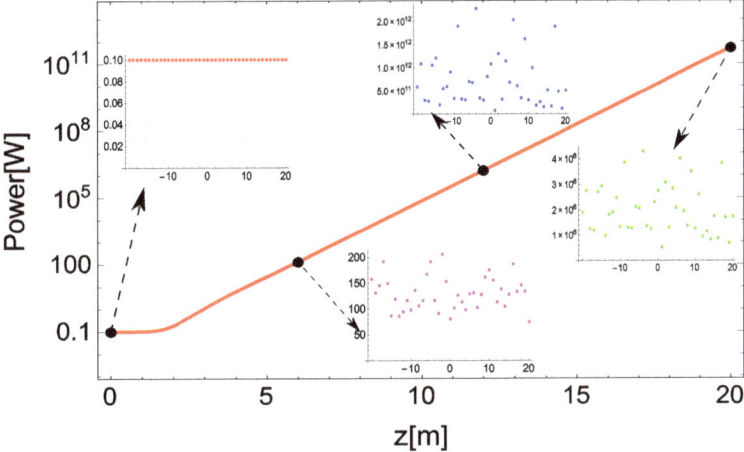

Figure 10. Same as Figure 9—all slices with the same energy spread and the maximum current associated with the rear part of the bunch ($s* = 1$). Slice evolution vs z and intensity evolution vs. z. The slices are characterized by the same amount of charge and different values of the energy spread with $\lambda_u = 0.015$, $\rho_0 = 0.0011$, $\sigma_\varepsilon = 0.05$, $\sigma_d = 0.002$, $\delta = 0.01$ and $I_0 = 10^{-1}$. The intensity growth does not refer to a single slice but to the relevant average. The slices have a flat distribution in z, and each is characterized by an initial seed of 0.1 W. The vertical axis is in log-scale; the insets are plotted in linear scale.

6. Final Remarks

This paper has treated different topics in the small signal evolution of high gain $SASE$ devices. We have just touched on the nonlinear effects leading to saturation. It has been underscored that the relevant pattern is accompanied by mechanisms of higher order bunching leading to the process of higher order harmonic emission.

From the phenomenological point of view, saturation can be included by modifying the small signal power evolution in Equation (29) as

$$I_s(\tilde{z}) = I_0 \frac{A(\tilde{z})}{1 + \frac{I_0}{I_F}(A(\tilde{z}) - 1)}, \quad I_F = \sqrt{2}\rho P_E \quad (63)$$

where P_E is the electron beam power intensity and I_0 is the input seed intensity. I_0 is usually specified by the rule of thumb that a value usually 10^8 below the saturated power density is chosen. The intensity I_F yields the saturated power. The term at the denominator accounts for the saturation mechanisms, using a kind of logistic model, as displayed in Figure 11. The last figure needs its own mention: it shows the power growth in the deep saturated regime. Equation (63) reproduces well the evolution up the maximum and then remains fixed without following the oscillations (see Figure 12) due to the post saturation dynamics, characterized by e-beam rotation in phase-space, induced by an exchange of power between laser field and electrons.

A more complete view is reported in Figure 13. The physical content can be noted as reported below.

The figure exhibits the first and third harmonics, along with the associated wave packet evolution (upper and lower panels). We have assumed the growth from a coherent seed, and no spiking appears before the saturation. With the onset of the power oscillations, the optical packets start to be characterized by the appearance of side bands, which degrade the laser pulse itself in correspondence with the minima of the oscillations [61–63]. The effects of beam qualities can be also included by replacing $A(z)$ with approximants discussed in the previous section.

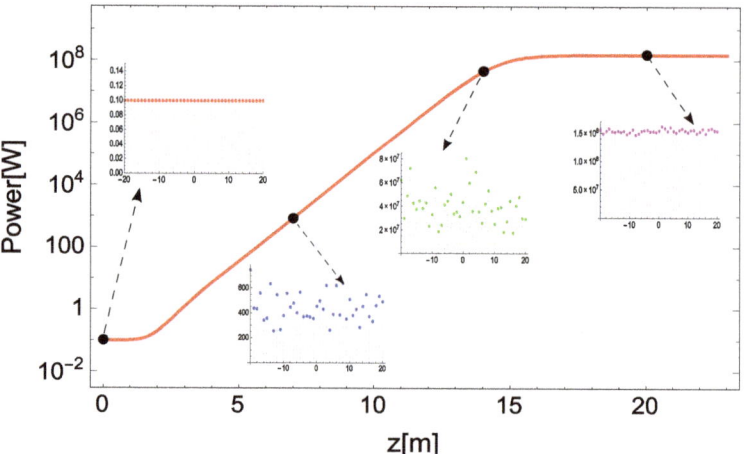

Figure 11. Same parameters as in Figure 10 with the inclusion of the saturation. The slices have a flat distribution in z, and each is characterized by an initial seed of 0.1 W. The vertical axis is in log-scale; the insets are plotted in linear scale.

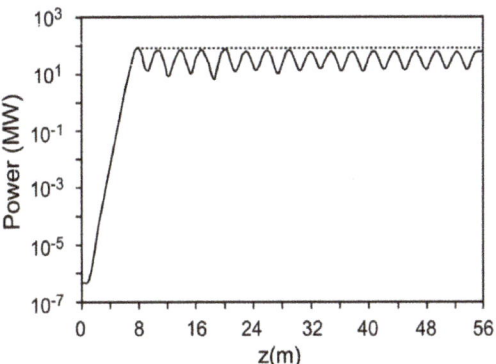

Figure 12. Power growth and oscillation after saturation (no specific parameters of the simulation have been inserted because we are just interested to the oscillating behavior, characterizing any $SASE$ FEL operating with constant parameters).

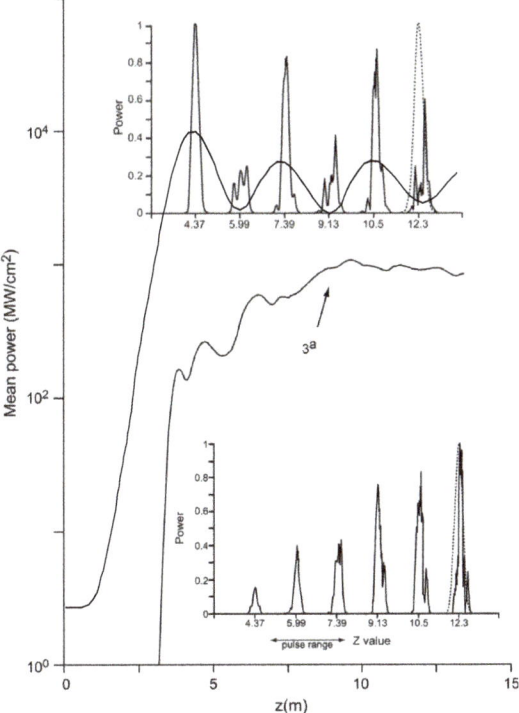

Figure 13. First and third harmonic power growth vs. z, along with the power oscillations and associated changes in the laser packet distribution.

The pivotal element of the discussion of this paper has been centered around the FEL high gain equation, which, including the necessary modifications, is able to describe different physical situations regarding the FEL phenomenology. The FEL high gain equation has been derived from the FEL pendulum equation after a suitable linearization. A different treatment can be, however, exploited: it employs a Hamiltonian picture and the associated Liouville equation. The by-product of this treatment (see, e.g., [9,10,17,18,49,50,52–60,64]) yields results not dissimilar from those discussed in the previous sections, and the bunching coefficient of the n-th harmonic induced by the fundamental behaves like $|a|^n$. Such an effect is of fundamental importance in the handling of the so-called segmented magnet configurations [50,65]. FEL adopting this type of solution exploits the growth of the bunching inside a first section, which is interrupted and connected to a second undulator, tuned at one of its harmonics. The result is the growth of a coherent signal emerging from the beam bunching acquired in the first section. Methods based on the joint use of the solution of the high gain FEL equation, on the study of the relevant Liouville equation and on the use of massive simulation codes, allow the possibility of deriving useful scaling relations concerning the onset and saturation of the FEL signal from a suitably pre-bunched beam [65].

$$\Pi_n(z) = \Pi_{0,n} \frac{e^{\frac{z}{L_g^{(n)}}}}{1 + \frac{\Pi_{0,n}}{\Pi_{F,n}}\left(e^{\frac{z}{L_g^{(n)}}} - 1\right)}, \qquad L_g^{(n)} = \frac{L_g}{n},$$

$$\Pi_{0,n} = c_n \left(\frac{P_0}{9\rho P_E}\right)^n \Pi_{F,n}, \qquad \Pi_{F,n} = \frac{1}{\sqrt{n}}\left(\frac{f_{b,n}}{n f_{b,1}}\right)^2 P_F$$

(64)

where the coefficients c_n are just numerical characteristics for each harmonic. Equation (64) yields the growth of the nonlinear part of the n-th harmonic. The relevant gain length is decreased by a factor corresponding to the order of the harmonics; $\Pi_{F,n}$ is the harmonic saturated power. The number of photons/seconds at the n-th harmonic can accordingly be calculated as

$$\dot{N}_n = \frac{\Pi_{F,n}}{n\hbar\omega} = E_n \dot{N}_1, \qquad E_n = \frac{1}{n\sqrt{n}}\left(\frac{f_{b,n}}{n f_{b,1}}\right)^2,$$

(65)

where E_n represents a kind of efficiency displaying how the fundamental harmonic contributes to the higher order harmonics.

We have so far given a general discussion of analytical and numerical methods to treat the FEL intensity evolution in the high gain/$SASE$ regime. We have just touched on the problems associated with short pulse effects, which will be treated elsewhere in a dedicated monography.

Author Contributions: Conceptualization, G.D., E.D.P., E.S.; methodology, G.D., E.D.P., E.S. software, E.D.P., E.S.; validation, G.D., E.D.P., S.L., E.S.; formal analysis, G.D., E.D.P., S.L., E.S.; data curation, G.D., E.D.P., S.L., E.S. writing–original draft preparation, G.D., E.D.P., E.S.; writing–review and editing, S.L.; visualization, G.D., E.D.P., S.L., E.S. supervision, G.D., E.D.P., S.L., E.S.; project administration, E.D.P. All authors have read and agreed to the published version of the manuscript.

Funding: This research received no external funding.

Acknowledgments: The work of S. Licciardi was supported by an Enea Research Center individual fellowship.

Conflicts of Interest: The authors declare no conflict of interest.

References

1. Madey, J.M.J. Stimulated Emission of Bremsstrahlung in a Periodic Magnetic Field. *J. Appl. Phys.* **1971**, *42*, 1906. [CrossRef]
2. Dattoli, G.; Di Palma, E.; Pagnutti, S.; Sabia, E. Free Electron coherent sources: From microwave to X-rays. *Phys. Rep.* **2018**, *739*, 1–51. [CrossRef]
3. Neyman, P.J.; Colson, W.B.; Gottschalk, S.C.; Todd, A.M.M.; Blau, J.; Cohn, K. Free Electron Lasers in 2017. In Proceedings of the 38th International Free Electron Laser Conference, FEL2017, Santa Fe, NM, USA, 20–25 August 2017. Available online: https://accelconf.web.cern.ch/fel2017/papers/mop066.pdf (accessed on 17 December 2020).
4. Rossbach, J.; Schneider, J.R.; Wurth, W. 10 years of pioneering X-ray science at the Free-Electron Laser FLASH at DESY. *Phys. Rep.* **2019**, *808*, 1–74. [CrossRef]
5. Topics. Available online: https://lcls.slac.stanford.edu/ (accessed on 17 December 2020).
6. Topics. Available online: https://www.elettra.trieste.it/lightsources/fermi/machine.html (accessed on 17 December 2020).
7. Topics. Available online: http://xfel.riken.jp/eng/ (accessed on 17 December 2020).

8. Colson, W.B. Free Electron Laser Theory. Ph.D. Thesis, Stanford University, Stanford, CA, USA, 1977.
9. Colson, W.B. *Classical Free Electron Laser Theory, Laser Handbook*; Colson, W.B., Pellegrini, C., Renieri, A., Eds.; North-Holland: Amsterdam, The Netherlands, 1990; Volume VI.
10. Saldin, E.L.; Schneidmiller, E.V.; Yurkov, M.V. *The Physics of Free Electron Lasers*; Springer: Berlin/Heidelberg, Germany, 2000; doi:10.1007/978-3-662-04066-9. [CrossRef]
11. Kim, K.J.; Huang, Z.; Lindberg, R. *Synchrotron Radiation and Free Electron Lasers*; Cambridge University Press: Cambridge, UK, 2017. [CrossRef]
12. Bergmann, U.; Yachandra, V.; Yano, J. *X-ray Free Electron Laser: Applications in Materials, Chemistry and Biology*; Royal Society of Chemistry: Cambridge, UK, 2017; ISBN 978-1-84973-100-3.
13. Dattoli, G.; Doria, A.; Sabia, E.; Artioli, M. *Charged Beam Dynamics, Particle Accelerators and Free Electron Lasers*; IOP Publishing Ltd.: Bristol, UK, 2017.
14. Szarmes, E.B. *Classical Theory of Free-Electron Lasers*; IOP Publishing Ltd.: Bristol, UK, 2017.
15. Jaeschke, E.; Khan, S.; Schneider, J.R.; Hastings, J.B. *Synchrotron Light Sources and Free-Electron Lasers*; Springer: Berlin/Heidelberg, Germany, 2016; ISBN 978-3-319-14393-4.
16. Behrens, C.; Schmüser, P.; Dohlus, M.; Rossbach, J. *Free-Electron Lasers in the Ultraviolet and X-ray Regime*; Springer: Berlin/Heidelberg, Germany, 2014.
17. Dattoli, G.; Ottaviani, P.L. *Fel Small Signal Dynamics and Electron Beam Prebunching*; ENEA Internal Report, RT/INN/93/10; ENEA: Frascati, Italy, 1993.
18. Dattoli, G.; Ottaviani, P.L.; Pagnutti, S. *Booklet for FEL Design: A Collection of Practical Formulae*; ENEA—Edizioni Scientifiche: Frascati, Italy, 2007.
19. Bonifacio, R.; Pellegrini, C.; Narducci, L.M. Collective instabilities and high-gain regime in a free electron laser. *Opt. Commun.* **1984**, *50*, 373–378. [CrossRef]
20. Haus, H. Quantum Electronics, Noise in Free Electron Laser Amplifier. *IEEE J. Quantum Electron.* **1981**, *17*, 1427–1435. [CrossRef]
21. Dattoli, G.; Marino, A.; Renieri, A.; Romanelli, F. Progress in the Hamiltonian picture of the free-electron laser. *IEEE J. Quantum Electron.* **1981**, *17*, 1371–1387. [CrossRef]
22. Petelin, M.I. On the theory of ultrarelativistic cyclotron self-resonance masers. *Radiophys. Quantum Electron.* **1974**, *17*, 686–690. [CrossRef]
23. Nusinovich, G. *Introduction to the Physics of Gyrotrons*; The John Hopkins University Press: Baltimore, MD, USA, 2004.
24. Bratman, V.L.; Ginzburg, N.S.; Petelin, M.I. Common properties of free electron lasers. *Opt. Commun.* **1979**, *30*, 409–412. [CrossRef]
25. Di Palma, E.; Sabia, E.; Dattoli, G.; Licciardi, S.; Spassovsky, I. Cyclotron auto resonance maser and free electron laser devices: A unified point of view. *J. Plasma Phys.* **2017**, *83*, 905830102. [CrossRef]
26. Caloi, R.; Ciocci, F.; Dattoli, G.; Torre, A. The High-Gain FEL Equation: An Inexpensive Numerical Algorithm. *Il Nuovo Cimento B* **1991**, *106*, 627–640. [CrossRef]
27. Dattoli, G.; Renieri, A.; Torre, A. *Lecture on Free Electron Laser Theory and Related Topics*; World Scientific: Singapore, 1990.
28. Tremaine, A.J.; Rosenzweig, B.; Anderson, S.; Frigola, P.; Hogan, M.; Murokh, A.; Pellegrini, C.; Nguyen, D.C.; Sheffield, R.L. Observation of Self-Amplified Spontaneous-Emission-Induced Electron-Beam Microbunching Using Coherent Transition Radiation. *Phys. Rev. Lett.* **1998**, *81*, 5816. [CrossRef]
29. Nguyen, D.C.; Sheffield, R.L.; Fortgang, C.M.; Kinross-Wright, J.M.; Ebrahim, N.A.; Goldstein, J.C. A High-Power compact Regenerative Amplifier FEL. In Proceedings of the 17th PAC Conference, Vancouver, BC, Canada, 12–16 May 1997; p. 897. Available online: https://cds.cern.ch/record/909415?ln=it (accessed on 17 December 1997).
30. Dattoli, G.; Cabrini, S.; Giannessi, L. Simple Model of Gain Saturation in Free Electron Laser. *Phys. Rev. A* **1991**, *44*, 8433. [CrossRef] [PubMed]
31. Dattoli, G. Logistic function and evolution of free-electron-laser oscillators. *J. Appl. Phys.* **1998**, *84*, 2393–2398. [CrossRef]
32. Dattoli, G.; Ottaviani, P.L. Semi-analytical models of Free Electron Laser Saturation. *Opt. Comm.* **2002**, *204*, 283–297. [CrossRef]
33. Dattoli, G.; Giannessi, L.; Ottaviani, P.L.; Ronsivalle, C. Semi-analytical model of self-amplified spontaneous-emission free-electron lasers, including diffraction and pulse-propagation effects. *J. Appl. Phys.* **2004**, *95*, 3206–3210. [CrossRef]
34. Shih, C.C.; Yariv, A. Inclusion of Space-Charge Effects with Maxwell's Equations in the Single-Particle Analysis of Free-Electron Lasers. *IEEE J. Quantum Electron.* **1981**, *17*, 1387–1394. [CrossRef]
35. Dattoli, G.; Torre, A.; Centioli, C.; Richetta, M. Free Electron Laser Operation in the Intermediate Gain Region. *IEEE J. Quantum Electron.* **1989**, *25*, 2327–2331. [CrossRef]
36. Elias, L.R.; Fairbank, W.M.; Madey, J.M.J.; Schwettman, H.A.; Smith, T.I. Observation of Stimulated Emission of Radiation by Relativistic Electrons in a Spatially Periodic Transverse Magnetic Field. *Phys. Rev. Lett.* **1976**, *36*, 717. [CrossRef]
37. Deacon, D.A.G.; Elias, L.R.; Madey, J.M.J.; Ramian, G.J.; Schwettman, H.A.; Smith, T.I. First Operation of a Free-Electron Laser. *Phys. Rev. Lett.* **1977**, *38*, 892–894. [CrossRef]
38. Colson, W.B. The nonlinear wave equation for higher harmonics in free-electron lasers. *IEEE J. Quantum Electron.* **1981**, *17*, 1417–1427. [CrossRef]
39. Dattoli, G.; Ottaviani, P.L.; Pagnutti, S. Non Linear Harmonic Generation in high gain free electron laser. *J. Appl. Phys.* **2005**, *97*, 113102. [CrossRef]

40. Dattoli, G.; Ottaviani, P.L.; Pagnutti, S. The PROMETEO Code: A flexible tool for Free Electron Laser study. *Il Nuovo Cimento C* **2009**, *32*, 283–287.
41. Gallardo, J.C.; Elias, L.R.; Dattoli, G.; Renieri, A. Integral equation for the laser field in a long-pulse free-electron laser. *Phys. Rev. A* **1987**, *36*, 3222. [CrossRef]
42. Colson, W.B.; Dattoli, G.; Ciocci, F. Angular-gain spectrum of free-electron lasers. *Phys. Rev. A* **1985**, *31*, 828. [CrossRef]
43. Giannessi, L. Seeding and Harmonic Generation in Free-Electron Lasers. In *Synchrotron Light Sources and Free-Electron Lasers*; Springer: Berlin/Heidelberg, Germany, 2016; pp. 195–223, ISBN 978-3-319-14393-4.
44. Lambert, G.; Hara, T.; Garzella, D.; Tanikawa, T.; Labat, M.; Carre, B.; Kitamura, H.; Shintake, T.; Bougeard, M.; Inoue, S.; et al. Injection of harmonics generated in gas in a free electron laser providing intense and coherent extreme-ultraviolet light. *Nat. Phys.* **2008**, *4*, 296–300. [CrossRef]
45. Colson, W.B.; Gallardo, J.C.; Bosco, P.M. Free-electron-laser gain degradation and electron-beam quality. *Phys. Rev. A* **1986**, *34*, 4875. [CrossRef]
46. Dattoli, G.; Ottaviani, P.L.; Segreto, A.; Altobelli, G. Free electron laser gain: Approximant forms and inclusion of inhomogeneous broadening contributions. *J. Appl. Phys.* **1995**, *77*, 6162. [CrossRef]
47. Dattoli, G.; Giannessi, L.; Torre, A.; Segreto, A. The pulse propagation problem in free electron lasers: Gain parametrization formulae. *J. Appl. Phys.* **1996**, *79*, 6729. [CrossRef]
48. Bonifacio, R.; McNeil, B.W.J.; Pierini, P. Superradiance in the high-gain free-electron laser. *Phys. Rev. A* **1989**, *40*, 4467. [CrossRef]
49. Saldin, E.L.; Schneidmiller, E.A.; Yurkov, M.V. Diffraction effects in the self-amplified spontaneous emission FEL. *Opt. Commun.* **2000**, *186*, 185–209. [CrossRef]
50. Saldin, E.L.; Schneidmiller, E.A.; Yurkov, M.V. Properties of the third harmonic of the radiation from self-amplified spontaneous emission free electron laser. *Phys. Rev. Spec. Top. Accel. Beams* **2006**, *9*, 030702. [CrossRef]
51. Dattoli, G.; Sabia, E.; Ottaviani, P.L.; Pagnutti, S.; Petrillo, V. Longitudinal dynamics of high gain free electron laser amplifiers. *Phys. Rev.Spec. Top. Accel. Beams* **2013**, *16*, 030704. [CrossRef]
52. Merminga, L.; Morton, P.L.; Seeman, J.; Spence, W.L. Transverse phase space in the presence of dispersion. In Proceedings of the 1991 Institute of Electrical and Electronics Engineers (IEEE) Particle Accelerator Conference (PAC), San Francisco, CA, USA, 6–9 May 1991; Volume 910506, pp. 461–463.
53. Dowell, D.H.; Bolton, P.R.; Clendenin, J.E.; Emma, P.; Gierman, S.M.; Graves, W.S.; Limborg, C.G.; Murphy, B.F.; Schmerge, J.F. Slice emittance measurements at the SLAC Gun Test Facility. *Nucl. Instrum. Meth. A* **2003**, *507*, 327–330. [CrossRef]
54. Ferrario, M.; Alesini, D.; Bellaveglia, M.; Benfatto, M.; Boni, R.; Boscolo, M.; Castellano, M.; Chiadroni, E.; Clozza, A.; Cultrera, L.; et al. Recent results of the SPARC FEL experiments. In Proceedings of the 31st FEL Conference Liverpool, Liverpool, UK, 23–28 August 2009.
55. Bettoni, S.; Aiba, M.; Beutner, B.; Pedrozzi, M.; Prat, E.; Reiche, S.; Schietinger, T. Preservation of low slice emittance in bunch compressors. *Phys. Rev. Accel. Beams* **2016**, *19*, 034402. [CrossRef]
56. Dattoli, G.; Giannessi, L.; Torre, A. Unified view of free-electron laser dynamics and of higher-harmonics electron bunching. *J. Opt. Soc. Am.* **1993**, *10*, 2136–2143. [CrossRef]
57. Dattoli, G.; Giannessi, L.; Ottaviani, P.L. Free electron laser small signal dynamics and inclusion of electron-beam energy phase correlation. *J. Appl. Phys.* **1999**, *86*, 1710–1715. [CrossRef]
58. Dattoli, G.; Giannessi, L.; Ottaviani, P.L.; Pagnutti, S. Energy Phase Correlation and Pulse Dynamics in Short Bunch High Gain FELs. *Opt. Commun.* **2010**, *285*, 710–714. [CrossRef]
59. Dattoli, G.; Sabia, E.; Ronsivalle, C.; Del Franco, M.; Petralia, A. Slice emittance, projected emittance and properties of the SASE FEL radiation. *Nucl. Instrum. Methods Phys. Res. Sect. A Accel. Spectrometers Detect. Assoc. Equip.* **2012**, *671*, 51–61. [CrossRef]
60. Bonifacio, R.; De Salvo, L.; Pierini, P. Large harmonic bunching in a high-gain free-electron laser. *Nucl. Instrum. Methods Phys. Res. Sect. A Accel. Spectrometers Detect. Assoc. Equip.* **1990**, *293*, 627–629. [CrossRef]
61. Dattoli, G.; Ottaviani, P.L.; Pagnutti, S. High gain amplifiers: Power oscillations and harmonic generation. *J. Appl. Phys.* **2007**, *102*, 033103. [CrossRef]
62. Giannessi, L.; Musumeci, P.; Spampinati, S. Nonlinear pulse evolution in seeded free-electron laser amplifiers and in free-electron laser cascades. *J. Appl. Phys.* **2005**, *98*, 043110. [CrossRef]
63. Yang, X.; Mirian, N.; Giannessi, L. Postsaturation dynamics and superluminal propagation of a superradiant spike in a free-electron laser amplifier. *Phys. Rev. Accel. Beams* **2020**, *23*, 010703. [CrossRef]
64. Gardelle, J.; Labrouche, J.; Marchese, G.; Rullier, J.L.; Villate, D. Analysis of the beam bunching produced by a free electron laser. *Phys. Plasmas* **1996**, *3*, 4197. [CrossRef]
65. Dattoli, G.; Ottaviani, P.L.; Pagnutti, S. Theory of High Gain Free Electron Laser, operating with segmented undulators. *J. Appl. Phys.* **2006**, *99*, 044907. [CrossRef]

MDPI
St. Alban-Anlage 66
4052 Basel
Switzerland
Tel. +41 61 683 77 34
Fax +41 61 302 89 18
www.mdpi.com

Applied Sciences Editorial Office
E-mail: applsci@mdpi.com
www.mdpi.com/journal/applsci

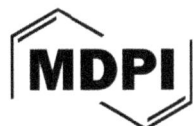

www.ingramcontent.com/pod-product-compliance
Lightning Source LLC
LaVergne TN
LVHW070656100526
838202LV00013B/975